Exercise Testing for Primary Care and Sports Medicine Physicians

T0180935

Corey H. Evans MD, MPH · Russell D. White MD
Editors

Exercise Testing for Primary Care and Sports Medicine Physicians

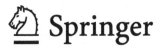 Springer

Editors

Corey H. Evans MD, MPH
Director of Medical Education
St. Anthony's Hospital
Private Practice Family Physician
Florida Institute of Family Medicine
St. Petersburg, FL, USA
email@coreyevansmd.com

Russell D. White MD
Professor of Medicine
Director, Sports Medicine Fellowship
Department of Community and Family
  Medicine
University of Missouri—Kansas City
Truman Medical Center Lakewood
Kansas City, MO, USA
jockdoc2000@hotmail.com

ISBN 978-1-4419-2630-2   e-ISBN 978-0-387-76597-6
DOI 10.1007/978-0-387-76597-6

Printed on acid-free paper

springer.com

This book is dedicated to Myrvin H. Ellestad, MD, and Victor F. Froelicher, MD. Their work and textbooks in the field of exercise and exercise testing are truly the bibles in this field and have helped countless physicians. We appreciate their guidance, friendship, and support over the years and their encouragement of exercise testing among primary care physicians.

Foreword

This book by Corey H. Evans, Russell D. White, and coauthors is a gem. There was a time when exercise testing was largely limited to cardiologists, but no more. Exercise testing, which provides information on fitness, the risk of coronary disease, and all around vitality, is now being performed in the offices of primary care physicians across the United States.

Although there is a significant risk in some populations, a careful doctor who takes the trouble to become knowledgeable in exercise physiology and the pathophysiology of coronary artery disease can use exercise testing to improve his ability to give excellent, preventive medicine.

Over the years I have read many books on this subject, and even contributed to some, and this one rates right up there with the best. Like many multiauthored books there is some repetition, but this is not all bad. A careful study of the various chapters will provide a depth of knowledge that will come in good stead when problems arise.

I can especially recommend the chapter on exercise physiology. When the reader has mastered the material presented in this chapter, he has acquired a knowledge base so that he can become an expert in exercise testing equal to almost anyone.

Over the years I have been privileged to know several of the authors and have followed their publications. Their contributions to our knowledge base in this field have been considerable. Acquiring this book and becoming familiar with its contents will set you apart in the field of exercise testing.

Myrvin H. Ellestad
Long Beach, CA
July 2008

Preface

With more than 40 years of experience between us teaching exercise testing on the national level, it is a pleasure for us to present a book on exercise testing for primary physicians. As primary care physicians, we both share strong interests in sports medicine, exercise promotion and testing, and prevention of cardiovascular disease. It is our desire to develop a text that primary care physicians can use to assess fitness, encourage and prescribe exercise, and discuss tools to evaluate our patients and athletes. We also wanted to share the basic and advanced concepts behind exercise testing so that readers can master the principles and use the exercise test in their practices. We strongly believe that the exercise test is invaluable for many of these purposes and should be widely used by primary care physicians.

Over the years we have been fortunate to teach and write with many of the national leaders in the field of exercise and exercise testing including Drs. Myrvin Ellestad, Victor Froelicher, and Nora Goldschlager. We have included these nationally recognized leaders as coauthors in this text and we appreciate their support.

It is our desire to help the reader know when statements are evidence based and the strength of the evidence. To that end, we have used a common rating system, used by the American College of Cardiology and others. When possible statements and recommendations will be categorized into three classes, based on the evidence and consensus of experts:

- Class I: There is evidence and/or general agreement that a given procedure, treatment, or recommendation is useful and effective.
- Class II: There is conflicting evidence and/or a divergence of opinions about the usefulness/efficacy of a treatment, procedure, or recommendation

  o Class IIa: Weight of evidence/opinion is in favor of usefulness/efficacy
  o Class IIb: Usefulness/efficacy is less well established.

- Class III: Conditions for which there is evidence and/or general agreement that the treatment/procedure is not useful/effective or actually harmful.

In addition, where applicable we use the following levels of evidence:

- Level of evidence A: Data were derived from multiple randomized clinical trials that involved large numbers of patients.

- Level of evidence B: Data were derived from a limited number of randomized trials that involved small numbers of patients or from careful analysis of nonrandomized studies or observational registries.
- Level of evidence C: Expert consensus was the primary basis for the recommendation.

The book is divided into initial chapters on the physiology of exercise and the performance of the exercise test. This includes the equipment, protocols, and interpretation. The next section discusses common abnormal examples, exercise testing coupled with imaging techniques, and the important area of risk stratification. This includes using the exercise test and other tests to stratify patients with chest pain, asymptomatic patients, preoperative patients, and those after angioplasty and coronary artery bypass graft (CABG) surgery.

Because health promotion is essential to improving our patients' lives, we included a chapter on using the exercise test and other tools in our practices to create lifestyle changes. The medical–legal aspects of exercise testing are also discussed.

The final section deals with fitness and sports medicine topics. It is important for primary physicians to understand how to evaluate and promote fitness. Since gas analysis is the best way to directly measure fitness, we felt it was important to introduce readers to gas analysis as an additional component of the exercise test. The last two chapters deal with testing both asymptomatic and symptomatic athletes. Finally, we have included a chapter using case studies to illustrate many of the important and interesting points. We certainly want to thank all of the authors for their contributions toward making this book a reality, for without their efforts we could never have finished this project. Also, many thanks to the help and patience of our editor, Margaret Burns.

We sincerely hope the readers find this text helpful in the day-to-day management of patients as we all strive to improve the lives of our patients. As we battle against obesity, diabetes, and heart disease in the US, we hope this reference enables the primary care physicians to promote fitness and exercise as well as to use tools herein to evaluate the diseases associated with obesity and inactivity.

On a personal note we would like to acknowledge our families for their support. I (RDW) would like to thank my wife, Dara, for her constant encouragement. And I (CHE) would like to thank my father, Paul Evans, for his loving support and lifelong commitment to a personal exercise program. Dad, you certainly set a great example, and now in your eighties, you are still reaping the benefits. May my boys and I continue this great tradition.

St. Petersburg, FL, USA   Corey H. Evans
Kansas City, MO, USA   Russell D. White
                                                                                      July 2008

Contents

Part IV   Case Studies

Contributors

Michael Altman Department of Family Medicine, University of Texas Health Science Center, Houston, TX, USA, Michael.A.Altman@uth.tmc.edu

Patricia A. Deuster Department of Military and Emergency Medicine, Uniformed Services University, Consortium for Health and Military Performance, Bethesda, MD, USA, pdeuster@usuhs.mil

Kevin Edward Elder HealthPoint Medical Group; Department of Family Medicine, University of South Florida, Tampa, FL, USA, kelder@tampabay.rr.com

Myrvin H. Ellestad Exercise Laboratory, Memorial Heart Institute; Department of Cardiology, University of California, Irvine School of Medicine, Long Beach, CA, USA, mellestad@memorialcare.org

Corey H. Evans St. Anthony's Hospital, St. Petersburg, FL; Florida Institute of Family Medicine, St. Petersburg, FL, USA, email@coreyevansmd.com

Karl B. Fields Moses Cone Health System, Greensboro, NC; Department of Family Medicine, University of North Carolina at Chapel Hill, Greensboro, NC, USA, bert.fields@mosescone.com

Grant Fowler Department of Family and Community Medicine, The University of Texas Health Science Center Houston, Houston, TX, USA, grant.c.fowler@uth.tmc.edu

Victor F. Froelicher Department of Cardiology, Stanford/Palo Alto Veterans Affairs Health Care Center, Palo Alto, CA, USA, vcimd@pabell.net

Nora Goldschlager Department of Medicine, Division of Cardiology, University of California San Francisco, San Francisco, CA, USA NGoldschlager@medsfgh.ucsf.edu

George D. Harris Department of Community and Family Medicine, University of Missouri-Kansas City, School of Medicine, Truman Medical Center—Lakewood, Kansas City, MO, USA, george.harris@tmcmed.org

David L. Herbert David L. Herbert and Associates, LLC, Canton, OH, USA, herblegal@aol.com

William G. Herbert Laboratory for Health & Exercise Science, Department of Human Nutrition, Foods, & Exercise, Virginia Tech, Blacksburg, Virginia; The Exercise Standards and Malpractice Reporter, Canton, OH, USA

Bryan C. Hughes Oak Grove Medical Clinic, Oak Grove, MO, USA, Big1500@hotmail.com

Joseph S. Janicki Department of Cell Biology and Anatomy, University of South Carolina School of Medicine, Columbia, SC, USA, jjanicki@gw.med.sc.edu

Ajoy Kumar Family Practice Training Program, Bayfront Medical Center, St. Petersburg, FL, USA, vsingh@health.usf.edu

Matthew T. Kunar 4th BCT, 82nd Airborne Division, Fort Bragg, NC, USA, kunar36@msn.com

Steven C. Masley University of South Florida, Tampa; Masley Optimal Health Center, St. Petersburg, FL, USA, steven@drmasley.com

Patricia Nguyen Department of Cardiology, Stanford University School of Medicine, Palo Alto, CA, USA, pknguyen1@yahoo.com

Francis G. O'Connor Department of Military and Emergency Medicine, Consortium for Health and Military Performance, Uniformed Services University of the Health Sciences, Bethesda, MD, USA, foconnor@usuhs.mil

David E. Price Department of Family Medicine, Carolinas Medical Center – Eastland, Charlotte NC, USA, david.price@carolinas.org

H. Jack Pyhel Department of Family Practice, University of South Florida Medical School at Bayfront Medical Center, St. Petersburg; Heart & Vascular Institute of Florida, St. Petersburg, FL, USA, Hjp@tampabay.rr.com

Vibhuti N. Singh Department of Medicine, Division of Cardiology, University of South Florida College of Medicine; Director, Clinical Research, Suncoast Cardiovascular Center, St. Petersburg, Florida, USA, vsingh@health.usf.edu or vnsingh@post.harvard.edu

Eric T. Warren Department of Family Medicine, Carolinas Medical Center – Eastland, Charlotte NC, USA, eric.warren@carolinas.org

Russell D. White Department of Community and Family Medicine, University of Missouri—Kansas City, Truman Medical Center Lakewood, Kansas City, MO, USA, Russell.White@tmcmed.org or jockdoc2000@hotmail.com

Part I
Performing the Exercise Test

Chapter 1
Exercise Physiology for Graded Exercise Testing: A Primer for the Primary Care Clinician

Francis G. O'Connor, Matthew T. Kunar, and Patricia A. Deuster

Exercise testing is an advanced clinical procedure used by providers to assess functional capacity for the purpose of guiding cardiovascular and pulmonary diagnoses and therapies. Numerous clinical guidelines, texts, and consensus statements have been published to assist clinicians in the identification of indications and criteria for treadmill stress testing, as well as procedures for test performance and interpretation [1–4]. However, the physiology of exercise testing, which is the foundation for exercise testing, is often overlooked in resource publications, as well as during the clinical training of providers. Education in exercise physiology is largely limited to the pre-clinical years, despite the fact that progress in cardiovascular exercise physiology is ongoing. This chapter functions as a primer for the primary care clinician who conducts exercise testing: core concepts pertaining to energy metabolism, skeletal muscle physiology, and cardiovascular and pulmonary physiology are reviewed. Additionally current concepts pertaining to testing for maximal aerobic power, factors that influence both test performance and results, and the physiology of myocardial ischemia and ST-segment depression are discussed.

Skeletal Muscle and Energy Production

Skeletal Muscle Physiology

The end-organ of exercise is skeletal muscle. Skeletal muscle can be subdivided anatomically into fascicles, which contain approximately 150 myofibers (muscle cells) (Fig. 1.1). Each muscle cell is composed of many myofibrils (5–10,000). Each myofibril in turn contains approximately 4,500 sarcomeres, which constitute

F.G. O'Connor (✉)
Department of Military and Emergency Medicine, Consortium for Health and Military Performance, Uniformed Services University of the Health Sciences, 4301 Jones Bridge Rd., Bethesda, MD 20814, USA
e-mail: foconnor@usuhs.mil

C.H. Evans, R.D. White (eds.), *Exercise Testing for Primary Care and Sports Medicine Physicians*, DOI 10.1007/978-0-387-76597-6_1
© Springer Science+Business Media, LLC 2009

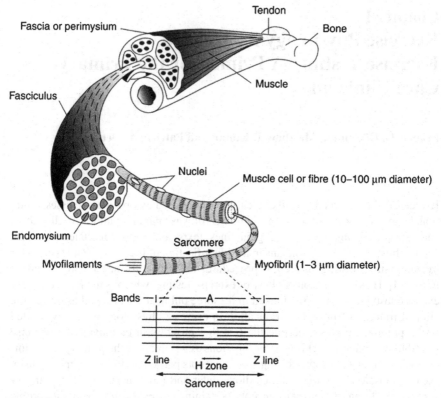

Fig. 1.1 Basic anatomy and structure of skeletal muscle physiology

the functional unit of the muscle cell. Sarcomeres are composed of two distinct myofilaments: thick and thin, with myosin and actin being the primary thick and thin myofilament proteins, respectively. Troponin, tropomyosin, titin, nebulin, and desmin are other important proteins that maintain the structure and function of the myofilaments.

Muscle Contraction

The dominant theory of muscle contraction is the sliding filament theory, which states that muscle contraction occurs when myosin heads bind to actin. The subsequent binding of adenosine triphosphate (ATP) to myosin breaks the actin–myosin bond and allows myosin to bind to another actin site farther along the thin filament. The process of myosin binding, releasing, and rebinding to actin forces the myofilaments to slide past each other in a ratchet-like fashion to create a series of cross-bridge linkages. This cross-bridging creates an oscillatory pattern with no more than 50% of the myosin heads attached to actin at any given moment.

Muscle Fiber Types

Skeletal muscle consists of two major fiber types: type I (slow twitch) and type II (fast twitch). Overall, type I fibers are characterized by lower force production, power, and speed, but greater endurance than type II fibers. Type I fibers have lower glycogen stores and myosin-ATP-ase activity and more mitochondria than their type II counterpart. The abundance of mitochondria and the high activities of enzymes involved in aerobic metabolism are associated with resistance to fatigue and ability to sustain submaximal activities. Type II muscle fibers, which can be classified into at least two other types (type IIa and type IIx), exhibit an approximately three to five times faster time to peak tension than type I fibers and are recruited preferentially during high-intensity exercise [5–12]. In fact, a hierarchical order of fiber activation with increasing intensity of exercise has been shown [13]. Type II fibers also have higher rates of cross-bridge turnover than type I fibers, and thus require more ATP per unit of time and are readily fatigued [5, 6]. Additionally, type II fibers exhibit greater activities of the enzyme lactate dehydrogenase (LDH) than type I fibers [14]. LDH, as discussed below, catalyzes the reversible reduction of pyruvate to lactate with accompanying oxidation of NADH to nicotinamide adenine dinucleotide (NAD+), in an effort to maintain ATP in the absence of oxygen.

The distribution of fiber types varies as a function of genetics and training. The proportions of type I and type II fibers in untrained persons are approximately 53 and 47%, respectively, whereas the proportion of type II fibers in resistance and endurance-trained individuals averages 67 and 50%, respectively [5, 6, 10–12]. The metabolic and mechanical profiles of fiber types can adapt in response to training, but the adaptations are training specific [11, 12].

Energy Metabolism

As indicated earlier, the process that facilitates muscular contraction is entirely dependent on the body's ability to provide and rapidly replenish ATP. Minimal amounts of ATP are stored for muscle contraction, but ATP can be derived from three specific energy systems: the immediate or creatine phosphate system; the short-term or glycolytic system; and the long-term or oxidative/aerobic system. Muscle fiber types at rest have intrinsically different contents of creatine phosphate (CP), ATP, and Inorganic Phosphate (Pi).

The immediate or phosphagen system consists of adenosine diphosphate (ADP), ATP, creatine (C), and CP. ATP is produced/regenerated when the enzyme creatine kinase catalyzes the transfer of phosphate from CP to ADP. Muscle fibers store approximately four times more CP than ATP, with type II fibers storing almost twice as much as type I fibers [15]. The CP system sustains energy during very short bursts of maximal power (Table 1.1).

The short-term or glycolytic system provides 1–1.6 min of energy for muscular activity. At the onset of any exercise, the oxygen demand is greater than the supply, so glucose from glycogen is converted to pyruvate for a net yield of 2 ATP. For glycolytic production of ATP to continue in the absence of oxygen, nicotinamide

Table 1.1 Energy systems

Energy systems	Mole of ATP per min	Time to fatigue
Immediate: phosphagen	4	5–10 s
Short-term: glycolytic	2.5	1–1.6 min
Long-term: aerobic	1	Unlimited

adenine dinucleotide (NADH), an important coenzyme, must reduce pyruvate to lactate to regenerate NAD+ [16]. It is the regeneration of NAO+ that allows gly-colytic production of ATP to continue. ATP synthesis through this anaerobic system is inefficient in that it yields only 2 ATP per molecule of glucose in contrast to 36 ATP from oxidative metabolism of glucose. Exercise at near maximal intensities results in a rapid breakdown of muscle PCr, predominantly in type IIx fibers [8]. In contrast, glycogen appears to be depleted similarly in type I and type II fibers at maximal intensities, but preferentially in type I fibers after submaximal exercise [17,18]. This evidence demonstrates the importance of type II fibers in maximal force generation.

The long-term or oxidative/aerobic system involves two major fuels: carbohydrates, in the form of glucose, and free fatty acids (FFA). At rest and during submaximal exercise both carbohydrates and FFA contribute to ATP synthesis. Although FFA are a more efficient source of energy (they yield 8 ATP per carbon compared to only 6.3 ATP for glucose) than carbohydrates, glucose is more readily available and can be metabolized more rapidly than FFA to generate ATP. Glucose can be stored as glycogen in liver and muscle and is readily available for energy; alternatively, glucose can be used in the synthesis of fatty acids and stored as triacylglycerol, primarily in adipocytes. Triacylglycerols must be hydrolyzed to release the free fatty acids before being available for energy.

Aerobic energy production takes place within the mitochondria. If pyruvate formed in the cytoplasm crosses the mitochondrial membrane, it is oxidized to acetyl coenzyme A (acetyl CoA), which enters the tricarboxylic acid (TCA/Krebs) cycle where it is oxidized to carbon dioxide. In the process three molecules of NADH and one molecule of reduced flavin adenine dinucleotide ($FADH_2$) are produced. It is these reduced coenzymes that present electrons to the electron transport chain to generate ATP in the mitochondria. As noted above, one molecule of glucose ultimately contributes a total of 36 ATP. Free fatty acids are sequentially oxidized to yield acetyl CoA, which enters the TCA cycle as noted above.

Acute Exercise and the Cardiopulmonary Response

Cardiovascular Physiology

The principal function of the cardiovascular system during exercise is to sustain delivery of oxygen (O_2) and vital nutrients to the target organ, skeletal muscle. The cardiovascular system consists of a pump, a high-pressure distribution circuit, exchange vessels, and a low-pressure collection and return circuit [19]. This system moves approximately 5 liters (L) of blood each minute at rest, so the heart pumps nearly 7,200 L (1,900 gallons) per day. The cardiovascular system's productivity can increase more than four to eight times ($\sim$40 L min^{-1}) above resting levels during strenuous exertion in the upright position, as a result of changes in heart rate, stroke volume, and peripheral resistance.

Maximal Oxygen uptake ($VO_{2\,max}$) is considered the "gold standard" of cardiopulmonary health and represents the body's ability to deliver and utilize oxygen. $VO_{2\,max}$ is a product of cardiac output and extraction of oxygen from the circulation by the peripheral skeletal muscles; $VO_{2\,max}$ is conveniently expressed by the Fick equation:

$VO_{2\,max}$ =   Maximal cardiac output $\times$ Maximal arteriovenous oxygen difference

Maximal cardiac output = Heart rate$_{MAX}$ $\times$ Stroke volume$_{MAX}$

Maximal arteriovenous oxygen difference = Capillary arterial O_2 $-$ Capillary venous O_2

The volume of blood moved by cardiac activity each minute is termed *cardiac output* and is typically expressed in L min^{-1}. Cardiac output is a function of heart rate (beats min^{-1}, bpm) and stroke volume (mL beat^{-1}) and is the principal, or central, component of an individual's $VO_{2\,max}$. The ability of the working muscles to extract oxygen from the blood is the peripheral component of $VO_{2\,max}$ determination; it is calculated from the arteriovenous oxygen difference (a $-$ vO_2). Each component of the Fick equation is critical to the performance and understanding of the exercise stress test and is subsequently reviewed in detail and summarized in Fig. 1.2.

$VO_{2\,max}$

By definition, *maximal oxygen uptake*, $VO_{2\,max}$, is the highest oxygen uptake (VO_2) achieved when a person is working at maximal capacity. Classically, VO_2 reaches a plateau and does not increase further, even with an increase in external workload. Absolute values, typically expressed in L min^{-1}, may range from as low as 1.0 L min^{-1} (or lower in persons with cardiovascular disease) up to 6 L min^{-1} (or possibly higher in large, well-trained individuals). One of the most predictable relationships in exercise physiology is that between oxygen uptake and cardiac output: VO_2 is directly related to cardiac output (Fig. 1.2) [4, 20].

Because two individuals of quite different sizes may have the same absolute values for $VO_{2\,max}$ it is often normalized for body weight to allow for between-subject comparisons. The most familiar unit of expression is milliliter (mL) kilogram (kg)$^{-1}$ min^{-1}. Values for $VO_{2\,max}$ range from a low of 10 to a high of 80^{+} mL kg^{-1} min^{-1}. For example, if two men both have absolute values of 4.2 L min^{-1} and one weighs 70 kg and the other 95 kg, then their $VO_{2\,max}$ values relative to body weight would be 60 mL kg^{-1} min^{-1} for the 70-kg man and 44.2 mL kg^{-1} min^{-1} for the 90-kg man. This relative $VO_{2\,max}$ provides an indication of an individual's potential for work, particularly running, swimming, cycling, and overall endurance. Clearly the man who weighs only 70 kg is in better shape for physical work because he could work with less relative effort at 40 mL kg^{-1} min^{-1} than the 90 kg man (66 vs. 90% of VO$_{2\,max}$).

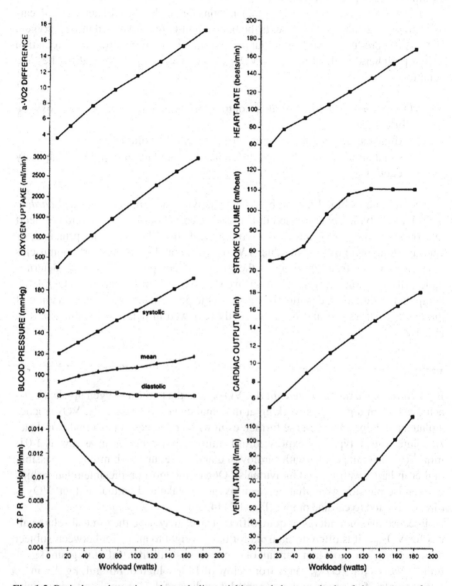

Fig. 1.2 Basic hemodynamic and metabolic variables and the magnitude of the response from rest to a moderately high level of exercise. TPR = total peripheral resistance. Units for a–VO$_2$ difference are mL O$_2$ per 100 mL blood. (From Myers JN. The physiology behind exercise testing. *Primary Care* 2001;28:5–14, with permission of Elsevier.)

VO_2, in addition to being normalized by weight, can also be normalized clinically. In the clinical setting VO_2 is normalized to metabolic equivalents (METs), which represent a multiple of an average value of resting energy expenditure of $3.5 \, mL \, kg^{-1} \, min^{-1}$. The VO_2 above rest required to perform recreational or occupational work can then be represented by the number of METs for a given activity. The determination of maximal MET capacity can be of use when risk-stratifying patients for clinical decisions. Most activities of daily living require less than 4 METs; patients with coronary artery disease or congestive heart failure who perform below this level have a guarded prognosis. In contrast, the ability to exercise at 10 METs without ischemia places the patient at low risk, with a 1-year mortality of <2% [21]. A maximal exercise capacity of 13 METs, regardless of other factors to include the presence and extent of ischemia, predicts an excellent short-term prognosis.

The American College of Sports Medicine (ACSM) has published normative values for $VO_{2\,max}$ by age and gender so that individual values can be classified into one of five groups: poor (well below average), fair (below average), average, good (above average), and excellent (well above average) [4] (Table 1.2). The importance of $VO_{2\,max}$ cannot be overemphasized with respect to health: low aerobic power, or low cardiovascular fitness, is associated with higher morbidity and earlier mortality for all causes [22]. Data from 1999–2000 to 2001–2002 National Health and Nutrition Examination Surveys (NHANES) showed that approximately 11.3% of non-Hispanic whites and 22.9% of non-Hispanic blacks between 20 and 49 years of age had estimated $VO_{2\,max}$ values in the ACSM's poor category (below $30 \, mL \, kg^{-1} \, min^{-1}$) [23]. Non-Hispanic black women had the lowest $VO_{2\,max}$ values such that 30.9% were in the poor category. Of note is the finding that 33.6% of adolescents have poor aerobic fitness [24]. Thus, despite the importance of maximal aerobic power, the distribution of estimated $VO_{2\,max}$ values from NHANES indicates low fitness among most of the US population.

Table 1.2 Normative values (percentile) for maximal aerobic power for men and women by age*

Age	Poor (≤10)	Fair (10–30)	Average (30–70)	Good (70–90)	Excellent (≥ 90)
			Men		
20–29	< 35	35–41	42–49	50–55	> 55
30–39	<33	33–39	40–47	48–52	> 52
40–49	<31	31–36	37–45	46–51	> 51
50–59	<30	30–35	36–41	42–49	> 49
≥ 60	<27	27–31	32–37	38–44	> 44
			Women		
20–29	< 28	28–33	34–41	42–49	> 49
30–39	<27	27–31	32–39	40–46	> 46
40–49	<25	25–30	31–36	37–43	> 43
50–59	<22	22–27	28–33	34–38	> 38
≥ 60	<20	20–23	24–31	32–35	> 35

*American College of Sports Medicine Aerobic Power Standards for men and women. Reprinted with permission from LLW.

Heart Rate

The cardiovascular control center that regulates heart rate, as well as stroke volume and the peripheral redistribution of blood to working muscle, is located in the ventrolateral medulla. Anticipation of exercise is processed in the brain and results in an inhibition of parasympathetic activity and an increase in sympathetic outflow, with cardio-acceleration actually preceding the onset of voluntary muscle contraction [25]. In addition to acceleration of heart rate, these neural activation responses result in a series of cardiovascular responses: increased myocardial contractility; vasodilation in skeletal muscle; vasoconstriction in non-exercising areas (e.g., gut); and an increase in arterial blood pressure. The redistribution of cardiac output to exercising muscle can be quite impressive, with greater than 85% of total blood flow directed to the skeletal muscle with peak exercise.

Heart rate acceleration with exercise is subject to a number of intrinsic and extrinsic factors, including age, fitness level, the presence of cardiac disease, blood volume, the type of activity, body position, and the environment. Maximum heart rate can be estimated from the formula 220 – age in years; however, there is a wide variation in maximal heart rate capability, with one standard deviation of 10–12 bpm. In addition, maximum heart rate and cardiac output are generally decreased in older individuals, secondary to intrinsic cardiac changes, including decreased beta-adrenergic responsivity [26,27]. Therefore, although the age-predicted maximum heart rate is a useful measurement for an initial estimation, the large standard deviation limits the usefulness of this parameter in estimating the exact age-predicted maximum for an individual patient [28]. In general, maximal heart rate is generally unchanged by exercise training, while resting heart rate frequently decreases with aerobic training, secondary to an enhanced vagal tone.

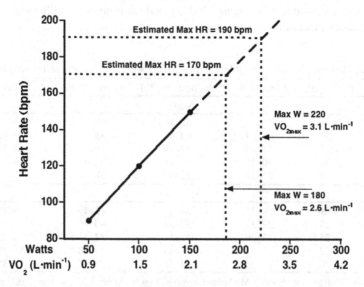

Fig. 1.3 The relationship between heart rate and $VO_{2\,max}$

Fitness level is also directly related to heart rate at a given workload. Individuals who are more fit and have a higher intrinsic $VO_{2\,max}$ can accomplish comparable workloads with lower heart rates. A trained runner may be able to run 6 mph on a treadmill at a heart rate of 110 bpm, whereas a less fit person may require a corresponding heart rate of 150 bpm to run at the same pace. The ability to produce a cardiac output to meet the demands of comparable workload and oxygen requirement is explained by the Fick equation: the well-trained runner has the advantage of a training-induced increase in stroke volume and more efficient peripheral extraction of oxygen by exercising muscle than the less fit non-runner.

Heart rate is known to increase with increasing VO_2. Åstrand and Ryhming were among the first to report this linear relationship between heart rate and VO_2 and, based on this relationship, recommended the use of heart rate to predict $VO_{2\,max}$ (Fig. 1.3) [29]. Because heart rate in a trained athlete can go from a resting rate of 40 bpm to over 200 bpm, heart rate is the principal driver for the increase in cardiac output.

Stroke Volume

The second principal component of cardiac output that changes with exercise is stroke volume. Enhanced sympathetic activity increases not only heart rate, which provides a chronotropic stimulus, but also an inotropic stimulus, which increases myocardial contractility. Stroke volume is determined by subtracting the volume of blood in the left ventricle at end-systole from that identified at end-diastole. Normal values for stroke volume range from 75 to 100 mL beat^{-1}, which can nearly double with exercise. Factors that can affect an individual's stroke volume include genetics (e.g., heart size); conditioning (e.g., contractility, preload, and afterload); and disease (e.g., valvular and wall motion abnormalities).

Filling pressure is instrumental in augmenting cardiac output by increasing the end-diastolic volume. The Frank–Starling law of the heart states that the force of contraction of cardiac muscle remains proportional to its initial resting length. As cardiac preload increases with an increased venous return, a more forceful contraction results. During exercise, stroke volume is principally augmented by increasing end-diastolic volume and reducing peripheral vascular resistance, which decreases cardiac afterload. Maximal stroke volume is achieved at relatively low exercise intensities, as pericardial constraint serves to limit left ventricular end-diastolic volume. Increasing cardiac output becomes dependent on an increase in heart rate.

Cardiac contractility also contributes to the increase in stroke volume, but not to the extent seen with changes in end-diastolic volume. Increasing cardiac contractility reduces end-systolic volume by increasing ejection fraction and thereby increasing stroke volume. Increased cardiac contractility has been observed in healthy hearts, whereas subjects with coronary artery disease or congestive heart failure have less predictable responses and may actually demonstrate increasing end-systolic volumes with an increasing exercise demand.

Cardiac afterload is a measure of the force required to eject blood from the heart into the peripheral circulation. An increase in afterload, or peripheral resistance, can result in a decreased ejection fraction. Systolic blood pressure represents the force of the blood against the arterial walls with ventricular contraction, whereas diastolic blood pressure reflects peripheral resistance during the relaxation phase of the cardiac cycle. During dynamic exercise, total peripheral resistance is normally decreased as a result of vasodilation of the skeletal muscle vasculature. Accordingly, despite a marked increase in cardiac output with peak exercise and a clear rise in systolic blood pressure, mean arterial pressure increases only moderately (Fig. 1.2).

Arterial-Venous Oxygen Concentration Difference

The peripheral contribution to $VO_{2\,max}$ is the difference between the O_2 concentration of the arteries and veins $(a - vO_2)$. At rest the $(a - vO_2)$ is typically 4–5 mL O_2 per 100 mL, which equates to 23% extraction. During dynamic exercise, this difference can increase as exercising muscle extracts oxygen more efficiently. At peak exercise the $(a - vO_2)$ may reach 18 mL O_2 per 100 mL, which is approximately 85% extraction [30]. In general, the $(a - vO_2)$ difference or the percent O_2 extracted does not explain differences in $VO_{2\,max}$ between subjects who are relatively homogeneous; the $(a - vO_2)$ difference appears to increase by a relatively fixed amount during exercise, such that differences in $VO_{2\,max}$ are principally explained by changes in cardiac output [30]. This observation supports the conclusion that O_2 supply, not muscle use, limits aerobic capacity.

Many factors can alter the $(a - vO_2)$ difference. Hemoglobin concentration, alveolar ventilation, partial pressure of O_2, and pulmonary diffusion capacity are important for the arterial component. In addition, the $(a - vO_2)$ difference is altered by conditions that shift the O_2 dissociation curve to the left, such as decreased carbondioxide (CO_2), decreased temperature, decreased 2,3-diphosphoglycerate (2,3-DPG), and an increased pH. Any increase in the affinity of O_2 for hemoglobin will reduce the O_2 released to the tissue at a given partial pressure of O_2. In contrast, conditions that shift the O_2 dissociation curve to the right (an increase in 2,3-diphosphoglycerate or temperature, a decreased pH) allow greater O_2 dissociation at the tissue level and thereby augment extraction [19]. It is important to note that arterial hemoglobin and O_2 saturation levels in healthy adults remain similar throughout exercise to resting levels.

As previously discussed, the ability to extract O_2 is not altered significantly by aerobic training. However, training appears to increase muscle capillary density, which serves to increase blood flow to working muscles. Studies have demonstrated that fit individuals have a tremendous ability to alter blood flow to exercising muscle and tend to have a greater muscle capillary density, which in turn facilitates greater oxygen delivery to working muscle [31].

Pulmonary Physiology

Exercise performance is dependent on the body's ability to deliver O_2 to the target organ of exercise, skeletal muscle. The ability to perform physical work is dependent upon a number of factors, with the initial step accomplished by the pulmonary system. The transport of O_2 from the external environment to the lung is a carefully orchestrated process, wherein air is ventilated from the lungs to the alveolus and O_2 diffuses across a pulmonary membrane to bind with hemoglobin, which resides inside a red blood cell traveling through a pulmonary capillary.

The cornerstone of understanding pulmonary aspects of exercise testing and physiology is a clear understanding of the nomenclature. The amount of air moving in and out of the lung per minute is defined as minute ventilation (VE). VE is a function of tidal volume (VT) and respiratory rate and is expressed in L min^{-1}. Maximal voluntary ventilation (MVV), a measure of the maximum breathing capacity, is the volume of air exchanged during repeated maximal respirations in a specified period of time; it too is expressed in L min^{-1}. The ventilatory threshold is defined as the point where ventilation increases disproportionately to VO_2.

Strenuous work requires the pulmonary system to move massive amounts of air into and out of the lungs. Accordingly there is an increase in the end-inspiratory and a decrease in the end-expiratory lung volume. In highly fit individuals, VE has been shown to increase from approximately 8 to 12–150 L min^{-1} at peak exercise. Pulmonary blood flow also increases two- to fourfold during exercise with a small increase in pulmonary artery pressure. These changes in flow and pressure are associated with significant reductions in pulmonary vasculature resistance.

Testing for Maximal Aerobic Power

Maximal aerobic power, or maximal oxygen uptake ($VO_{2\,max}$), is a measure of the maximum amount of oxygen that an individual can use per unit of time during strenuous physical exertion at sea level. It is an important measure for several reasons: (1) it serves as an index of cardiovascular and pulmonary function; (2) it characterizes the functional capacity of the cardiopulmonary system to transport oxygen to the working muscles; and (3) it is one of the limiting factors in endurance performance. An individual's $VO_{2\,max}$ can be estimated by a variety of techniques to include treadmill running, cycle ergometry, arm cranking, stair stepping, rowing, or walking. However, the gold standard is progressive treadmill testing by running to exhaustion. The most common way to measure $VO_{2\,max}$ is by open-circuit spirometry, whereby the individual breathes in ambient air and the exhaled air is measured and analyzed. The amount of oxygen consumed (VO_2) can be computed based on knowing the composition of the inspired air and by quantifying the volume (V) and oxygen (O_2) content of the expired air.

When a maximal aerobic power test is conducted, it is important to document whether a true $VO_{2\,max}$ has been achieved. Such a determination begins with understanding the physiologic responses to severe exercise and assessing selected parameters that have been designated as criteria for a $VO_{2\,max}$ test. The criteria allow the tester to decide whether the obtained value should be considered $VO_{2\,max}$ or a peak VO_2 (VO_{2peak}). As noted above, a plateau in VO_2, or only a small increase in VO_2 with an increase in external workload, is considered the primary criterion. Secondary criterion includes measures of blood (or plasma) lactate, respiratory exchange ratio (RER), heart rate, and perceived exertion [4, 32, 33].

Criteria for Maximal Aerobic Power

A Plateau in Oxygen Uptake

A plateau in oxygen intake, despite an increase in workload, is considered the primary criterion for $VO_{2\,max}$. If a plateau in VO_2 is observed, $VO_{2\,max}$ has been achieved. However, this criterion is not always achieved. Various factors influence quantification of $VO_{2\,max}$, to include between-subject variability and absolute increases in grade and speed. Meyers et al. [34] suggested that a plateau phenomenon is not always seen with various protocols because of the sampling interval selected (e.g., breath-by-breath, 5, 10, or 15 s averages) and magnitude of work increments for each exercise stage. Many efforts have been undertaken to define a precise criterion for attaining a plateau. In one of the early studies, performed by Taylor et al., 115 subjects ran at a speed of 7 mph on a given grade (0–12.5%) for 3 min; the grade was increased 2.5% until the subject could go no longer; grade increases were typically carried out on different days or after a period of rest [35]. With this protocol, they showed that a 2.5% grade increase typically resulted in a rise of approximately 300 mL min^{-1} in VO_2. However, at a certain point, higher levels of exercise, which were different for each person, did not elicit the 300 mL min^{-1} increase. Based on this information, it was determined that an increase of less than 150 mL min^{-1} or 2.1 mL kg^{-1} min^{-1} in VO_2 at the next higher work rate marked a plateau. They concluded that a grade increase was preferable to speed increases for achieving a plateau. Further, they demonstrated that 93.9% of persons tested achieved the designated plateau [35].

Importantly, other investigators have not always found that such a high percentage of persons achieve plateau. The percentage of adults achieving plateau ranges from 25% of men and women to 72.5% of men [36–38]. The numbers are similar for children with 25–33% of prepubertal children achieving a plateau during treadmill exercise and cycle ergometry, respectively [37, 39]. For most studies, VO_{2peak} values do not differ from $VO_{2\,max}$ values. Thus, although a plateau is not seen in many people, due to various factors, VO_{2peak} may be considered a valid index of $VO_{2\,max}$. Although no consensus has been reached over the years, this criterion is still considered by many to be the gold standard or the primary criterion. Because a plateau is not consistently observed, secondary criteria described below have evolved.

Blood Lactate Levels

In the absence of a true plateau in VO_2, a rise in blood lactate has been used to demonstrate a maximal effort [4, 40]. As the workload continues to rise and the person nears a maximal effort, blood lactate levels increase due to accelerated glycolysis, an increase in the recruitment of fast-twitch muscle fibers, a reduction in liver blood flow, and/or an elevation in plasma epinephrine concentration [3, 14, 40, 41]. These observations were first made by Åstrand, who noted that in the absence of a visible plateau, lactate values, along with a subject-reported stress level, could be used to document attainment of a true $VO_{2\,max}$ [40, 42].

Although identifying a standard cutoff for blood lactate levels has been difficult, the values derived from Åstrand's earliest studies suggesting a cutoff of 7.9–8.4 mmol L^{-1} are still accepted today [40, 42]. Subsequent investigators have noted that 8 mM is a reasonable criterion value [32, 33, 43, 44]. Cumming and Borysyk [43] and Stachenfeld [44] found that 78% of their test subjects achieved lactate levels greater than 8 mmol L^{-1}. Moreover, 8 mmol L^{-1} was the best criterion in terms of specificity and positive predictive value as compared to other secondary criteria [44]. Current standards vary, but a value greater than or equal to 8 mmol L^{-1} appears to be consistent with research studies and is well accepted by researchers in general.

Respiratory Exchange Ratio

The respiratory quotient (RQ) and respiratory exchange ratio (RER) are both calculated as the ratio of the volume of CO_2 produced to the volume of O_2 used, or VCO_2/VO_2. The RQ, which typically ranges between 0.7 and 1.0, is an indicator of metabolic fuel or substrate utilization in tissues; it must be calculated under resting or steady-state exercise conditions. A ratio of 0.7 is indicative of mixed fat utilization whereas a ratio of 1.0 indicates exclusive use of carbohydrates [45]. Thus, during low-intensity, steady-state exercise, the RQ and RER are typically between 0.80 and 0.88, when fatty acids are the primary fuel.

As the intensity of the exercise increases, and carbohydrate becomes the dominant or primary fuel, the RQ and RER increase to between 0.9 and 1.0. Because the RQ reflects tissue substrate utilization, it cannot exceed 1.0. In contrast, the RER, which reflects respiratory exchange of CO_2 and O_2, commonly exceeds 1.0 during strenuous exercise. During non-steady-state strenuous exercise, the volume of CO_2 production rises because of hyperventilation and increased buffering of blood lactate derived from skeletal muscles; thus, RER no longer reflects substrate usage, but rather high ventilation rates and blood lactate levels [33, 42, 45].

Because RER reproducibly increases during exercise, it is considered a parameter that can document maximal effort. Issekutz, the first to propose the use of RER as a criterion for $VO_{2\,max}$, noted that it must exceed 1.15 [45]. A higher value may suggest a more accurate assessment of $VO_{2\,max}$. The 1.15 value appears to be reasonable, although not all persons are able to achieve it. Studies have noted values of 1.00, 1.05, 1.10, and 1.13 as criterion for maximal performance, but at present no clear consensus has been reached [32, 33].

Age-Predicted Maximal Heart Rate

The widely recognized linear relationship between heart rate and VO_2 has encouraged the use of estimated maximal heart rate as a criterion for achieving $VO_{2\,max}$. Attaining a target percentage of the age-predicted maximal heart rate is one of the most widely recognized criterion [32]. Unfortunately, the traditional equation used to estimate maximal heart rate (220 – Age) was derived from approximately 10 different studies and most of these studies tested subjects younger than 65 years [28]. Additionally, the equation was never validated for adults over 60 years, and thus, it may underestimate maximal heart rate in older adults by more than 20 bpm. For this reason, the ACSM and others have recommended that heart rate should not be used alone, but rather in combination with other secondary criteria [4, 32, 33]. In 2001, Tanaka et al. published a new equation for estimating age-predicted maximal heart rate (208 – 0.7 × Age), but whether it will prove to be less variable at all ages remains to be determined [28].

Borg Scale or Rating of Perceived Exertion

The Borg scale is the most widely used method for quantifying perceived exertion. It was designed to increase in a linear fashion as exercise intensity increased and parallel the apparent linearity of VO_2 and heart rate with work load [46, 47]. The original Borg scale ranges from 6 to 20, with each number anchored by a simple and understandable verbal expression. The specific numbers of the scale were intended to be a general representation of actual heart rate, such that when a person was exercising at 130 bpm, a perceived exertion of 13 should be reported. Similarly, if the perceived exertion were 19, a heart rate of around 190 would be expected. The scale was not intended to be exact, but rather an aid in the interpretation of perceived exertion.

Studies have demonstrated a good correlation between RPE and VO_2 [48, 49]. Eston et al. [48] obtained RPE values during a graded exercise test and reported a good correlation between heart rates and VO_2 when the reported RPE was between 13 and 17. An RPE value of 17 or greater should be accepted as meeting the criterion for achieving $VO_{2\,max}$.

Since the initial scale was developed, a variant scale that uses 0–10 as the numeric ratio has been proposed. This non-linear scale, which has not been widely accepted, is suitable for examining subjective symptoms, such as breathing difficulties [46]. However, the original 15-point RPE scale remains the standard for use as a criterion for $VO_{2\,max}$.

Recommended Criteria for Testing

The criteria for $VO_{2\,max}$ were initially established for a discontinuous treadmill test that used 2.5% increases in grade. To date, the criteria for a plateau have not been redefined for other specific tests, but the $150\,mL\;min^{-1}$ increase continues to be used. Since attainment of a true plateau is not an absolute prerequisite, some combination of secondary criterion may be preferable. The criteria presented in Table 1.3 are offered as a guide, and it is suggested that three of the four secondary criteria be met. If a true plateau is noted, then this alone would be sufficient for documenting $VO_{2\,max}$. If the criteria are not met, then the test would be considered $VO_{2\,peak}$.

Table 1.3 Criteria for documenting a maximal effort test*

↑ in VO_2 < 150 mL•min^{-1} or 2.1 mL•kg^{-1}•min^{-1} with a 2.5% grade ↑
Blood lactate ≥ 8 mmol L^{-1}
RER ≥ 1.15
↑ in HR to maximal estimated for age ± 10
Borg scale ≥ 17

* If the first criterion is not met, then at least three of the remaining four should be met.

Factors Affecting Maximal Exercise Performance

Intrinsic Factors

Although many factors determine exercise capacity, the most influential intrinsic factors that influence maximal exercise performance are age, gender, and genetics. Clearly age is one of the most important predictors of exercise capacity. Age is inversely related to $VO_{2\,max}$: $VO_{2\,max}$ declines approximately 10% per decade in the absence of regular activity. Regular aerobic exercise can assist in attenuating this decline. Women tend to have lower $VO_{2\,max}$ levels when compared to men; values are approximately 15% lower even when matched by activity status. Lower values reflect intrinsic differences in body composition, including a greater percent body fat, less muscle mass, smaller hearts, lower vital capacity and lower hemoglobin levels. Genetic endowment may be an important predictor of performance, as both $VO_{2\,max}$ and skeletal muscle adaptations to training appear largely genotype dependent [50].

Extrinsic Factors

In addition to individual intrinsic factors, extrinsic factors, including type of exercise, environment, and postural position can significantly affect performance. $VO_{2\,max}$ is highly dependent on the quantity of skeletal muscle engaged during the exercise. Studies have demonstrated that exercise performed on a treadmill elicits higher $VO_{2\,max}$ values than those elicited by cycle or arm ergometry. However, the specificity of the test is also important: higher $VO_{2\,max}$ values are achieved in swimmers and cyclists when tested while swimming and cycling, respectively. In contrast, persons who have never cycled will typically not do as well on a cycle ergometer as on a treadmill.

Environmental extremes can challenge peak exercise performance; heat and cold produce competing demands for blood flow to accommodate temperature control, whereas altitude compromises peak performance through lower partial pressures of oxygen. Supine and upright exercise can produce significantly different results; upright exercise tends to be more familiar and produces a greater driving force for tissue perfusion, whereas exercise in the supine position elicits higher stroke volumes and cardiac output. These are just a few of the extrinsic factors to be discussed. Others include dietary supplements, prescription medications, clothing, and the like.

Physiology of Ischemia

Myocardial Oxygen Uptake

In order to meet the increasing O_2 demands of external work, the heart must correspondingly increase its own O_2 requirements. The increase in the internal work of the heart is identified as myocardial oxygen uptake (MO_2). Although direct measurements can only be performed in a laboratory setting, MO_2 can be estimated by multiplying systolic blood pressure by heart rate to yield the "double product" or "rate pressure product". The O_2 supply to the heart is augmented primarily by increasing coronary blood flow.

A healthy heart has the capacity to augment coronary blood flow at least fivefold, principally through vasodilation of large and small arterioles. This "coronary flow reserve" is the principal determinant of whether or not the exercise load will result in myocardial ischemia. Ischemia will ensue when the ability of the coronary arteries to augment coronary blood flow is compromised, e.g., atherosclerosis.

ST-Segment Depression

The principal indicator of myocardial ischemia during a graded exercise test is the presence of ST-segment depression. The phenomenon of ST-segment depression reflects an imbalance between myocardial O_2 supply and demand. The normal myocardial action potential has four distinct phases (Fig. 1.4). The fast depolarization (phase 0) is shown by the abrupt upstroke, which is related to the rapid entry of sodium (Na^+) into the cell through the fast Na^+-channels. The fast Na^+-influx initiates atrial, ventricular, and Purkinje action potentials. Phase 0 is terminated at about +30 mV when the fast Na^+-channels are inactivated/closed because of voltage threshold. Phase 1 marks the early repolarization from the upstroke due to potassium (K^+)-outflow. Phase 2 designates the plateau of the action potential, wherein the slow calcium (Ca^{2+})-Na^+-channels remain open for up to 300 ms. Phase 3 is the terminal repolarization and occurs when all the K^+-channels open so that large amounts of K^+ can diffuse out of the ventricular fibers. Phase 4 is recognized by restoration of the resting membrane potential to $-$ 90 mV. This is brought about by the Na^+-K^+ pump, which restores ionic concentrations by exchanging Na^+ for K^+ in a ratio of 3:2.

Ischemia, with a resultant change in deflection of the ST-segment, reflects complex alterations in the electrical properties of the myocardial cell. Under normal conditions, the ST-segment is isoelectric since all myocardial cells repolarize at the same rate to the same resting potential. Ischemia causes a loss of the resting membrane potential, a shortened duration of repolarization, and a decrease in the amplitude and rate of rise for the action potential of phase 0 (Fig. 1.4) [51]. These changes create a voltage gradient between normal and abnormal myocardial cells

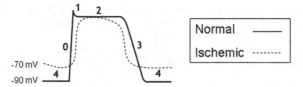

Fig. 1.4 Ventricular ischemia may alter the myocardial action potential by creating a lower resting membrane potential, decreased amplitude of phase 0, and an abbreviated repolarization in phases 2 and 3. The differential repolarization patterns between the epicardium and the endocardium can result in shifts in the ST-segment. (Adapted from Mirvis DM GA. Electrocardiography. In Zipes DP LP, Bonow RO, Braunwald E, ed., *Braunwald's Heart Disease: A Textbook of Cardiovascular Medicine*. Philadelphia: Elsevier; 2005, with permission of Elsevier.)

that leads to changes in repolarization of the cardiac vector and resultant changes in ST-segment deviation on the surface electrocardiogram.

Summary

Exercise testing is an invaluable tool for the primary care clinician. This resource provides a wealth of clinical information pertaining to the cardiopulmonary system, in particular, about how to identify patients with potential heart disease. Knowledge of exercise physiology and its application allows the clinician to create a more accurate picture of the patient's cardiovascular health. In turn, the clinician should be able to more accurately diagnose and manage the patient in health and disease.

References

1. Gibbons RJ, Balady BG, Bricker JT, et al. ACC/AHA 2002 guideline update for exercise testing. Summary article: A report of the ACC/AHA task force on practice guidelines. J Am Coll Cardiol 2002;40:1531.
2. Fletcher GF, Balady GJ, Amsterdam EA, Chaitman B, Eckel R, Fleg J, Froelicher VF, Leon AS, Pina IL, Rodney R, Simons-Morton DA, Williams MA, Bazzarre T. Exercise standards for testing and training: A statement for healthcare professionals from the American Heart Association. Circulation 2001;104:1694–740.
3. Balady GJ, Berra KA, Golding LA, editors. ACSM's Guidelines for Exercise Testing and Prescription. 6th ed. Philadelphia: Lippincott, Williams & Wilkins; 2000.
4. Whaley MH, Brubaker PH, Otto RM, editors. ACSM's Guidelines for Exercise Testing and Prescription. 7th ed. Baltimore: Lippincott, Williams & Wilkins; 2006.
5. Tesch PA, Thorsson A, Essen-Gustavsson B. Enzyme activities of FT and ST muscle fibers in heavy-resistance trained athletes. J Appl Physiol 1989;67:83–7.
6. Li JL, Wang XN, Fraser SF, Carey MF, Wrigley TV, McKenna MJ. Effects of fatigue and training on sarcoplasmic reticulum Ca(2+) regulation in human skeletal muscle. J Appl Physiol 2002;92:912–22.
7. Beltman JG, de Haan A, Haan H, Gerrits HL, van Mechelen W, Sargeant AJ. Metabolically assessed muscle fibre recruitment in brief isometric contractions at different intensities. Eur J Appl Physiol 2004;92:485–92.

8. Beltman JG, Sargeant AJ, Haan H, van Mechelen W, de Haan A. Changes in PCr/Cr ratio in single characterized muscle fibre fragments after only a few maximal voluntary contractions in humans. Acta Physiol Scand 2004;180:187–93.

9. Sargeant AJ, de Haan A. Human muscle fatigue: the significance of muscle fibre type variability studied using a micro-dissection approach. J Physiol Pharmacol 2006;57 Suppl 10:5–16.

10. Kosek DJ, Kim JS, Petrella JK, Cross JM, Bamman MM. Efficacy of 3 days/wk resistance training on myofiber hypertrophy and myogenic mechanisms in young vs. older adults. J Appl Physiol 2006;101:531–44.

11. Putman CT, Xu X, Gillies E, MacLean IM, Bell GJ. Effects of strength, endurance and combined training on myosin heavy chain content and fibre-type distribution in humans. Eur J Appl Physiol 2004;92:376–84.

12. Neary JP, Martin TP, Quinney HA. Effects of taper on endurance cycling capacity and single muscle fiber properties. Med Sci Sports Exerc 2003;35:1875–81.

13. Beltman JG, Sargeant AJ, van Mechelen W, de Haan A. Voluntary activation level and muscle fiber recruitment of human quadriceps during lengthening contractions. J Appl Physiol 2004;97:619–26.

14. Whaley MH, Brubarker PH, Otto RM, editors. ACSM's Guidelines for Exercise Testing and Prescription. 7th ed. Baltimore: Lippincott, Williams & Wilkins; 2006.

15. Kushmerick MJ, Moerland TS, Wiseman RW. Two classes of mammalian skeletal muscle fibers distinguished by metabolite content. Adv Exp Med Biol 1993;332:749–60; discussion 60–1.

16. Stallknecht B, Vissing J, Galbo H. Lactate production and clearance in exercise. Effects of training. A mini-review. Scand J Med Sci Sports 1998;8:127–31.

17. Bell DG, Jacobs I. Muscle fiber-specific glycogen utilization in strength-trained males and females. Med Sci Sports Exerc 1989;21:649–54.

18. Jacobs I, Kaiser P, Tesch P. Muscle strength and fatigue after selective glycogen depletion in human skeletal muscle fibers. Eur J Appl Physiol Occup Physiol 1981;46:47–53.

19. McArdle WD, Katch FI, Katch VL. Exercise Physiology: Energy, Nutrition & Human Performance. 6th ed. Baltimore: Lippincott, Williams and Wilkins; 2007.

20. Levine BD. Exercise physiology for the clinician. In Thompson PD. editor. Exercise and Sports Cardiology. New York: McGraw Hill; 2001.

21. DeBusk RF, Blomqvist CG, Kouchoukos NT, Luepker RV, Miller HS, Moss AJ, Pollock ML, Reeves TJ, Selvester RH, Stason WB, et al. Identification and treatment of low-risk patients after acute myocardial infarction and coronary-artery bypass graft surgery. N Engl J Med 1986;314:161–6.

22. Blair SN, Kohl HW, 3rd, Paffenbarger RS, Jr., Clark DG, Cooper KH, Gibbons LW. Physical fitness and all-cause mortality. A prospective study of healthy men and women. Jama 1989;262:2395–401.

23. Duncan GE, Li SM, Zhou XH. Cardiovascular fitness among U.S. adults: NHANES 1999–2000 and 2001–2002. Med Sci Sports Exerc 2005;37:1324–8.

24. Carnethon MR, Gulati M, Greenland P. Prevalence and cardiovascular disease correlates of low cardiorespiratory fitness in adolescents and adults. JAMA %R 101001/jama294232981 2005;294:2981–8.

25. Victor RG, Secher NH, Lyson T, Mitchell JH. Central command increases muscle sympathetic nerve activity during intense intermittent isometric exercise in humans. Circ Res 1995;76:127–31.

26. Correia LC, Lakatta EG, O'Connor FC, Becker LC, Clulow J, Townsend S, Gerstenblith G, Fleg JL. Attenuated cardiovascular reserve during prolonged submaximal cycle exercise in healthy older subjects. J Am Coll Cardiol 2002;40:1290–7.

27. Williams MA, Fleg JL, Ades PA, et al. Secondary prevention of coronary heart disease in the elderly (with emphasis on patients > or =75 years of age): An American Heart Association scientific statement from the council on clinical cardiology subcommittee on exercise, cardiac rehabilitation, and prevention. Circulation 2002;105:1735–43.

28. Tanaka H, Monahan KD, Seals DR. Age-predicted maximal heart rate revisited. J Am Coll Cardiol 2001;37:153–6.
29. Astrand PO, Ryhming I. A nomogram for calculation of aerobic capacity (physical fitness) from pulse rate during sub-maximal work. J Appl Physiol 1954;7:218–21.
30. Myers JN. The physiology behind exercise testing. Prim Care 2001;28:5–14.
31. Andersen P, Henriksson J. Capillary supply of the quadriceps femoris muscle of man: adaptive response to exercise. J Physiol 1977;270:677–90.
32. Duncan GE, Howley ET, Johnson BN. Applicability of VO2max criteria: Discontinuous versus continuous protocols. Med Sci Sports Exerc 1997;29:273–8.
33. Howley ET, Bassett DR, Jr., Welch HG. Criteria for maximal oxygen uptake: Review and commentary. Med Sci Sports Exerc 1995;27:1292–301.
34. Myers J, Walsh D, Sullivan M, Froelicher V. Effect of sampling on variability and plateau in oxygen uptake. J Appl Physiol 1990;68:404–10.
35. Taylor HL, Buskirk E, Henschel A. Maximal oxygen intake as an objective measure of cardiorespiratory performance. J Appl Physiol 1955;8:73–80.
36. Day JR, Rossiter HB, Coats EM, Skasick A, Whipp BJ. The maximally attainable VO2 during exercise in humans: The peak vs. maximum issue. J Appl Physiol 2003;95:1901–7.
37. Kyle SB, Smoak BL, Douglass LW, Deuster PA. Variability of responses across training levels to maximal treadmill exercise. J Appl Physiol 1989;67:160–5.
38. Fielding RA, Frontera WR, Hughes VA, Fisher EC, Evans WJ. The reproducibility of the Bruce protocol exercise test for the determination of aerobic capacity in older women. Med Sci Sports Exerc 1997;29:1109–13.
39. Gürsel Y, Sonel B, Gok H, et al. The peak oxygen uptake of healthy Turkish children with reference to age and sex: A pilot study. Turk J Pediatr 2004;46:38–43.
40. Astrand PO. Quantification of exercise capability and evaluation of physical capacity in man. Prog Cardiovasc Dis 1976;19:51–67.
41. Astrand PO, Saltin B. Maximal oxygen uptake and heart rate in various types of muscular activity. J Appl Physiol 1961;16:977–81.
42. Astrand PO, Rodahl K. Textbook of work physiology: Physiological bases of exercise. 4th ed. Canada: Human Kinetics; 2003.
43. Cumming GR, Borysyk LM. Criteria for maximum oxygen uptake in men over 40 in a population survey. Med Sci Sports 1972;4:18–22.
44. Stachenfeld NS, Eskenazi M, Gleim GW, et al. Predictive accuracy of criteria used to assess maximal oxygen consumption. Am Heart J 1992;123:922–5.
45. Issekutz BJ, Birkhead NC, Rodahl K. Use of respiratory quotients in assessment of aerobic work capacity. J Appl Physiol 1962;17:47–50.
46. Borg GA. Psychophysical bases of perceived exertion. Med Sci Sports Exerc 1982;14:377–81.
47. Borg GA, Noble B. Perceived exertion. In Wilmore J editor. Exercise and Sport Science Reviews. Wilmore JH ed. New York: Academic Press; 1974, 131–53.
48. Eston RG, Davies BL, Williams JG. Use of perceived effort ratings to control exercise intensity in young healthy adults. Eur J Appl Physiol Occup Physiol 1987;56:222–4.
49. Glass SC, Knowlton RG, Becque MD. Accuracy of RPE from graded exercise to establish exercise training intensity. Med Sci Sports Exerc 1992;24:1303–7.
50. Hamel P, Simoneau JA, Lortie G, et al. Heredity and muscle adaptation to endurance training. Med Sci Sports Exerc 1986;18:690–6.
51. Mirvis DM GA. Electrocardiography. In Zipes DP LP, Bonow RO, Braunwald E editor. Braunwald's Heart Disease: A Textbook of Cardiovascular Medicine. Philadelphia: Elsevier Saunders; 2005.

Chapter 2
Performance of the Exercise Test

George D. Harris and Russell D. White

Each year, over 1 million Americans experience a nonfatal or fatal myocardial infarction or sudden death from coronary heart disease (CHD) [1]. Unfortunately, death or myocardial infarction is the first symptom in 55% of patients with coronary artery disease [2] and is usually due to dislodgement of a plaque causing acute coronary occlusion. However, about 30% of these patients present with ischemia and have concurrent chest pain. In these individuals, exercise treadmill testing is a practical and the most commonly performed test to identify or confirm the presence of latent coronary artery disease [2]. In addition, an abnormal test has been shown to have definite predictive value. It is well known that when symptoms of typical angina are present, coronary disease can be predicted with considerable reliability. Even when there is no history of pain, there is still a strong possibility of significant coronary disease in patients with specific risk factors. Also, the reliability of the test in asymptomatic patients is improved when testing patients with a higher prevalence of the disease.

Exercise testing may also be used to measure functional capacity, assess the patient's prognosis in coronary artery disease, and evaluate the patient's treatment for hypertension, certain arrhythmias, angina, and congestive heart failure. It can be beneficial for patients who will be involved in exercise rehabilitative programs.

It may be useful for predicting mortality risk among patients who plan to start an exercise program, whose job affects public safety (airline pilot), or who have specific medical conditions (diabetes or chronic renal insufficiency).

The inherent accuracy of the test is defined by the sensitivity and specificity. The results of the test when applied to an individual depend on the prevalence of disease in the population to which the patient belongs. So, the two most important factors in the analysis of patients undergoing stress testing are the pre-test prevalence of disease and the sensitivity and specificity of the test. Various types of chest pain affect the probability of disease in each patient. By dividing the patients into one

G.D. Harris (✉)
Department of Community and Family Medicine, University of Missouri-Kansas City, School of Medicine, Truman Medical Center—Lakewood, 7900 Lees Summit Rd., Kansas City, MO 64139, USA
e-mail: george.harris@tmcmed.org

C.H. Evans, R.D. White (eds.), *Exercise Testing for Primary Care and Sports Medicine Physicians,* DOI 10.1007/978-0-387-76597-6_2

Table 2.1 Pre-test probability of coronary artery disease by age, gender, and symptoms

Age	Gender	Typical/definite angina pectoris	Atypical/probable angina pectoris	Nonanginal chest pain	Asymptomatic
30–39	Men	Intermediate	Intermediate	Low	Very low
	Women	Intermediate	Very low	Very low	Very low
40–49	Men	High	Intermediate	Intermediate	Very low
	Women	Intermediate	Low	Low	Very low
50–59	Men	High	Intermediate	Intermediate	Low
	Women	Intermediate	Intermediate	Low	Very low
60–69	Men	High	Intermediate	Intermediate	Low
	Women	High	Intermediate	Intermediate	Low

From Institute for Clinical Systems Improvement. Health Care Guideline: Cardiac Stress Test Supplement, 6th ed. 2004.

of four groups (typical angina, atypical angina, nonanginal chest pain, or no chest pain), one can predict the probability of heart disease in individuals (Table 2.1; see Chapter 5 on interpreting the exercise stress test).

The pre-test evaluation becomes very important when deciding when and how to study an asymptomatic patient. An estimated 1–2 million middle-aged men have asymptomatic but physiologically significant coronary artery obstruction, placing them at increased risk for coronary heart disease events [3,4] Unfortunately, multiple cohort studies have demonstrated that screening exercise tolerance testing identifies only a small proportion of asymptomatic persons (up to 2.7% of those screened) with severe coronary artery obstruction who may benefit from revascularization [1]. In addition, several large prospective cohort studies suggest that exercise tolerance testing can provide independent prognostic information about the risk for future

Table 2.2 Coronary artery risk factors for risk stratification

Hypertension Systolic > 140 mmHg
Diastolic > 90 mmHg
Currently on antihypertensives
Hyperlipidemia
Serum cholesterol > 200 mg%
LDL cholesterol > 130 mg%
HDL cholesterol < 35 mg%
Impaired glucose intolerance
Fasting blood glucose > 100 mg%
Cigarette smoking
Current smoker
Quit smoking 6 months or less
Sedentary lifestyle
Not exercising
Exercising < minimal activity level
Family history
Myocardial infarction
Sudden death
Coronary revascularization

coronary heart disease events (relative risk with abnormal exercise tolerance testing, 2.0–5.0). Thus, evaluation of the exercise test as a prognostic rather than a diagnostic test suggests that the prognostic value of the screening exercise test may have been underestimated.

However, when the risk for CHD is low, there is an increase in false-positive findings resulting in unnecessary further testing or patient anxiety [1]. Therefore, when deciding how to study an asymptomatic patient for coronary disease each patient must be properly evaluated by a history and physical examination as well as stratified by age, gender, symptoms (typical angina, atypical angina, nonanginal chest pain, no symptoms), and major risk factors (diabetes mellitus, hypertension, dyslipidemias, smoking) (Table 2.2).

Indications

The three major cardiopulmonary indications for performing exercise testing are (1) to diagnose the presence or absence of heart disease; (2) to determine the prognosis (risk) in assessing the severity of previously diagnosed disease; and (3) to develop a therapeutic prescription or test the adequacy of the patient's therapy.

Since cardiovascular disease is the leading cause of death in patients with diabetes and diabetes is a coronary artery disease equivalent (the risk of myocardial infarction in patients with diabetes is similar to that of patients without diabetes who have had a previous myocardial infarction), the American College of Cardiology, the American Heart Association, and the American Diabetes Association have recommended graded exercise testing in asymptomatic patients with diabetes who plan to begin a moderate- to high-intensity exercise program and are at increased risk for coronary heart disease (CHD) based on one or more risk factors [2, 5]. The risk factors include age >35 years; age >25 years and type 2 diabetes of > 10 years duration or type 1 diabetes of >15 years duration; any additional risk factors for CHD; and the existence of microvascular disease (retinopathy, neuropathy, nephropathy) or peripheral arterial occlusive disease (PAOD) [6].

However, this level of evidence is based on opinion and not on well-established medical evidence [2, 5]. Furthermore, there are limitations for recommending a screening exercise treadmill testing (ETT) in asymptomatic patients with diabetes. ETT in this population can only identify a small proportion of asymptomatic persons with severe coronary artery obstruction who may benefit from revascularization [7].

The American Heart Association/American College of Cardiology and US Preventive Services Task Force guidelines also acknowledge the possible value of exercise testing in men 45 years old and women 55 years old who plan to start vigorous exercise programs or are involved in high-risk occupations [1, 8].

The American College of Sports Medicine (ACSM) has developed recommendations for exercise testing prior to beginning an exercise program [9]. Patients are categorized according to low-, moderate-, and high-risk groups based on age, sex, presence of coronary artery disease risk factors, major symptoms of disease, or known heart disease [9]. A low-risk individual is an asymptomatic person (man

<45 years or woman <55 years) with no more than one risk factor. An individual at moderate risk is older (man >45 or woman >55) or has more than two risk factors. The individual at high risk has one or more symptoms/signs of CAD or has either known cardiovascular disease, pulmonary disease, or metabolic disease (diabetes mellitus, thyroid disorder, renal disease, liver disease) [9]. Their activity level is divided into moderate (3–6 METs or 40–60% $VO_{2 max}$) and vigorous (> 6 METs or >60% $VO_{2 max}$) exercise. An individual who wants to perform moderate activity and is at high risk or wishes to perform vigorous activity levels and is at moderate or high risk needs an exercise test performed prior to starting that level of exercise [9]. Exercise testing in low-risk, asymptomatic males is usually not recommended unless there are specific cardiac risk factors. There is no chronological age for routine screening of individuals, but the ACSM recommends that low-risk men and women (age < 45 years and 55 years, respectively) be exempted from routine screening [9].

Exercise treadmill testing is indicated for evaluating a patient with chest pain, determining the prognosis and severity of disease, evaluating the effects of medical and surgical therapy, evaluating a patient after myocardial infarction for risk stratification and for the early detection of labile hypertension, and evaluating arrhythmias, congestive heart failure, and a patient's functional capacity. It can also be used to formulate an exercise prescription or to evaluate an individual training program for an athlete.

Contraindications

Absolute Contraindications

Absolute contraindications include those situations in which the risks involved in performing the procedure outweigh any benefit [1]. Some of these patients should be referred directly to a cardiologist while others should be further evaluated prior to cardiac testing.

The absolute contraindications [10] to performing exercise testing include the following:

1. A recent significant change in the resting electrocardiograph (ECG) suggestive of significant ischemia or other recent cardiac event
2. Recent myocardial infarction (within 2 days) or other acute cardiac event
3. Unstable angina
4. Uncontrolled cardiac arrhythmias causing symptoms or hemodynamic compromise
5. Patients with known severe left main disease
6. Severe symptomatic aortic stenosis
7. Uncompensated congestive heart failure
8. Acute pulmonary embolus or pulmonary infarction (within 3 months)
9. Suspected or confirmed dissecting aneurysm
10. Acute infection

11. Hyperthyroidism
12. Severe anemia
13. Acute myocarditis or pericarditis
14. Uncooperative patient
15. Neuromuscular, musculoskeletal, or rheumatoid disorders that prohibit exercise or are exacerbated by exercise

Relative Contraindications

Relative contraindications include those situations in which the risks involved from performing the procedure may exceed the benefits. These patients require careful evaluation, and cardiology consultation may be indicated in some cases. Some of these conditions require correction or stabilization before testing. Relative contraindications [10] to exercise testing include

1. Known left main artery stenosis
2. Moderately stenotic valvular heart disease
3. Electrolyte abnormalities (e.g., hypokalemia, hypomagnesemia)
4. Severe arterial hypertension (systolic greater than 200 mmHg or diastolic greater than 110 mmHg) [10]
5. Asymmetrical septal hypertrophy
6. Hypertrophic cardiomyopathy or other forms of outflow tract obstruction
7. Compensated heart failure
8. Ventricular aneurysm
9. Uncontrolled metabolic disease (e.g., diabetes mellitus, thyrotoxicosis, or myxedema)
10. Patients with high-degree atrioventricular heart block
11. Tachy- or brady-arrhythmias
12. Mental or physical impairment leading to inability to exercise adequately

Special Considerations for Exercise Testing

There are special situations in which the physician must evaluate the patient carefully before undertaking exercise testing or consider an alternative test. An alternative to exercise stress testing is chemical (pharmacological) stress testing, e.g., those unable to exercise on the treadmill. With either chemical or exercise stress testing one may couple imaging studies such as echocardiography or nuclear scanning. With chemical stress testing a specific medication, such as dobutamine, dipyridamole, or adenosine, is administered with the patient resting supine to chemically stimulate the heart and increase the heart rate. For example, a post-cerebrovascular accident patient may be unable to exercise and may require a pharmacological stress test for evaluation.

Other special situations will usually fall into one of three groups: (1) conduction disturbances, (2) medication effects, and (3) special clinical situations.

Conduction Disturbances

Conduction disturbances involving atrioventricular (AV) blocks must be evaluated from the baseline ECG. Patients with first-degree AV blocks and some second-degree AV blocks (Mobitz type I) may undergo exercise stress testing. However, testing those with high-degree AV blocks (second-degree Mobitz type II and third-degree AV block), especially in older individuals, is not recommended [2]. With the high incidence of coronary artery disease in these persons one may see progression to or exacerbation of third-degree heart block with marked bradycardia, resulting in serious hemodynamic changes.

The presence of left bundle branch block or Wolff–Parkinson–White syndrome precludes diagnostic exercise testing for coronary artery disease. The distorted ST-segment changes seen on baseline ECGs cannot be interpreted accurately during exercise testing. Instead, one should consider nuclear imaging and chemical stress tests in these individuals [2, 5]. In contrast, those individuals with the presence of right bundle branch block can usually be studied. Because the ST-segment distortion is usually limited to leads $V_1–V_3$, one can generally diagnose ischemia based on the lateral chest leads.

Medication Effects

Many patients selected for stress testing may be under treatment for other medical problems. Medication effects may influence the exercise test and either preclude testing or alter results. It is not uncommon for the physician to see a patient who develops chest pain while under treatment for hypertension or coronary artery disease with beta blockers or calcium channel blockers. Some controversy exists as to whether the beta blockers should be stopped or continued at the time of exercise testing. One may choose to test patients while receiving beta blocker therapy to test drug efficacy. If they are continued, the heart-rated response may be blunted. When the test is done for diagnosis of coronary artery disease, most clinicians stop beta blockers prior to the test, tapering short-acting agents to avoid a rebound phenomenon [11]. If a short-acting agent (e.g., metoprolol) is prescribed, one may hold the medication on the test day, but long-acting agents should be held 1–2 days prior to the test. Beta blockers not only will decrease the maximal heart rate achieved in a given patient but may also improve exercise capacity in cardiac patients. Some clinicians use a stress-imaging test to diagnose coronary artery disease in those patients when beta blockers cannot be stopped. Ellestad feels these agents will not obscure ischemic ST-segment depression seen in those with epicardial coronary artery disease [5].

Calcium channel blockers, in contrast, often delay the time of onset of ST-segment depression. Furthermore, the antianginal properties of these agents decrease the sensitivity of the exercise test. Specific agents, such as high-dose verapamil, may alter the heart rate response to exercise similar to that seen with beta blockers. Excessive doses of nifedipine may produce hypotension with exercise and reduce the exercise tolerance of the patient [12, 13]. While high doses of diltiazem may also block the heart rate response, moderate doses are often well tolerated. Second-generation dihydropyridine agents (e.g., felodipine, nicardipine, isradipine) do not produce tachycardia, do not alter heart rate response, and extend the ischemic threshold [5].

Cardiac glycosides are known to produce ST-segment depression and inhibit the chronotropic response during exercise in both normal persons and patients with known coronary artery disease [5]. Because exercise-induced changes may persist for 14 days after digoxin is discontinued, many patients are tested while receiving the medication [14]. If marked depression (4–5 mm) occurs, ischemic heart disease is confirmed. In patients with enhancement of rest ST-segment depression, one must evaluate the degree of change that occurs to determine the presence of ischemia. Marked ST-segment changes due to ischemia will improve with nitroglycerin administration while those changes due to digitalis will not. Thus, patients receiving digitalis who experience mild ST-segment changes with exercise may need a stress-imaging study or angiography to determine whether these changes are due to drug effect.

Tricyclic antidepressants are known to alter ECGs, but there are no reports of ST-segment depression with exercise testing. However, these agents may depress left ventricular function, produce hypotension, and create increasing degrees of heart block. Thus, caution is warranted when testing persons treated with these medications [15–17]. While serotonin uptake inhibitors (SSRIs) may reduce the capacity to perform prolonged exercise, no metabolic or cardiorespiratory responses to exercise have been reported and they should not affect exercise test results [18].

The common use of diuretics must be evaluated carefully. Moderate ST-segment depression may be induced if hypokalemia from diuretics is severe. Thus, serum potassium should be measured in patients receiving potassium-depleting diuretics. In contrast, angiotensin-converting enzyme inhibitors would produce neither hypokalemia nor significant ST-segment changes [19, 20]. During exercise testing in patients receiving angiotensin-converting enzyme inhibitors (ACEIs), the systolic blood pressure is lower during exercise than in controls with no change in heart rate response. In addition, ACEIs have been reported to reduce exercise-induced ischemia [2, 21]. In many ways the physiology of the angiotensin II receptor blockers (ARBs) parallels the ACEIs. Hamroff et al. have shown that ARBs also improve exercise capacity and prolong the time to ischemia [22].

Special Clinical Situations

Testing hypertensive patients in clinical practice is common. However, one should not test patients with severe resting hypertension (blood pressure recordings greater than 240/130 mmHg) until their hypertension is under control [2]. In addition, labile hypertension often becomes manifest during exercise testing following a normotensive resting blood pressure. This hypertensive response to exercise requires either initiation or augmentation of antihypertensive therapy.

Another special consideration in exercise testing is aortic stenosis. The presence of valvular outflow obstruction is worrisome and may precipitate serious complications including syncope, acute myocardial infarction, and lethal ventricular dysrhythmias. Thus, testing patients with severe aortic stenosis is contraindicated. Patients with moderate disease require pre-test echocardiography, careful consideration, and possible cardiology consultation before undergoing exercise testing.

Finally, someone who suffers from severe arthritis or marked exogenous obesity may be unable to exercise for cardiac evaluation. Pharmacologic stress testing or coronary angiography may be indicated in these individuals.

The Setting

The exercise treadmill area should be a pleasant, professional environment properly air-conditioned and regulated at a comfortable temperature and humidity. The individuals in the room should be limited to only the physician, an advanced cardiac life support (ACLS) certified nurse, and the patient to provide for maximum patient safety.

The Equipment

Exercise testing equipment includes an exercise device, a monitor, an electrocardiography (ECG) recorder, and resuscitative equipment. Vendors are listed in Table 2.3. The treadmill is the most common exercise device used in the United States. Most Americans are familiar with walking and are comfortable with this testing method. It allows the patient to walk, jog, or run at measured speeds and grades of incline to regulate the workload or stress to the body. Current computerized systems control these parameters while an ECG monitor records cardiovascular changes with exercise. While standard testing programs have been developed, individual protocols can be designed by the physician but this is not encouraged since individual self-developed protocols may not be verified in large numbers of patients. In addition, the ramp protocol can be individualized for specific individuals.

The four features of the treadmill include the speed, grade or slope, controls, and safety features. The speed commonly begins with a warm-up rate of 0.5–1.5 mph and increases to testing speeds ranging from 2.0 to 5.0 mph. Most individuals can

Table 2.3 Equipment and supplies

GE Marquette CASE Stress System	Milwaukee, WI	http://www.gehealthcare.com/worldwide.html
Medgraphics Cardio Perfect Stress System	St. Paul, MN	http://www.medgraph.com/datasheet_cardio_perfect.htm
Quinton Q-Stress Cardiac Stress System	Bothell, WA	www.quinton.com
Spacelabs Burdick Quest Stress Test System	Deerfield, WI	www.spacelabsburdick.com
Welch Allyn PCE PC-Based ECG System	Skaneateles Falls, NY	www.welchallyn.com

be tested within this range. For the testing of endurance or elite athletes, the speed may be increased to 7.0 mph or greater.

The treadmill incline determines the slope or grade of the treadmill. Most systems start at 0% grade and range up to 20% grade. The standard Bruce protocol begins at a grade of 10%, while protocols for elite athletes range up to 25% grade. The stage in a specific stress protocol is defined by the time interval (usually, 2 or 3 min), the speed and slope of the treadmill during that interval. By changing the speed and slope of the treadmill during a defined interval (stage), one is able to vary the workload presented to the patient.

Controls for treadmill testing are computer-assisted but can be manually overridden. Standard protocols with specific speed and grade intervals are available. Systems are equipped with stage-advance and stage-hold controls which permit the physician to customize a stress test to the individual patient. Safety features include front and side rails as well as emergency stop features. Most motors are quiet, powerful, and self-calibrating. An adequate running surface is necessary to accommodate tall subjects and allow them to maintain a normal stride and not affect their performance.

In contrast, most Europeans are more familiar with cycling and this testing device is more common there. The two basic bicycle ergometers include manual and electric models. The manual type is inexpensive but requires mechanical adjustment of the resistance while maintaining a constant pedaling speed. Electronically braked models include a computerized system that compensates for a decrease in speed with increasing resistance or workload. These models are more expensive. The workload from the cycle ergometer is measured in kiloponds (1 W equals 6 kiloponds) and increases by 150 kiloponds for each 2 min stage of exercise.

Compared to treadmill systems ergometers require less space, less expense or cost, and produce less artifact on the ECG due to less torso movement. Some individuals may have lower test results on the bicycle due to less-developed muscles required for cycling. Niederberger et al. found that bicycle testing elicits a greater stress on the cardiovascular system than does treadmill testing for specific level of oxygen uptake [23]. An individual performing on the treadmill may or will have a peak $VO_{2\,max}$ 5–10% higher than on a cycle ergometer [24]. The greatest disadvantage of the treadmill is the difficulty in quantifying work rate because any connections between the patient and the treadmill decrease the expected energy requirement for body movement at that grade and speed [24]. With the bicycle, the weight must be considered and calculated to determine the METs achieved. With the treadmill the weight occurs in both the numerator and the denominator of the calculation and is thus not considered in the final calculation.

The monitors have computer programs that can present the ECGs in a neatly arranged form. Most monitors display three simultaneous leads (e.g., II, V_1, and V_5) although all 12 leads can be monitored. These three leads, together with the speed, slope, stage, time, METs, and recorded blood pressure measurements, are displayed on the screen for continuous review by the physician.

The recording device is a 12-lead ECG recorder for producing a permanent record of the ECG tracing in addition to a digital record. These records include the digitally processed ECG complexes, degree of ST-segment abnormalities, and workload accomplished together with blood pressure response, heart rate response, METs achieved, and any clinical symptoms.

While the computer-generated report may be useful, the physician must still over-read the ECG hard copy and not rely on the signal-averaged data and complexes.

Blood pressure monitoring needs to be done before, during, and after the test. The standard cuff method is still preferred even though a number of automated devices are available but not recommended [2].

Other equipment that may be utilized includes ventilation-measuring equipment to determine the oxygen uptake (VO_2) during exercise. The development of newer equipment has made this less cumbersome and less costly. In addition, this can be utilized in the outpatient setting. Gas analysis enhances the accuracy of the estimated $VO_{2\,max}$ from exercise stress testing.

The Preparation

The objective should be to learn the maximum about the patient's pathophysiological causes of exercise limitation with the greatest accuracy, with the least stress to the patient, and in the shortest timeframe [24].

Physician's Responsibilities

The physician's responsibilities include (1) pre-test patient evaluation and clearance; (2) selection of the proper protocol; (3) performing the test, including (a) patient preparation, (b) patient monitoring, (c) test termination; (4) recovery of the patient; and (5) interpretation of the test.

Pre-test Patient Evaluation and Clearance

Obtaining a careful history of the patient's symptoms and past medical problems is the most important aspect of patient evaluation. Chest pain symptoms should be defined and characterized as angina, atypical angina, or atypical chest pain. One should be aware of any history or symptoms of exercise-induced syncope or near-syncope, significant left ventricular outflow obstruction, uncontrolled congestive heart failure or unstable angina as well as symptoms suggestive of viral myocarditis or pericarditis. These pathological processes may produce chest pain syndromes but are situations in which exercise testing is contraindicated. One should note any major risk factor for coronary artery disease, including a history of smoking, hypertension, hyperlipidemia, diabetes mellitus, obesity, as well as family history. Any family history of sudden death during exercise is particularly worrisome. Results from any previous exercise test should be reviewed and the patient queried of any problems with prior testing. It is especially important to discuss any recent interval change in the chest pain pattern or medical history before initiating exercise testing. Some patients may experience progression of atypical chest pain to unstable angina following initial scheduling of the exercise test a few days earlier.

Physical Examination

At some point before exercise testing, a pre-test cardiovascular examination should include (1) bilateral blood pressure measurements, (3) notation of pulse pressure, (3) simultaneous radial–femoral pulse evaluation, (4) carotid upstroke evaluation, and (5) careful auscultation of the second heart sound. The examiner should note any systolic murmurs suggestive of aortic stenosis or hypertrophic cardiomyopathy. One should search for any signs of uncompensated congestive heart failure or extra heart sounds.

Patient Informed Consent

The examiner should explain the test once again to the patient and then obtain written consent. Risks of the procedure are explained, and other options for evaluation are reviewed. Safety equipment and trained personnel as described in the 2007 ACLS guidelines should be available [25]. Studies have shown that risks from submaximal testing and the testing of low-risk individuals are very minimal. In some large centers, testing is completed by properly trained health professionals in consultation with physicians [9]. It is recommended that family physicians be physically present when doing exercise testing in their office.

Selecting the Protocol

Bruce, Ellestad, Naughton, and other cardiologists have developed several treadmill protocols for inducing and detecting ECG changes consistent with myocardial ischemia [24]. With each protocol, the measurement of performance is expressed in basal metabolic equivalents (METs). One MET equals the resting oxygen consumption rate of $3.5\,ml\,O_2/kg/min$. The maintenance of life in the resting state (lying or sitting) requires one MET of energy. Multiples of this basal energy rate are required for different activities. Most exercise testing systems automatically estimate the METs, and maximum workload attained is best expressed in these units. All test results stated in this manner can be compared with a previous or subsequent test of a given patient. With treadmill stress testing the MET level at each stage of the exercise test is the same for a given weight of the study person and requires no correction. In contrast, the patient's weight must be factored into results when utilizing the cycle ergometer.

There are clear advantages in customizing the protocol to the individual patient to allow 8–12 min of exercise. Exercise capacity should be reported in estimated metabolic equivalents (METs) of exercise. If exercise capacity is also reported in minutes, the nature of the protocol should be specified clearly [10].

Prior to selecting the exercise protocol, one must decide whether to choose a maximal or submaximal exercise test. Most information is usually obtained from a maximal exercise test in which a patient performs true maximum effort and reaches the point of exhaustion. In this manner a true peak maximal effort is achieved rather than a level defined from age-determined heart rate tables. If one chooses a symptom-limited maximal stress test, the patient is in control and ultimate information is obtained. If the ECG and blood pressure are normal and the patient follows the Borg Scale of perceived exertion, very little risk is posed for the patient. The use of rating of perceived exertion scales is often helpful in assessment of patient fatigue [10, 26]. One can instruct the patient in using either the Borg RPE Scale (the classic 15-grade scale) or the nonlinear 10-grade scale (the Borg CR10 Scale; Borg's Perceived Exertion and Pain Scales, Human Kinetics, Champaign, IL) [27, 28]. The selected protocol should provide an optimal test duration of 8–12 min [5].

Symptom-limited tests are maximal tests that may be terminated easily if the patient develops a significant symptom based on either subjective or objective parameters. These parameters include the patient's appearance and breathing rate, the Borg Scale of perceived exertion, the age-predicted maximum heart rate, exercise capacity, and the blood pressure response. When choosing exercise protocols the clinician should be familiar with both an easy protocol and a more vigorous one.

The Bruce protocol is the most common protocol for exercise testing and is used in 66% of all routine clinical tests performed [7]. This protocol begins with 3 min stages of walking at 1.7 mph and 10% grade. The grade is incremented 2% every 3 min and the speed is incremented 0.8 mph every 3 min until the treadmill reaches 18% grade and 5 mph. This is a vigorous approach involving large jumps in workloads between stages reaching high exertional levels rapidly. Stage four of this protocol is frequently awkward, and it is sometimes difficult for the patient to choose between running and walking, which results in differing oxygen consumption rates. In some studies, it has been found to have a poor correlation with measured gas analysis.

There are several ways to achieve an easy protocol for less fit or elderly persons. A Naughton 2.0 or modified Bruce protocol may be chosen when the patient may require a warm-up phase or is less fit. The patient begins with 3 min of exercise at 0% grade at 1.7 mph and then increases to 3 min of 5% grade at 1.7 mph. The patient then enters the standard Bruce protocol.

Submaximal heart rate-limited tests involve terminating exercise when the patient reaches some predetermined minimal heart rate. For diagnostic testing, this target heart rate is commonly 85% of the maximum predicted heart rate (MPHR). By convention, calculation of the MPHR is 220–240 beats/min minus the person's age in years. This calculated MPHR has a standard deviation of $\pm$ 12 beats. The heart rate-limited tests have a lower sensitivity due to the large range in the age-predicted maximal heart rates [5]. For example, two persons of the same age may have a calculated predetermined heart rate of 170 while one may exercise maximally to 160 and the other at 182 with formal testing. This system may result in a failure to gain all of the information available in comparison with a symptom-limited exercise test. By using submaximal tests, one will usually over-test the fit, low-risk patient and under-test the unfit, high-risk patient. This can lead to false-negative results.

Submaximal tests are also used to evaluate patients' status post-myocardial infarction before discharge from the hospital to ensure that they can safely perform activities of daily living. Testing of these patients is usually terminated when the patient achieves 5 METs of work or approximately 65% of the maximum predicted heart rate. Often, the Naughton or USAFSAM 2.0 treadmill protocol is utilized as the submaximal test protocol.

With the USAFSAM or Balke–Ware protocols, the speed remains constant while the grade is gradually increased. This is quite useful for older individuals who cannot tolerate rapid walking or running. However, these persons can tolerate an increasing grade, and, in this fashion, their workload can be increased and measured. With these protocols there are smaller but equal workload changes between stages. For those patients requiring a protocol between the low-level USAFSAM and the standard Bruce protocol, a 3.3-mph modified Balke–Ware protocol might be utilized [5]. These exercise protocols are summarized in Fig. 2.1.

Incremental exercise protocols obtain continual measurements while the work rate is increased continuously (ramp protocol) or by a uniform amount each minute until the patient is limited by symptoms or the clinician feels the protocol cannot be continued safely [24].

Incremental exercise protocols are considered more physiologic and involve a continuous steady increase in workload without the abrupt, unequal changes seen in the stage protocols. The gradual increases in both speed and slope can be individualized to the testing situation. Typically, one estimates and then enters the maximum MET level for a given individual, the desired test duration, and the test speed. The ramp protocol then derives the increases in grade to achieve this predetermined maximum MET level at the desired finishing time. Alternatively, one may utilize

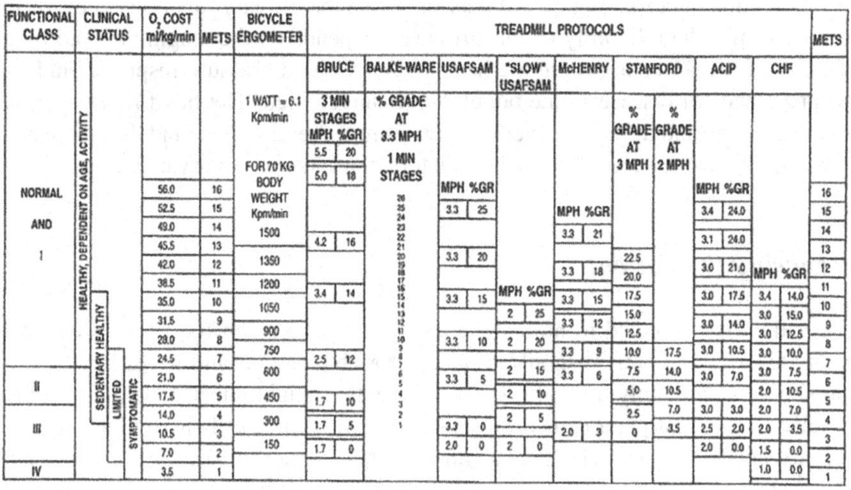

Fig. 2.1 Summary of protocols (From White RD, Evans EH [32], with permission of *Primary Care Clin*, with permission of Elsevier.)

a ramped Bruce protocol which is designed to complete Stage IV in 12 min and has been preferred by patients [29]. Ramp protocols correlate well with measured gas analysis [5].

Some patients may benefit from proceeding directly to exercise testing coupled with echocardiography or a nuclear imaging study, such as thallium-201 or technetium [(technetium-99m sestamibi [*Cardiolite*] or technetium-99m tetrofosamine {*Myoview*}]. When choosing an imaging procedure for primary evaluation, the examiner should consider the following:

1. Imaging testing greatly adds to the expense of the procedure.
2. Imaging testing may increase time for the procedure, e.g., two-phase technetium imaging.
3. One should consider radionuclide testing if there are resting ECG changes of left bundle branch block; pre-excitation syndrome, such as Wolff–Parkinson–White; marked ST-segment changes secondary to hypertension, digoxin, or quinidine; Q-wave evidence of prior large infarctions; or an inability to attain target heart rate.
4. Stress echocardiography is helpful if one suspects a wall-motion abnormality.
5. Some investigators may choose to perform cardiac catheterization directly due to a high probability of severe coronary artery disease.
6. Some patients requiring cardiac catheterization may still benefit from exercise testing for prognostic (risk stratification analysis) or exercise prescription but not for diagnostic considerations.

The Procedure

The prediction of coronary artery disease is one of the primary functions of exercise stress testing. The reliability of the stress test depends on the magnitude and time of onset of the ST changes, on the heart rate and blood pressure response, and on the prevalence of disease in the population being studied. The heart rate response during exercise and during recovery, the maximum exercise time, and the frequency of ventricular ectopy are additional predictors of a future coronary event.

Preparing the Patient

The patient is instructed to not smoke and to eat little or no food for at least 2 h before testing. The patient should wear comfortable clothes and shoes for the test and should avoid applying body oils or lotions that might interfere with attaching the electrodes. Lastly, patients are usually reminded to take their routine medications except their beta blockers or calcium channel blockers prior to exercise testing. The exception to this recommendation deals with those patients with documented CAD. These individuals do better during exercise with beta blockers, achieving a higher workload [2]. Patients taking calcium channel blockers also perform at higher workloads even though their systolic blood pressure and heart rate decrease for a given level of exercise [2, 30].

For ECG monitoring, the skin must be prepared properly. Hair must be shaved in the appropriate locations, an abrasive rub applied to the skin to remove the superficial dead skin cells (which act as insulators), and any oils or other chemicals removed with an alcohol wipe. Although these steps can be time-consuming, they are very important to ensure an adequate tracing for data analysis. The goal is to reduce the skin resistance between any two electrodes to less than 5,000 ohms. When the prep steps have been completed, the silver chloride electrodes are applied. A simple "tap test" can be done by striking the electrodes to see whether any artifact is produced. A well-prepared electrode should display no artifact. Objective testing of the electrode prep with commercial impedance meters or a simple ohmmeter is recommended.

Electrodes are then placed in the standard positions for obtaining a resting 12-lead ECG. This tracing is compared with a previous tracing to determine if any recent ECG change has occurred. Next a Mason–Likar torso-mounted lead system is utilized by placing modified arm leads on the lateral front edge of the shoulders bilaterally. The modified right leg electrode (ground lead) is placed over the backbone on the lower back while the left leg electrode (bottom of Einthoven's triangle) is placed directly below the umbilicus [5] (Fig. 2.2).

In 1999, Michaelides et al. published an article on the use of right ventricular leads to increase the sensitivity of the standard exercise test [31]. Michaelides et al. tested 275 patients referred for evaluation of angina-type symptoms. Each patient underwent exercise testing with the standard leads and right ventricular leads, thallium-201 scintigraphy, and cardiac catheterization. They found that using the right ventricular leads increased the sensitivity of the exercise test to detect significant coronary artery disease from 66 to 92%, creating sensitivity equal to that of thallium scanning (93%). There is some disagreement on the significance of these findings since this study has never been replicated. Some feel that right precordial leads should not be routinely used until the findings of Michaelides are validated in larger studies, while others feel using right precordial leads is of proven value both in diagnosing right ventricular infarctions and in standard exercise testing [32].

To use right precordial leads, the precordial areas of the chest on the right side that correspond to the left precordial lead of V_4, V_5, and V_6 are prepped and electrodes placed in these corresponding areas. The additional electrode lead wires are attached to these new leads which are labeled V_4R, V_5R, and V_6R. Once these leads are in place, the test is performed as usual and the ECG recorder prints a 15-lead electrocardiogram at each stage and in recovery, with the right precordial leads appropriately labeled. This 15-lead ECG monitoring requires special equipment and programs with an increased cost.

Finally, an appropriately sized blood pressure cuff is placed snugly on the patient's arm and secured in place for serial measurements during the testing process. Although commercial automatic blood pressure manometers have been developed, none can be recommended [5]. Indications for any additional monitoring at that time can be reviewed, including pulse oximetry measurements in selected individuals

12-lead ECG Electrode Placement

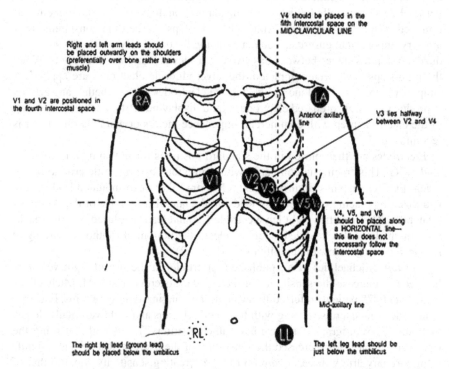

Fig. 2.2 Mason–Likar lead placement (From White RD, Evans EH [32], with permission of *Primary Care Clin*, with permission of Elsevier.)

with chronic obstructive pulmonary disease or in those in whom exercise-induced hypoxemia is suspected. In addition, a pre-test blood glucose measurement can be obtained and repeated at intervals in selected diabetic patients. Also, peak flow measurements or spirometry are done in those with suspected exercise-induced asthma (EIA), which is the most common cause of atypical chest pain associated with exercise in younger groups.

Monitoring the Patient

At this time, the pre-test checklist can be reviewed and final instructions given [32] (Table 2.4). One may obtain the baseline ECG tracings, blood pressure recordings, and heart rate. These resting measurements are obtained in the supine as well as standing positions. First, a standard resting supine ECG is obtained with

Table 2.4 Pre-test checklist

1. Equipment and safety check (including defibrillator and resuscitative medications)
2. Obtain informed consent
3. Pre-test history and physical examination
4. Enter patient information into exercise test system
5. Electrode skin preparation and placement
6. Connect exercise testing monitor to electrodes
7. Place blood pressure cuff on appropriate arm and secure in place
8. Place patient supine and obtain resting blood pressure and ECG
9. Review resting 12-lead ECG for any recent changes
10. Change electrode positions to Mason–Likar torso-mounted limb lead position
11. Have patient stand and obtain blood pressure and ECG
12. Hyperventilation ECG is no longer recommended and may be omitted
13. Instruct and demonstrate appropriate treadmill walking method

    a. Instruct patient to neither hold tightly onto nor grip hand rails; use light touch for balance
    b. Encourage upright position and long stride length
    c. Remind patient that blood pressure will be checked during each stage
    d. Remind patient regarding use of Borg scale
    e. Remind patient to notify examiner when within one minute of maximum effort

14. Complete any other tests, e.g., fingerstick glucose, pulse oximetry, peak flow measurement
15. Ask if there are any final questions prior to testing

Adapted from White RD, Evans EH: Performing the exercise test. Primary Care 21:455, 1994, with permission of Elsevier.

the extremity leads placed on the wrists and ankles for comparison with the patient's previous standard supine tracing. With this important step the examiner can evaluate any recent ECG changes that might preclude exercise testing. These extremity leads are then moved to the modified positions as described previously in the Mason–Likar lead system and a second tracing obtained. The patient is then placed in the standing position, and an ECG utilizing the modified leads is obtained. One may note a change in the R vector (usually lead aV_L) with a change in the standing position. One should compare the modified standing baseline ECG, which now becomes the baseline tracing, against ECGs obtained during the exercise test. One is now ready to begin the exercise testing mode.

Exercise Testing Mode

Once the patient has completed a low-level warm-up and has adapted to the treadmill, the chosen test protocol is begun. When the patient is comfortable, the exercise phase should be initiated and the patient checked constantly. The patient is cautioned to avoid tightly gripping the safety side or front rails. This practice alters the workload and measured performance.

The electrocardiogram (ECG), heart rate, and blood pressure should be monitored and recorded during each stage of exercise and during ST-segment abnormalities and chest pain. The patient should be monitored continuously for transient rhythm disturbances, ST-segment changes, and other electrocardiographic manifestations of myocardial ischemia [10].

The physician should observe the ECG monitor carefully. A 12-lead ECG tracing should be obtained during the last minute of each stage of exercise, at the point of maximum exercise testing, at 1 min in recovery, and then every 2 min during the recovery phase. The blood pressure is obtained and recorded with each ECG tracing. This includes a blood pressure reading with the patient resting supine, standing at rest, during the last minute of each stage of the exercise protocol, at the point of maximum exercise, immediately post-exercise, at 1 min in recovery and then every 2 min during the recovery phase (1, 3, 5, 7 min, etc.). During the testing procedure, the examiner should communicate frequently with and warn the patient of upcoming stage changes. The examiner should stop the exercise test when the patient has reached maximal effort (Borg Scale) or exhibits clinical signs to terminate. It has been found that symptom-limited testing with the Borg CR10 Scale as an aid is very important when the test is used to assess functional capacity.

Terminating the Test

The patient should be informed that he/she is in charge and can stop the test at any time. Otherwise, test termination requires clinical evaluation and judgment concerning the status of the patient. Absolute indications to terminate exercise testing include the following:

1. Acute myocardial infarction or suspicion of myocardial infarction
2. Onset of progressive angina or anginal equivalents
3. Exertional hypotension – decrease of systolic blood pressure (20 mmHg) with increasing workload or a decrease below the baseline standing systolic blood pressure prior to test, accompanied by signs or symptoms indicating poor left ventricular function and poor cardiac output
4. Serious dysrhythmias, e.g., ventricular tachycardia
5. Signs of poor perfusion (pallor, cyanosis, nausea or cold, clammy skin)
6. Central nervous system symptoms (ataxia, vertigo, visual or gait problems, and confusion)
7. Failure of increasing heart rate response with increasing workload
8. Technical problems with monitoring the ECG or equipment failure
9. Patient requests to stop

Relative indications to terminate exercise testing include the following:

1. Pronounced ECG changes from baseline, including more than 2 mV of horizontal or downsloping ST-segment depression or 2 mV of ST-segment elevation
2. Progressive or increasing chest pain
3. Pronounced fatigue or shortness of breath

4. Wheezing
5. Leg cramps or intermittent claudication
6. Hypertensive response (systolic blood pressure greater than 250 mmHg or diastolic blood pressure greater than 115 mmHg) [5]
7. Less serious dysrhythmias such as supraventricular tachycardia
8. Exercise-induced bundle branch block that cannot be distinguished from ventricular tachycardia

Recovery of the Patient

During the recovery phase, the patient should be placed immediately in the supine position or allowed a "cool-down walk" and then placed in a chair. The examiner should auscultate the patient immediately for any abnormal heart findings such as a new-onset heart murmur or third heart sound. In addition, one should auscultate the lungs for any evidence of exercise-induced bronchospasm, which might be a cause of chest pain complaints. During the recovery phase the blood pressure and ECG recordings should be obtained at 1 min and then every 2 min. The heart rate recording at 1 min post-graded exercise and the 3 min systolic BP:peak BP ratio have been correlated with overall mortality and prognosis [33]. The patient is observed carefully until he/she is stable and any observed ST-segment changes have returned to baseline. This usually requires 8–10 min. It is important to watch carefully for any "recovery-only" ST-segment depression [34].

Some debate exists as to whether the patient should be immediately placed supine or allowed a cool-down walk. The consensus opinion is that a cool-down walk will delay "recovery-only" ST-segment depression, and thus the patient should be monitored in recovery for at least 10 min with this method. If, instead, the patient is immediately placed supine after maximal exercise and the legs elevated, recovery monitoring can be limited to 6–8 min. Maximal test sensitivity is achieved with the patient supine post-exercise. If any ST-segment depression persists in the recovery period, one may consider administration of sublingual nitroglycerin. If nitroglycerin is given, one should place the patient supine and monitor the blood pressure and other vital signs until the ST-segment changes have resolved.

Once the patient is stable, the ECG monitoring equipment can be removed, the information interpreted, the patient informed of the results, and a formal dictation of the procedure completed.

Hazards and Complications of Exercise Testing

Serious complications include acute myocardial infarction, ventricular fibrillation, or death. To deal with these possible complications, one must be trained in cardiopulmonary resuscitation (CPR) as well as advanced cardiac life support (ACLS) protocols. ACLS equipment, including proper medications and a defibrillator, should be available at all times. The most important safety precaution is careful pre-test patient evaluation and selection of the proper protocol in light of the contraindications.

Table 2.5 CPT codes

CPT code	Description
93000	ECG with interpretation and report
93005	ECG, without interpretation and report
93010	ECG interpretation and report only
93015	CV stress test with supervision, interpretation, and report
93016	CV stress test supervision only
93018	CV stress test interpretation and report only
94760	Pulse oximetry, single determination
94761	Pulse oximetry, multiple determination
94620	Pulmonary stress testing with pre- and post-spirometry and oximetry

The Report

Current computer treadmill systems produce tabular and graphical analysis of the results of the study. ECG, heart rate, and blood pressure data provide the information leading to pathophysiologic diagnosis. The report should include a brief summary of relevant clinical information, medications, specific exercise-related complaints, a brief description of the methods and procedure, and a narrative analysis and interpretation. In addition, recommendations regarding the results are included [24]. CPT codes are listed in Table 2.5.

Summary

With proper training, exercise testing is a useful procedure for the primary care physician in the outpatient as well as the inpatient setting. By careful pre-test evaluation, one is able to study patients safely, obtain both diagnostic and prognostic information concerning the risk of cardiovascular disease, formulate appropriate treatment plans, and develop therapeutic prescriptions for exercise.

References

1. Fowler-Brown A, Pignone M, Pletcher M, et al. Exercise tolerance testing to screen for coronary heart disease: A systematic review for the technical support for the U.S. preventive services task force. Ann Intern Med. 2004;140:W9–W24.
2. Ellestad MH. Stress testing: Principles and practice, 5th ed. Oxford University Press. 2003.
3. Thaulow E, Erikssen J, Sandvik L, Erikssen G, Jorgensen L, Cohn PF. Initial clinical presentation of cardiac disease in asymptomatic men with silent myocardial ischemia and angiographically documented coronary artery disease (the Oslo Ischemia Study). Am J Cardiol. 1993;72:629–633.
4. Institute for clinical systems improvement. Health Care Guideline: Cardiac Stress Test Supplement, 6th ed. 2004.
5. Froelicher VF, Myers JN. Exercise and the Heart, 5th ed. Philadelphia, Elsevier, Inc., 2006, 15.

6. Diabetes mellitus and exercise. ADA standards of medical care in diabetes—2007. Diabetes Care. 2007;30:S4–S41.

7. Stuart RJ, Ellestad MH. National survey of exercise stress testing facilities. Chest. 1980;77:94–97.

8. Gibbons RJ, Balady GJ, Bricker JT, et al. American College of Cardiology/American Heart Association Task Force on Practice Guidelines (Committee to Update the 1997 Exercise Testing Guidelines). ACC/AHA 2002 guideline update for exercise testing: summary article: A report of the American College of Cardiology/American Heart Association Task Force on Practice Guidelines (Committee to Update the 1997 Exercise Testing Guidelines). Circulation. 2002;106:1883–1892.

9. American College of Sports Medicine. Guidelines for Exercise Testing and Prescription, 6th ed. Baltimore, Lippincott Williams & Wilkins, 2000, 26.

10. ACC/AHA 2002 Guideline Update for Exercise Testing. A report of the American College of Cardiology/American Heart Association Task Force on Practice Guidelines (Committee on Exercise Testing). Circulation J Am Coll Cardiol. 2002.

11. Fletcher GF, Froelicher VF, Hartley LH, Haskell WL, Polluck ML. Special report of exercise standards: A statement for health professionals from the American Heart Association. Circulation. 1990;82:2286–2322.

12. De Ponti C, De Biase AM, Cataldo G, et al. Effects of nifedipine, acebutolol, and their association on exercise tolerance in patients with effort angina. Cardiology. 1981;68: 195–199.

13. Fox KM, Deanfield J, Jonathan A, et al. The dose-response effects of nifedipine on ST- segment changes in exercise testing: Preliminary studies. Cardiology. 1981;68:209–212.

14. Sundqvist K, Atterhog JH, Jogestrand T. Effect of digoxin on the electrocardiogram at rest and during exercise in healthy subjects. Am J Cardiol. 1986;57:661–665.

15. Gibbons RJ, Balady GJ, Beasley JW, et al. ACC/AHA guidelines for exercise testing: A report of the American College of Cardiology/ American Heart Association Task Force on Practice Guidelines (Committee on Exercise Testing). J Am Coll Cardiol. 1997;30:260–315.

16. Smith RB, Rusbatch BJ. Amitriptyline and heart block. Br Med J. 1967;3:311.

17. Vohra J, Burrows GD, Sloman F. Assessment of cardiovascular side effects of therapeutic doses of tricyclic anti-depressant drugs. Aust NZ J Med. 1975;5:7–11.

18. Wilson WM, Maughan RJ. Evidence for a possible role of 5-hydroxytryptamine in the genesis of fatigue in man: Administration of paroxetine, a 5-HT re-uptake inhibitor, reduces the capacity to perform prolonged exercise. Exp Physiol. 1992;77:921–924.

19. Fagard R, Amery A, Reybrouck T, et al. Effects of angiotensin antagonism on hemodynamics, renin, and catecholamines during exercise. J Appl Physiol. 1977;43:440–444.

20. Pickering TG, Case DB, Sullivan PA, et al. Comparison of antihypertensive and hormonal effects of captopril and propranolol at rest and during exercise. Am J Cardiol. 1982;49: 1566–1568.

21. Dickstein, K, et al. Comparison of the effects of losartan and enalapril on clinical status and exercise performance in patients with moderate or severe chronic heart failure. J Am Coll Cardiol. 1995;26:438.

22. Hamroff, G, et al. Addition of angiotensin II receptor blockade to maximal angiotensin-converting enzyme inhibition improves exercise capacity in patients with severe congestive heart failure. Circulation. 1999;99:990.

23. Niederberger M, Bruce RA, Kusumi F, et al. Disparities in ventilatory and circulatory responses to bicycle and treadmill exercise. Br Heart J. 1974;36:377.

24. Wasserman K, Hansen JE, Sue DY, Stringer WW, Whipp BJ. Principles of Exercise Testing and Interpretation, 4th ed. Lippincott Williams & Wilkins. 2005.

25. ACC/AHA Guideline Revision. ACC/AHA 2007 Guidelines for the Management of Patients with Unstable Angina/Non–ST-Elevation Myocardial Infarction—Executive Summary. J Am Coll Cardiol. 2007;50:652–726.

26. Borg GA. Psychophysical bases of perceived exertion. Med Sci Sports Exerc. 1982;14: 377–381.

27. Borg G. Perceived exertion as an indicator of somatic stress. Scand J Rehabil Med. 1970;23:92–93.
28. Borg G, Holmgren A, Lindblad I. Quantitative evaluation of chest pain. Acta Med Scand. 1981;644:43–45.
29. Will PM, Walter JD. Exercise testing: Improving performance with a ramped Bruce protocol. Am Heart J. 1999;138:1033–1037.
30. Rice, KR, et al. Effects of nifedipine on myocardial perfusion during exercise in chronic stable angina pectoris. Am J Cardiol. 1990;65:1097.
31. Michaelides AP, Psomadake ZD, Divaveris PE, et al. Improved detection of coronary artery disease by exercise electrocardiography with the use of right precordial leads. N Engl J Med. 1999;340:340–345.
32. White RD, Evans EH. Performing the exercise test. Primary Care. 2001;28(1):44.
33. Cole CR, Blackstone EH, Pashkow FJ, et al. Heart-rate recovery immediately after exercise as a predictor of mortality. N Engl J Med. 1999;341:1351–1357.
34. Lachterman B, Lehmann KG, Abrahamson D, Froelicher VF: "Recovery only" ST segment depression and the predictive accuracy of the exercise test. Ann Intern Med. 1990;112:11–16.

Chapter 3
Exercise Testing Special Protocols

George D. Harris

In the United States, exercise treadmill testing remains the most commonly performed test to identify or confirm the presence of latent coronary artery disease. In contrast, most Europeans are more familiar with cycling and this testing device is more common there. However, standard protocols with specific speed and grade intervals are available for each type of testing.

Exercise stress testing performed in the United States tends to use a continuous instead of an intermittent format, using a treadmill, a bicycle, or a stepping device, each varying in the amount of work applied and the duration of effort required. This approach does not permit the patient to rest. Instead, they experience a progressively increasing workload during the procedure, allowing for the patient's peak aerobic capacity or endpoint to be attained earlier [1].

When considering the selection of the protocol, several factors should be considered. These factors include the person's cardiac risk factors and how they affect the person's daily activities; consider the patient's cognitive status, age, weight, nutritional status, mobility, and the patient's preference, if feasible.

This chapter discusses selecting a protocol to correspond to a specific patient type (the patient with several cardiovascular risk factors, the poorly fit and conditioned patient, the post-myocardial infarction patient, the high-risk patient, and the well-trained athlete) and benefits as well as differences between each protocol.

The protocol for exercise stress testing should include (1) continuous electrocardiogram (ECG) monitoring; (2) a pre-test, during testing, and post-test ECG recording; (3) a type of activity to match the patient's ability; (4) a varied workload; (5) repeated frequent blood pressure measurements; (6) a way to estimate the aerobic requirements of individuals tested; (7) maximum safety and minimum discomfort; (8) the highest possible specificity and sensitivity; (9) sufficient amount of information; (10) a first stage to allow for warm-up phase; and (11) a practical and short program [1].

G.D. Harris (✉)
Department of Community and Family Medicine, University of Missouri-Kansas City, School of Medicine, Truman Medical Center—Lakewood, 7900 Lees Summit Rd., Kansas City, MO 64139, USA
e-mail: george.harris@tmcmed.org

C.H. Evans, R.D. White (eds.), *Exercise Testing for Primary Care and Sports Medicine Physicians*, DOI 10.1007/978-0-387-76597-6_3
© Springer Science+Business Media, LLC 2009

Bruce, Ellestad, Naughton, and other cardiologists have developed several tread-mill protocols for inducing and detecting ECG changes consistent with myocardial ischemia [2]. There are graded protocols for both treadmill and bicycle ergometers for clinical evaluation of patients with cardiovascular disease. Treadmill protocols tend to produce higher maximal oxygen consumption than do bicycle ergometer protocols. Multiple studies have shown that these standard treadmill protocols are hemodynamically comparable [3].

With each protocol, the measurement of performance is expressed in basal metabolic equivalents (METs). One MET equals the resting oxygen consumption rate of 3.5 ml O_2/kg/min. The maintenance of life in the resting state (lying or sitting) requires one MET of energy. Multiples of this basal energy rates are re-quired for different activities. Most exercise testing systems automatically estimate the METs, and maximum workload attained is best expressed in these units. All test results stated in this manner can be compared with a previous or subsequent test of a given patient.

Protocol Selection

No matter the protocol selected the total exercise time needs to be at least 8–12 min. The patient needs to be able to perform exercise. So, matching a protocol with the individual patient is imperative. Prior to selecting the exercise protocol one must decide whether to choose a maximal or submaximal exercise test. Most information is usually obtained from a maximal exercise test in which a patient performs true maximum effort and reaches the point of exhaustion. In this manner a true peak maximal effort is achieved rather than a level defined from age-determined heart rate tables.

Post-myocardial infarction (MI) patients, who need to be tested prior to discharge from the hospital, will require a low-level protocol (a submaximal test) to evaluate for dysrhythmias or ischemia. The goal for this test is a 65% of maximum predicted heart rate (MPHR) or 5 METs.

Bruce Protocol

Bruce developed the standardized treadmill test for diagnosing and evaluating heart and lung diseases. The Bruce protocol, developed in 1963, is used worldwide and is the most common protocol for exercise testing. It is used in 66% of all routine clinical tests performed [1] and has a large research database. This protocol begins with a 3-min stage of walking at 1.7 mph at 10% grade (Stage 1) (Table 3.1). Energy expenditure is estimated to be 4.8 METs during this stage. An individual requires an exercise intensity of at least 5 METs to carry out the activities of daily living. The speed and incline increase with each stage; the incline is incremented 2% every 3 min and the speed is incremented 0.8 mph every 3 min until the treadmill reaches 18% grade and 5 mph. This amounts to 2–3 METs increase per stage.

Table 3.1 Bruce protocol*

Stage	Speed (mph)	Grade (%)
1	1.7	10
2	2.5	12
3	3.4	14
4	4.2	16
5	5.0	18
6	5.5	20
7	6.0	22

*Each stage is 3 min.

This vigorous approach involving large jumps in workloads between stages reach high exertional levels rapidly. These changes are not physiologic. In addition, there is poor correlation with gas analysis in some studies. Stage 4 of this protocol frequently is awkward, and it is sometimes difficult for the patient to choose between running and walking, which results in differing oxygen consumption rates.

Modified Bruce Protocol

The Modified Bruce protocol has a lighter initial increment, but decreases moderately the capacity of peak exercise due to peripheral fatigue secondary to the first stage of low intensity. In comparison, the difference with the standard Bruce protocol is that it inserts two 3-min stages before entering the standard Bruce protocol which have the patient at the same speed as the grade is increased during Stage 0 and Stage 1/2 (Table 3.2). At Stage 1, the patient is at the same grade and speed as present in the standard Bruce protocol. It is ideal for those patients who are less fit or less active. Many persons can perform METs of work but not speed and this protocol allows them to exercise 8–12 min and achieve the METs needed to make a proper assessment.

Table 3.2 The modified Bruce protocol*

Stage	Speed (mph)	Grade (%)
1	1.7	0
2	1.7	5
3	1.7	10
4	2.5	12
5	3.4	14
6	4.2	16
7	5.0	18
8	5.5	20
9	6.0	22

*Each stage is 3 min.

Rapid Bruce Protocol

The difference in this protocol with the standard Bruce protocol is that it uses 1-min stages instead of 3-min stages (Table 3.3). Otherwise, the speed and grade remain the same as the standard Bruce protocol. The participant can achieve maximum workload in 3–7 min. Unfortunately, there are no significant data correlating this protocol with ischemic heart disease.

Table 3.3 Recommendations and level of evidence for the Bruce and modified Bruce protocols

Recommendations	Class	Level of evidence	References
The Bruce protocol is the most common protocol for exercise testing	I	A	[3, 7]
A ramped modified Bruce protocol achieves equivalent hemodynamic goals with better duration and the METS achieved	I	A	[7, 9]

Balke–Ware Protocol

In 1959, Balke and Ware developed a new exercise protocol and established a formula for the calculation of oxygen consumption based on the velocity and inclination of the treadmill [4]. The protocol allows the patient to be tested at the same speed (constant at 3.3 mph) while the grade changes for each stage (1-min stages) increasing from 0 to 26% grade, in 1% grade change intervals (Table 3.4). This protocol is ideal for those who can attain higher grade but not faster speed and still allow for an increase in METs from 4 to 26 METs. This works well for older patients who cannot tolerate rapid walking or running (0.5 METs increase per stage).

Table 3.4 Balke or Balke–Ware protocol*

Stage	Speed (mph)	Grade (%)
1	3.3	0
2	3.3	1
3	3.3	2
4	3.3	3
5	3.3	4
6	3.3	5
7	3.3	6
8	3.3	7
9	3.3	8
10–26	3.3	9–25
27	3.3	26

*Each stage is 1 min.

Naughton Protocol

The Naughton protocol [5] is a submaximal study which is used for high-risk patients. It uses 10 exercise periods of 3-min duration with each exercise period separated by rest periods of 3 min (Table 3.5). The modified Naughton protocol has 2-min stages and starts at a lower MET workload increasing by 1 MET per stage. Patients stop because of either fatigue or dyspnea. It contains a 4-min warm-up and a set speed of 2.0 mph. The grade increases 3.5% every 2 min until maximum effort is achieved. This approach allows for a better tolerated gradual progression in exercise. Also, it is a more accurate assessment of exertional capacity.

Table 3.5 Naughton protocol

Stage	Grade	Speed
1 Warm-up for 4 min	0.0	2.0
2*	3.5	2.0
3	7.0	2.0
4	10.5	2.0
5	14.0	2.0
6	17.5	2.0
7*	21.0	2.0

* Stages 2 and 7 are 2 min each.

United States Air Force Space and AeroMedicine

The United States Air Force Space and AeroMedicine (USAFSAM) – 2.0 mph protocol has similar indications to the Balke–Ware and is used for those individuals who are less fit and conditioned. It is a continuous treadmill protocol designed using a constant treadmill speed (2.0 mph) and regular equal increments in treadmill grade (5%/3 min). The constant treadmill speed requires only initial adaptation in patient stride. There are 3-min stages with a constant speed at 2.0 mph and the grade increasing with each stage: 0, 5, 10, 15, 20, 25%. The range is 2.5–9.8 METs. This protocol is ideal for those who can attain higher grade but not faster speed.

USAFSAM – 3.0 mph

This protocol has similar indications to 2.0 mph protocol but with a greater workload being achieved. There are also 3-min stages and a constant speed at 3.0 mph with grade increases at each stage: 0, 5, 10, 15, 20, 25%. The range is 4.0–14.8 METs.

Ellestad Protocol

Ellestad's protocol uses seven periods each of 2- or 3-min duration, at progressively increasing speeds (1.7, 3, 4, 5, 6, 7, and 8 mph) [6]. The grade is 10% for the first

Table 3.6 Ellestad protocol

Stage	Speed (mph)	Grade (%)	Time (min)
1	1.7	10	3
2	3	10	2
3	4	10	2
4	5	10	3
5	6	15	2
6	7	15	2
7	8	15	2

four periods and 15% for the last three periods (Table 3.6). Ellestad et al. [6] published this protocol for treadmill testing with a fixed inclination which also included follow-up electrocardiograms and measurements of the heart rate, blood pressure, and the presence of thoracic pain at each stage. This protocol is a more aggressive protocol than those previously discussed and the workload progresses from 4 to 20 METs in a total elapsed time of 13 min.

Modified Astrand Protocol

Modified Astrand protocol is a protocol which is ideal for well-trained athletes whose training includes running. The participant is able to select the ideal *speed* at which to test and then is tested at a constant speed (5.0–8.5 mph). The initial stage is 3 min with a 0% grade, then the grade is increased 2.5% with each stage (2.5, 5.0, 7.5, 10.0, 12.5, 15.0, 17.5%) every 2 min [1].

Costill Protocol

This is another protocol that is ideal for athletes. Following a 10-min warm-up the participant is placed at a speed which is set at 8.9 mph while the grade increases 2% every 2 min until exhaustion. This specialized protocol allows the individual to achieve a high MET level.

Harbor Protocol

The Harbor protocol uses a constant treadmill speed and increments the grade by a constant amount each minute. Under this protocol, after a 3-min warm-up at 0 grade and a comfortable walking speed (0.8–4.5 mph, depending on the patient's level of fitness), a constant grade increment of 1, 2, or 3% each minute is used until the patient's maximum tolerance is reached. The speed and grade are scaled and so the test ends in approximately 10 min after the treadmill is incremented [2].

Ramp Protocol

The Ramp protocol is a protocol that correlates well with VO_2 gas analysis. Once a target MET workload is selected, the total time is set at 10–12 min and then the computer selects the speed and grade to achieve the target workload. This allows for a more physiologic assessment and an unperceivable change with is stage by the participant. The grade and speed can be programmed to increase every 6 seconds in alternating fashion.

This protocol is used more by the cardiologists than the primary care physicians only because of lack of knowledge about it or limited experience. The Bruce protocol can be programmed into a Ramp protocol. So, at the end of 6 min, one is at the end of Stage 2 instead of completing two stages in that time frame. A ramped modification of the Bruce protocol seems to achieve equivalent hemodynamic goals but with better duration and the METS achieved. Since the patients exercised longer with the ramp than with the Bruce protocol they achieved an optimal duration for the exercise test of approximately 10 min [7] and met the criteria for an optimal exercise test. It was also recommended for serial exercise tests for assessment of chronic stable angina [8]. In addition, the patients preferred the ramp protocol with respect to comfort and ease to perform.

The ramp protocol's exercise data are correlated easily with standard protocols [9]. The differences evident between the Bruce and ramp protocols were in duration of exercise and METs achieved, with the patients exercising longer with the ramp than with the Bruce protocol. Myers et al. [10] demonstrated hemodynamic comparability among protocols, but marked variations in maximal oxygen uptake and the dynamics of gas exchange in conventional protocols compared with ramp protocols. Their study demonstrated that the ratio of oxygen uptake to work rate is greater in ramp protocols than in conventional protocols that involve large increments in work. In addition the study suggested that an optimal exercise test should be individualized to achieve test duration of approximately 10 min.

Revill et al. compared the peak exercise response and determined the limits of agreement between the ramp and the 1-min step cycle protocols in a representative population of patients with exertional breathlessness attending a respiratory outpatient clinic. There were no significant differences found between the two protocols for the peak physiologic responses and both are good choices for the measurement of maximal exercise capacity [11].

Storer–Davis Maximal Bicycle Protocol

Storer–Davis maximal bicycle protocol is a protocol used for the bicycle ergometer. It is an aerobic test which follows the Astrand maximal graded bicycle protocol. This test consists of a 4-min warm-up at 0 W after which the participant pedals at a constant rate of 60 rpm while the workload and ergometer settings are increased each minute. The workload is increased by 15 W while the ergometer kg setting is increased by 1/4 kg each minute [12]. The metronome is set at 120 (or 100) with a cycle rate of 60 (or 50) rpm (one foot down with each beat). The ergometer belt tension (resistance) is set at 1 kg 300 kg m/min, 2 kg 600 kg m/min, 3 kg 900 kg m/min, etc.

Wingate Anaerobic Test

The Wingate anaerobic test (WAnT) was developed in 1974 in Israel at the Wingate Institute for Physical Education and Sports Center and is generally used to evaluate anaerobic cycling performance. It has been used worldwide in both athletic and research settings and is considered the most popular test of anaerobic muscle performance [13]. It is considered a reliable and valid means to assessing endurance, power, and fatigue and is considered suitable for testing a variety of subpopulations (Table 3.7) [13]. It is used worldwide in both athletic and research settings and is considered the most popular test of anaerobic muscle performance [13].

The Wingate test uses an exercise bike that can be weighted with resistance based on a percentage of your body weight as well as a computer. It tests for maximal anaerobic power and measures supramaximal mechanical power and is designed to induce fatigue within seconds. The test is based on cycling at maximal speed, for 30 seconds, against a high braking force. There are two portions to the test: an aerobic portion of test (22–29%) with an accepted value of 27% and an anaerobic portion.

The protocol requires pedaling or arm cranking for 30 seconds to allow for a maximal speed against a constant force. Using the formula power (watts) = kp × rpm, computerized equipment counts the revolutions while a predetermined force is applied (adults – 0.100 kp/kg body weight and non-adults – 0.090 kp/kg body weight). This *force* remains constant throughout the test but, because it is so high, the subject cannot maintain the initial *velocity* for more than a few seconds, before starting to slow down. Mechanical power is measured during the 30 seconds using the equation power = force × velocity. The work generated by the subject is calculated by the equation work = power × time. There are three indices that describe the person's performance in the Wingate test: peak power, mean power, and fatigue index. Peak power is the highest mechanical power that is elicited during the test. The mean power corresponds to the average power sustained throughout the 30-second period. The fatigue index is a percent fatigue based on the degree of power drop-off during the test and. indicates the rate at which power output declines for an athlete.

Table 3.7 Recommendations and level of evidence for the Wingate anaerobic test

Recommendations	Class	Level of evidence	Reference
Wingate anaerobic test used worldwide in both athletic and research settings and is considered the most popular test of anaerobic muscle performance	I	A	[15]
WAnT requires the use of more anaerobically derived energy than previously estimated	I	B	[12]

The decline in power output from the beginning to the end of the test represents this percent fatigue. This fatigue can be an indicator of anaerobic power. A high peak power and a low fatigue factor may indicate a person with good anaerobic power.

Beneke et al. demonstrated that WAnT requires the use of more anaerobically derived energy than previously estimated, that anaerobic metabolism is dominated by glycolysis, and that WAnT mechanical efficiency is lower than that found in aerobic exercise tests [14].

Using an arm WanT instead of the bicycle for testing has been found to be a reliable measurement tool for the assessment of upper extremity muscular power in persons with complete paraplegia [15].

References

1. Stress Testing: Principles and Practice. 5th ed. Ellestad MH. Oxford University Press. 2003.
2. Wasserman K, Hansen JE, Sue DY, Stringer WW, Whipp BJ. Principles of Exercise Testing and Interpretation. 4th ed. Lippincott Williams & Wilkins 2005.
3. Pollock ML, Bohannon RL, Cooper KH. A comparative analysis of four protocols for maximal treadmill stress testing. Am Heart J. 1976;92:39–46.
4. Balke B, Ware RW. An experimental study of fitness of physical fitness of Armed Forces personnel. US Armed Forces Med J. 1959;10:675–688.
5. Naughton J, Balke B, Nagle F. Refinements in method of evaluation and physical conditioning before and after myocardial infarction. Am J Cardiol. 1964;14:837–843.
6. Ellestad MH, Allen W, Wan MCK, Kemp G. Maximal treadmill stress testing for cardiovascular evaluation. Circulation. 1969;39:517–522.
7. Buchfuhrer MJ, Hansen JE, Robinson TE, Sue DY, Wasserman K, Whipp BJ. Optimizing the exercise protocol for cardiopulmonary assessment. J Appl Physiol. 1983;55:1558–1564.
8. Webster MWJ, Sharpe DN. Exercise testing in angina pectoris: The importance of protocol design in clinical trials. Am Heart J. 1989;117:505–508.
9. Will PM, Walter JD. Exercise testing: Improving performance with a ramped Bruce protocol. Am Heart J. 1999;138(6):1033–1037.
10. Myers J, Buchanan N, Walsh D, Kraemer M, McAuley P, Hamilton-Wessler M. Comparison of the ramp versus standard exercise protocols. J Am Coll Cardiol. 1991;17:1334–1342.
11. Revill SM, Beck KE, Morgan MDL. Comparison of the peak exercise response measured by the ramp and 1 min step cycle exercise protocols in patients with exertional dyspnea. Chest. 2002;121:1099–1105.
12. Pate RR, Blair SN, Durstine JL, Eddy DL, Hanson P, Painter P, Smith LK, Wolfe LA. Guidelines for Exercise Testing and Prescription. 4th ed. RR Pate (ed). Philadelphia, PA, Lea & Febiger, 1991.
13. The Wingate Anaerobic Test (Paperback) by Omri Inbar, Oded Bar-Or, and James S. Skinner. Human Kinetics Europe Ltd (Sep 1996).
14. Beneke R, Pollman C, Bleif I, Leithauser RM Hutler M. How anaerobic is the Wingate Anaerobic Test for humans? Eur J Appl Physiol. 2002 Aug;87(4–5):388–392.
15. Jacobs PL, Mahoney ET, Johnson B. Reliability of arm Wingate Anaerobic Testing in persons with complete paraplegia. J Spinal Cord Med. 2003 Summer;26(2):141–144.

Chapter 4
Testing Special Populations

Bryan C. Hughes and Russell D. White

Much of the evidence for recommendations regarding electrocardiogram (ECG) treadmill stress testing has come from studies involving middle-aged men. Special consideration must be given when deciding who, when and how to screen for cardiovascular disease in patients who fall outside of this category. There is less data on noninvasive testing in women, older adults and people with diabetes, although this issue is being recognized and addressed through recent studies and literature. The previous conception that coronary artery disease is only a disease found in men is quickly being replaced. Clinicians are recognizing that different standards must be used for identification of patients at risk, testing protocols and test interpretation. This chapter addresses the use of ECG treadmill stress testing in women, the elderly and persons with diabetes.

Testing in Women

Cardiovascular disease is the leading cause of death for all women in the United States. It kills over 240,000 women annually, more than breast cancer or stroke [1]. Yet, the majority of studies done on cardiovascular disease defining its diagnosis and treatment have been done on men. Recommendations for ECG treadmill stress testing have been largely based on studies involving middle-aged men, and very few women. It is evident that not only is there a relative lack of supporting evidence for noninvasive diagnostic testing in women, but it has been demonstrated that women are less likely than men to be referred for such testing. Part of this disparity between genders may be due to the fact that women often present with different symptoms of cardiovascular disease than men, and these differences must be taken into consideration for diagnosis and screening for this lethal disease.

B.C. Hughes (✉)
Family Physician, Oak Grove Medical Clinic, 1900 S. Broadway, Oak Grove, MO 64075, USA
e-mail: Big1500@hotmail.com

C.H. Evans, R.D. White (eds.), *Exercise Testing for Primary Care and Sports Medicine Physicians*, DOI 10.1007/978-0-387-76597-6_4
© Springer Science+Business Media, LLC 2009

Epidemiology

The overall incidence of cardiovascular disease in women is less than the incidence in men, 42 million women compared to 79 million men in 2004. However, this is only true until the seventh decade of life, when women are more likely to have coronary artery disease. By age 79, the overall cardiovascular mortality rate for women starts to sharply rise, while the overall mortality rate for men sharply falls [1]. The prevalence of coronary artery disease (CAD) is decreased in premenopausal women compared to menopausal women. However, one in nine women aged 45–69 will have heart disease.

The morbidity and mortality for women with cardiovascular disease (CVD) is significantly higher than in men. Since 1984, the number of CVD deaths for women has exceeded those for men, mostly due to later age at onset, higher incidence of comorbid conditions and lack of screening women with subtle symptoms [2].

Clinical Presentation

A different approach must be taken in delineating the clinical history for cardiovascular disease in women than in men. Women tend to have more atypical symptoms that must be carefully evaluated. The differences in symptoms are due in part to less common causes of ischemia, such as microvascular angina, vasospastic ischemia and chest pain that is nonischemic, such as mitral-valve prolapse [3].

Typical symptoms common to both sexes include pain or pressure, described as squeezing or stabbing. Pain radiating to neck, shoulder, back, arm or jaw can be described. Dyspnea, nausea, diaphoresis and dizziness are other associated symptoms that can be seen in both sexes. Women tend to have atypical symptoms that are more generalized in nature. These include non-chest pain symptoms such as nausea, back pain and jaw pain. Generalized fatigue, weakness or dyspnea may also be reported. Women who have stable typical angina are also more likely than men to have pain during rest, sleep or during emotional stress (Table 4.1).

It is important to note that women are more likely to have comorbid conditions upon presentation with CAD, including hypertension, diabetes mellitus and dyslipidemia. This contributes to the overall poor prognosis for women with cardiovascular disease. Of these comorbidities, diabetes has been shown to have the

Table 4.1 Differences associated with coronary artery disease in women

Higher incidence of comorbidities	Common atypical symptoms
• Diabetes mellitus	• Nausea
• Obesity	• Back pain
• Hypertension	• Jaw pain
• Dyslipidemia	• Dyspnea
	• Generalized weakness

largest association with coronary artery disease [4]. Meta-analysis date suggests that women with diabetes have a higher relative risk for cardiac-related deaths than men [5]. Other factors such as poor social support and environmental stressors are associated with an increased risk for cardiovascular disease and poor prognosis. Obesity was found to be an independent risk factor in the Buffalo Health Study. Women with a body mass index (BMI) in the highest quartile had a three times greater risk of CAD than women in the lowest quartile [6].

The relationship between estrogen levels and cardiovascular disease remains controversial. For years, it was widely believed that estrogen provided a protective effect on the heart. The Nurses Health Study provided some evidence that estrogen replacement is beneficial, possibly through vasodilatation and digitalis-like effect due to similar chemical structure. The Heart and Estrogen/Progestin Replacement Study (HERS) demonstrated that hormonal therapy had neither a beneficial nor a harmful effect on coronary heart disease (CHD) events. There was a trend toward an increased risk of CHD events during year one of hormone therapy and a decreased risk during years three through five of therapy [7]. Recent data from the Women's Health Initiative Study has demonstrated that estrogen replacement is not long-term cardioprotective and is possibly associated with a small increase in the risk of cardiac death after 1 year [8].

Risk Stratification

Risk stratification for cardiovascular disease is an important process to determine which women to screen with ECG treadmill stress testing. The pretest probability will change the incidence of false-positive results. The Framingham risk score has been used as a way to identify patients at low, intermediate or high risk of cardiovascular events. This can be used to help determine the pretest probability before testing. The scoring system ranges from −17 to +25 with points awarded for age, total cholesterol, high-density lipoprotein (HDL), blood pressure, diabetes mellitus and tobacco use. Major risk factors in women include typical angina pectoris, hormonal status, diabetes mellitus and peripheral arterial disease. Intermediate risk factors include hypertension, tobacco abuse and dyslipidemia. Minor risk factors include age greater than 65, obesity, sedentary lifestyle and family history.

Women with a low risk of cardiac disease based on clinical assessment have a low incidence of cardiac disease. Thus, they generally have a good long-term prognosis, and noninvasive cardiac testing may not be appropriate for this group of women. The United States Preventative Services Task Force (USPSTF) and the American College of Cardiology/American Heart Association (ACC/AHA) both recommend against screening asymptomatic women who are at low risk for coronary heart disease. Instead, focus should be on monitoring and treating risk factors. In women with intermediate to high pretest probability, screening with ECG treadmill stress testing can be beneficial. ACC/AHA guidelines recommend that women with an intermediate pretest risk for CAD, a normal resting ECG and who are capable of maximal exercise should be screened with ECG treadmill stress testing.

In general, there has been a higher threshold to refer women for ECG stress testing because of preconception that coronary artery disease is a condition found in men. Clinical assessment of risk may not be completely accurate, but it is a way to stratify women who are appropriate for ECG stress testing, so that screening for CAD is appropriate, beneficial and cost-effective.

Performing the Test

For most cases, the procedural protocol for performing the treadmill stress test is the same for women and men. If a woman can safely exercise, the Standard Bruce Protocol may be used. In a meta-analysis by Kwok, of 19 studies using exercise stress testing (EST) in women, all but five successfully used the Bruce protocol exclusively [9]. If a woman has decreased exercise tolerance, the modified Bruce protocol is an alternative, since it begins with a lower metabolic equivalent (MET) level. Other protocols can be used depending on the pretest condition of the subject. The outcome goal for testing is for the participant to achieve approximately 85% of maximal heart rate. In most cases, maximum exercise capacity in women is achieved at 8–12 min into testing. It is best to use a protocol which reaches the participant's maximal MET at 10 min.

There is some evidence that modifications in lead placement may improve accuracy of testing. Michaelides et al. used right precordial leads (V_3R, V_4R and V_5R) in addition to standard 12 leads [10]. This modification improved sensitivity in women from 71 to 88%, with no change in the specificity of 80%.

Interpretation of the Test

Interpretation of the results of ECG treadmill testing for women requires focus on different variables of the test than are used in men. The sensitivity and specificity of ECG stress testing in women is less than that for men [9]. Various theories about differences in sensitivity and specificity of the test as compared to men involve lower pretest probability in women, digitalis-like effect of estrogen and higher incidence of single-vessel coronary disease as opposed to three-vessel disease.

Using standard interpretation for testing in women has decreased accuracy because women tend to have more frequent resting ST–T wave changes and decreased overall voltage on the ECG. Thus, ST-segment depression has a lower specificity for diagnosing coronary disease in women than in men [11]. Traditional interpretation of an ECG treadmill stress test as being positive or negative has relied on the presence of ST-segment depression. Other parameters must then be used in conjunction with ST-segment depression to determine overall posttest risk for coronary disease.

Studies have shown that exercise capacity and heart rate recovery are just as important if not *more* important than ST-segment depression for determining risk of significant coronary artery disease in women. This is due to certain physiologic changes seen in women during exercise that make these factors more important in the interpretation of the stress test. Up to age 13–14, the volume of oxygen (VO_2) in women is similar for that in men. After that age, the values diverge through adult life. Vital capacity for males is about 40% higher and heart volume is 30% larger. At any given VO_2 in women, the following changes are observed: lower tidal volume, higher respiratory rate, lower stroke volume and higher heart rate.

It has been established that exercise capacity is an independent predictor of cardiovascular events and all-cause mortality in men. Since vital capacity is 30% higher in men, one would expect that decreased exercise capacity in women is an even larger predictor or death in women, and this was demonstrated in a 2003 study by Gulati et al. [3] For each 1 MET increase in exercise capacity, there was a 17% reduction in mortality rate. Patients who fail to reach 5 METs during the test are at higher risk of cardiac disease. Patients must reach 4.7 METs during the Bruce protocol to be considered an adequate test. Those who fail to reach this level should be referred for pharmacologic cardiac stress imaging [12].

One consequence of these physiologic changes, coupled with the more frequent resting ECG changes in women, is a higher false-positive rate for coronary artery disease when testing women compared to men. Pratt demonstrated that false-positive tests were more common when a patient was able to exercise through Stage 3 Bruce protocol, and there was rapid normalization of ST-segment after cessation of exercise ($\leq 4 \min.$) [13]

Use of scores to determine the posttest analysis of testing is similar to men, with some exceptions. The Duke Treadmill Score is a tool used to assess the results of testing in assigning a risk for coronary artery disease. The score is as follows:

$$Exercise\ time - (5 \times ST\ deviation) - (4 \times chest\ pain)$$

Exercise time is in minutes, ST elevation is the largest measured net deviation, chest pain is measured using a score of 0 for no angina, 1 for nonlimiting angina and 2 for exercise-limiting angina. The score is then totaled where a negative score equals more risk. -25 is the highest risk and $+15$ is the lowest risk. This score was formulated using men as the subjects. The question must be raised, then, if the score can be used in women with equal accuracy. A study by Alexander et al. [11] determined that the Duke Treadmill Score was very helpful in women to exclude coronary disease, even better than in men. Women with a higher score had much less coronary artery disease. The score overall demonstrated equivalent accuracy in diagnosing women as it did with men.

The next steps in the diagnosis of coronary disease depend on the outcome of the test. Women with a high pretest and posttest probability warrant coronary angiography for accurate determination of disease. Women with intermediate test results, in most cases, should be referred for cardiovascular stress imaging for further diagnosis. Women with low pretest probability and low posttest probability after testing can, in most cases, be managed with risk factor modification alone and not be subject to the risk of more invasive testing. While coronary angiography is generally considered safe, it still carries risk, and discretion must be used to determine risk–benefit ratio.

Table 4.2 Recommendations for exercise stress testing in women

Recommendation	Class	Level of evidence	Reference
1. Women with an intermediate pretest risk for CAD and a normal resting ECG who are capable of maximal exercise should be screened with EST	I	B	2
2. Women who are at low risk for CAD and asymptomatic should be screened with EST	III		2

Summary

Despite the disparity of data regarding its accuracy in women, the ECG treadmill stress test can be effectively used to determine risk and prognosis for coronary heart disease in this population (Table 4.2). Clinicians should perform a more careful assessment of women who are at risk because women often do not present with classic symptoms of heart disease, and as a result, there is often a higher threshold for physicians to refer women for testing. Testing protocols are similar for women as in men, but interpretation is different. Because of higher incidence of resting ECG abnormalities and comorbid conditions, emphasis must be placed on exercise capacity and symptoms during testing more than ST-segment deviation to accurately determine risk for angiographic coronary artery disease. The ACC/AHA recommends that women who have a pretest intermediate risk for CAD, are able to exercise, and have no resting ECG abnormalities should be screened with ECG treadmill testing [14]. Women at low risk with no symptoms should not be routinely screened.

Testing in the Elderly

The prevalence of cardiovascular disease in older population continues to increase with the rise in number of adults over the age of 65. In this population, heart disease is still the leading cause of mortality in the United States. Treadmill ECG stress testing is an appropriate test for evaluating coronary disease in adults over 65. Over 800,000 tests are performed annually in the United States. However, special considerations must be given to performance of the test and interpretation of results due to the changes that aging imposes on physiology, higher incidence of comorbid conditions and general tendency for these patients to be less physically conditioned.

Epidemiology

The incidence of coronary artery disease continues to increase in older adults, partly due to the rapid growth of that segment of the population. In 2007, statistics from the AHA indicates that if all cardiovascular diseases were to be eliminated, the average life expectancy for an adult in the United States would increase by 10 years. This is because 68% of all deaths from cardiovascular disease occur over the age of 75 (close to the age of average life expectancy). An estimated 500,000 coronary artery bypass grafts are performed on adults in the United States each year, and approximately 30% of those procedures are performed on patients over 70 years of age [15]. Before age 75, a higher proportion of death from coronary disease occurs in men, but after age 75, mortality is higher in women [1].

Clinical Presentation

Careful clinical history must be taken in older adults to evaluate for heart disease. These patients have more comorbid conditions because of their age, and may present with symptoms that are less typical. Older adults may have compensated for coronary ischemia by adapting physical activity that does not rise above the threshold for producing typical angina. Therefore, they may not present with typical chest pain and may not have the ability to finish the required activity if they do not regularly exert themselves at a level to produce symptoms. Instead, they may present with more generalized symptoms of fatigue, malaise, back pain or neck pain. Dyspnea is often the only symptom found in an older adult with cardiovascular disease. Clinicians generally have a lower threshold for evaluation of older adults because of the increased incidence of cardiovascular disease in this population.

Performing the Test

Safety must be considered when choosing which testing protocol to use in an older adult. Vision, hearing and balance regulation in the elderly are often compromised, and care must be taken to make sure that the participant can safely walk on the treadmill without falling. Pretest assessment of normal daily activities and level of functioning may help predict if a patient will be able to safely walk on a treadmill up to required MET level. Exercise on a cycle may be a safer alternative to treadmill in some patients. Other considerations of comorbid conditions must be accounted for, such as higher incidence of pulmonary disease and chronic obstructive pulmonary disease (COPD), osteoarthritis, peripheral arterial disease or prior cerebrovascular accident (CVA). These conditions may affect the ability of the person to engage in higher levels of activity.

The protocol selected for use in the older adult must address the physical limitations of the person. The goal is to be able to attain approximately 85% of maximal workload and heart rate before skeletal muscle fatigue occurs. A less vigorous protocol may be needed to achieve this. The modified Bruce protocol is one example, which increases the exercise grade of incline at intervals of 3 min, but the overall speed is constant for the first two stages. The Balke–Ware is similar, but it increases the grade of incline at 1 min intervals while keeping a steady speed. The Naughton protocols increase both speed and incline at regular intervals. Any protocol may be used as long as it accomplishes the goal for maximal value of the test. Subjects should reach maximal predicted heart rate within 8 and 12 min from start of testing.

Interpretation of the Test

There are few studies that have assessed the value of predicting coronary risk with ECG treadmill stress testing in adults over 65. The studies that have been done demonstrate that ST changes during testing are NOT an accurate predictor of risk in older adults. More data must be collected from the results of EST in the elderly to calculate risk of coronary artery disease due to physiologic changes in exercise response, higher prevalence of comorbid conditions and the higher overall pretest probability of coronary artery disease in the elderly. Because of these factors, the sensitivity of EST in older adults is higher than in younger adults, but the specificity is lower, 84 and 70%, respectively.

Exercise capacity in older adults is typically reduced. Aerobic capacity generally decreases by 8–10% for each decade of life, the difference in exercise capacity between ages 30 and 80 reaches approximately 50%. Also, the elderly population is generally less active due to loss of muscular tone, degenerative disease of joints or other factors. This decreased exercise capacity has been shown in studies to be independently associated with overall death rates for coronary heart disease, and must be taken into consideration when performing exercise stress tests. Goroya et al. found that ST-segment changes were not as predictive of mortality as exercise capacity [16]. Messinger-Rapport et al. took this a step further to address not only exercise capacity but heart rate recovery as a predictor of death from cardiovascular events [17].

Heart rate recovery after exercise is affected by vagal nerve tone. Impaired vagal reactivation after heart rate has increased from exercise has also been associated with increased risk of death in persons with heart disease. When performing exercise stress testing in older populations, the heart rate should be carefully monitored after the exercise portion of the test is complete. In general, the inability of the heart rate to drop by 12 beats per minute in the first minute of recovery has been shown to be prognostic of an overall increase in mortality [18].

The accuracy of interpretation of results may be limited due to other comorbid and confounding conditions that affect ECG interpretation. Resting ECG changes such as ST-segment depression and atrial fibrillation are more common in older adults. Lai et al. found that all the major exercise ECG abnormalities were more prevalent in the elderly. ST-segment depression induced by exercise was much more common, with 31.5% of the elderly population studied versus 19.2% of the younger population [19]. The occurrence of ST-segment depression without chest pain was almost doubled in elderly subjects tested. Also, inability to achieve age-predicted heart rate occurred in almost half of the subjects tested.

The Duke Treadmill Score (DTS) can be used in the determination of risk after the ECG treadmill stress test, but may be limited. The DTS was developed in a population of mostly males with a mean age of 49. Because of increased incidence of CAD, decreased exercise capacity and the higher incidence of ST-segment changes without symptoms, the calculation of the score may not as accurately reflect the true risk for coronary disease.

It may be more beneficial to use a different scoring system in the elderly that includes correction for the other conditions mentioned previously. Lai et al. found that using the Veterans Affairs/University of West Virginia Score for diagnosing angiographic coronary artery disease was more prognostic than using the Duke Treadmill Score in adults over 65 [19]. This score calculates risk based on maximal heart rate, exercise ST-segment depression, age, angina history, hypercholesterolemia, diabetes and exercise-induced angina during the test.

Summary

Coronary artery disease is quite prevalent in adults over the age of 65 and will continue to be a leading cause of mortality. Appropriate steps can be taken to help identify patients at risk, because older adults tend to present with symptoms that are less typical than those seen in younger adults. EST is recommended as first-line testing for older adults with risk factors for CAD, no resting ECG changes that would affect interpretation of the test and who are able to perform the test (Table 4.3). Care must be taken to ensure that the ECG treadmill stress test be performed safely in older adults due to poor vision, hearing or balance problems. Exercise tolerance and heart rate recovery are important predictors for posttest risk of coronary disease in the elderly. Alternative scoring systems such as the Veterans Affairs/University of West Virginia Score may be more accurate to interpret the results of testing.

Table 4.3 Evidence-based recommendations for exercise stress testing in the elderly

Recommendation	Class	Level of evidence	Reference
Evaluation of men older than 45 and women older than 55 who plan to start vigorous exercise, who are at high risk for CAD due to other diseases	IIb	C	2
Routine screening of asymptomatic adults	III	C	2

Testing Persons with Diabetes

Diabetes mellitus is a group of metabolic disorders characterized by hyperglycemia and glucose intolerance resulting from defects in insulin secretion, insulin action or a combination of both. When not controlled, this chronic disease state causes complications within the vascular system. These complications include macrovascular (coronary artery disease, cerebrovascular disease, peripheral arterial disease) and microvascular disease (retinopathy, nephropathy, neuropathy). Uncontrolled diabetes also results in early death and cardiovascular disease is the most common cause [20]. For years it was felt that patients with type 1 diabetes suffered more complications from microvascular disease while patients with type 2 diabetes experienced more complications from macrovascular disease. In a prospective study of 23,751 patients from the United Kingdom, Laing et al. found that while the incidence of coronary artery disease in type 1 patients was significantly lower than in patients with type 2 diabetes, the incidence was several fold higher compared to a matched nondiabetic population [21]. This study confirmed the increased incidence of coronary artery disease in type 1 diabetes.

Epidemiology

The incidence of diabetes mellitus in the United States is increasing at a dramatic rate with the current estimate of 23.6 million persons with diabetes (7.6% of the population) [22]. Of this total number 17.9 million persons are currently diagnosed while 5.7 million are undiagnosed. In addition, 54 million persons have prediabetes [23] which leads to type 2 diabetes if there is no intervention. The Framingham Heart Study showed that the incidence of diabetes mellitus has doubled over the past 30 years [24].

Type 1 diabetes accounts for 5–10% of these patients while the remaining patients have type 2 diabetes. All too often the diagnosis of type 2 diabetes is made in patients following a diagnosis of heart disease. In fact, 14% of patients presenting to an urban hospital with acute coronary syndrome were diagnosed with new-onset diabetes mellitus [25]. In another study from Sweden, 31% of patients admitted with acute myocardial infarction were diagnosed with new-onset diabetes mellitus [26]. In contrast, following a diagnosis of diabetes mellitus adults have heart disease at 2–4 times higher rates than those without diabetes [22,27,28]. A recent article found that the impact of type 1 and type 2 diabetes on cardiovascular mortality in middle-aged subjects was similar. In fact, the long-term effect of hyperglycemia was more pronounced in type 1 than in type 2 patients [29]. An additional alarming trend is the marked increase in type 2 diabetes in the adolescent age group. If complications in these patients occur within 20 years following the disease onset, these patients will be encountering serious disease states while approaching their peak performance in the workforce and their contribution to society. With complications of cardiovascular disease occurring in the prime of their lives an economic and societal stress will be levied upon the population as a whole. As a result of these trends it is estimated that there will be 48.3 million persons in the United States with diabetes by the year 2050 [30].

Obesity is present in 80% of patients with type 2 diabetes [31] and visceral obesity and hypertriglyceridemia contribute to the release of cytokines and adipokynes. These substances, in turn, initiate a general inflammatory state that damages blood vessels and contributes to dyslipidemia, hypertension and further insulin resistance.

The major consequence of this cascade is microvascular and macrovascular disease including coronary artery disease.

The prevalence of coronary artery disease in the general population is 2–4% compared to 55% in adult patients with diabetes [32]. It is no surprise that coronary artery disease is so prevalent in those with diabetes when one analyzes our success in treating this disease process. In the NHANES 1999–2000 study only 7% of adult patients with diabetes mellitus achieved an A1C < 7%, blood pressure < 130/80 and a plasma cholesterol < 200 mg/dl [33, 34].

Heart disease and stroke are responsible for the majority of deaths in those with diabetes, and as many as 80% of patients with type 2 diabetes will die of macrovascular disease [22, 34, 35]. In comparison to those without diabetes, heart disease in person with diabetes affects women nearly as often as men, appears earlier in life and is more often fatal.

Clinical Presentation

When a patient with diabetes presents with possible symptoms of coronary artery disease, further evaluation is warranted. Unfortunately, some patients may suffer a cardiac event without preceding cardiac symptoms or before they are diagnosed with diabetes [36, 37]. Thus, the complication of coronary artery disease may actually precede the diagnosis of diabetes mellitus.

Once a person with diabetes suffers a primary cardiac event, the prognosis is worse than in those patients without diabetes. Initial myocardial infarction persons with diabetes are more likely to die from sudden cardiac death compared to persons without diabetes [38]. In addition, persons with treated diabetes (insulin or oral agents) are more likely to die from or suffer a subsequent myocardial infarction following percutaneous coronary angiography compared to coronary artery bypass surgery [39].

Finally, while there has been a decreasing trend in mortality from coronary artery disease in the overall population [40] and in the incidence of cardiovascular events in those with diabetes [35], problems with prevention and diagnosis persist. This lack of dramatic improvement is attributed to (1) diabetes mellitus as an independent risk factor for heart disease, (2) onset of diabetes producing coronary complications before the clinical diagnosis of diabetes and (3) atypical or absent symptoms of coronary disease in those with diabetes. An international prospective epidemiological study indicates that hyperglycemia poses an independent adverse effect on subsequent cardiovascular risk in both type 1 and type 2 diabetes. Furthermore, these risks are related to postprandial hyperglycemia and elevated A1C measurements [41]. This trend in cardiovascular mortality can only be improved by the early diagnosis and aggressive treatment of diabetes and careful screening for subclinical significant coronary artery disease.

Patients with diabetes may present with typical angina but variant symptoms are often presenting complaints (Table 4.4). One must be alert to changing or variant symptoms in someone with diabetes who presents with complaints that are related to

Table 4.4 Atypical or variant symptoms of angina in persons with diabetes mellitus

1. Difficulty completing usual tasks
2. Dizziness with activity
3. Dyspnea with minimal exertion
4. Easy fatigability
5. Lack of energy
6. Neck or jaw discomfort
7. Shoulder pain with a history similar to bursitis and related to activity
8. Upper back pain

activity. These complaints may represent the earliest subtle manifestations of coronary artery disease. Finally, patients with diabetes may present with an acute major cardiac event and remain asymptomatic until immediately prior to its onset [42]. Thus, while diagnosing and treating patients with diabetes and associated coronary artery disease is important, the proper screening for disease and evaluation remains difficult.

Indications for Testing

According to the American Diabetes Association and the American College of Cardiology [43] exercise stress testing (with or without imaging) is recommended in both symptomatic and asymptomatic patients with specific criteria listed in Table 4.5. In addition, diabetic patients with microalbuminuria and patients older than 35 years with evidence of autonomic neuropathy should undergo testing, since these two markers have been associated with a high risk of cardiovascular disease. If these initial tests are normal, repeat testing is recommended in 2 years. In 2006, the American Diabetes Association recommended that persons with type 2 diabetes undergoing activity level greater than the activity of daily living (ADL) undergo exercise stress testing [44].

Table 4.5 Exercise stress testing recommendations for symptomatic and asymptomatic patients with specific criteria

Perform exercise stress testing (with or without imaging) in patients with diabetes plus any of the following criteria:

1. ≥ 2 Cardiac risk factors
2. Peripheral artery disease
3. Carotid artery disease
4. Abnormal resting ECG
5. Symptomatic coronary artery disease
6. Initiating vigorous exercise program

Copyright © 1998 American Diabetes Association [43]. Reprinted with permission from The American Diabetes Association.

The American Heart Association has not recommended routine testing in diabetic patients who are asymptomatic [45–47]. Furthermore, if cardiac stress testing is done, individuals with diabetes at a low risk are difficult to identify [35]. Since diabetes mellitus is a cardiovascular disease equivalent, aggressive treatment of the diabetes and other cardiac risk factors is indicated regardless of the results of exercise testing with or without imaging. Furthermore, there are no objective data indicating the use of interventional therapy to improve subsequent outcome in asymptomatic patients with diabetes.

It is somewhat difficult to recommend exercise testing in those with diabetes since the results may not determine differential treatment following testing. If an asymptomatic patient with diabetes undergoes screening and the results are negative for cardiovascular disease, the patient would, nevertheless, be regarded as high risk for the presence of cardiac disease. On the other hand, if the results were positive for cardiovascular disease, the results would not necessarily alter subsequent management due to the patient's high-risk status. In short, there are no data showing benefit of treating asymptomatic diabetic patients with interventional therapy or anti-ischemic medications. Thus, there is no evidence to support risk stratification in these patients with diabetes. Exercise testing in patients with diabetes is given a IIb classification by the American Heart Association and the American College of Cardiology. This IIb classification states that "usefulness or efficacy is less well established by evidence or opinion"; the guideline also states that exercise treadmill testing in general "might be useful in people with heightened pretest risk" [46–48].

Some physicians recommend patients with diabetes for exercise testing to determine if (1) there are severe ischemic electrocardiogram changes present with exercise that are not present at rest, (2) clinical symptoms do occur with exercise (but not at limited activity) or (3) significant arrhythmias occur with exercise. The results may then prompt the physician to pursue further evaluation and management. However, this approach is not supported by evidence-based studies.

Other physicians utilize scoring systems for risk factor assessment. This usually involves either the Framingham Heart Study scoring system (www.statcoder.com), the United Kingdom Prospective Diabetes Study (UKPDS) risk engine [49,50] or the American Diabetes Association's Diabetes Personal Health Decisions (PHD) [51,52]. Those at increased risk for coronary artery disease are then studied.

The Framingham Heart Study has been adopted for persons with diabetes and renders a cardiac risk score based on 15 risk factors (Table 4.6) [53]. This score is limited by (1) a specific patient population of white subjects, (2) older population data and (3) limited risk factors. However, one strength of this prospective study is that individuals have now been followed for more than 50 years [54].

The United Kingdom Prospective Risk Engine renders a cardiovascular risk score based on multiple factors pertinent to persons with type 2 diabetes mellitus (Table 4.7) [49,50]. This risk engine considers duration of diabetes, A1C and ethnicity in addition to the usual risk factors for future cardiovascular risk. While this risk engine is limited to those diagnosed with type 2 diabetes, it is based on 4,540 patients with a total of 53,000 patient-years of data [50].

Table 4.6 Framingham cardiac risk scoring system

Age (Years)
Sex (M/ F)
Systolic blood pressure (mmHg)
Diastolic blood pressure (mmHg)
Smoking Hx. (Yes/No in the past month)
Diabetes (ADA guidelines or under treatment)
Total cholesterol (mg/dl)
HDL-cholesterol (mg/dl)
LDL-cholesterol (mg/dl)
Triglycerides (mg/dl)
Hypertension treatment (Yes/No receiving medicine for hypertension)
CHD equivalent (Clinical CHD, symptomatic carotid artery
   disease or 50% stenosis, Peripheral arterial disease, abdominal
   artery aneurysm, diabetes mellitus, calculated 10 year CHD risk
   of > 20%)
Family history of premature CHD (Yes/ No CHD in male
   first-degree relative < 55 years; CHD in female first-degree
   relative < 65 years)
Abdominal obesity (Yes/ No men > 40 inches; women > 35 inches)
Fasting glucose (> 110 mg/dl)

Data from Wilson PW, D'Agostino RB, Levy D, et al. Prediction of coronary
heart disease using risk factor categories. Circulation 1998;97:1837–47.

Table 4.7 United Kingdom Prospective Diabetes Study risk engine factors

Age (years)
Duration of diabetes mellitus (years)
Sex (M/F)
BMI (kg/cm^2)
Atrial fibrillation (Yes/No)
Ethnicity (White Caucasian/Afro-Caribbean/Asian-Indian)
Smoking (Yes/No)
A1C (%)
Systolic BP (mmHg)
Cholesterol (mm/l or mg/dl)
HDL-cholesterol (mm/l or mg/dl)

Data from Stevens RJ, Kothari V, Adler AI, et al. The UKDPS risk engine:
A model for the risk of coronary artery disease in Type II diabetes (UKDPS
56). Clinical Sciences 2001;101:671–9.

The Archimedes Diabetes Model includes 45 factors and markers for disease
states associated with diabetes mellitus (Table 4.8). This model can be used for all
types of diabetes, both genders, all age groups and all ethnicity groups. The model
then calculates the 30-year risk for diabetes mellitus, myocardial infarction, stroke,
renal failure, eye disease and foot problems. The Archimedes Diabetes Model has
been validated against clinical trials with excellent confirmation data (correlation
coefficient $r = 0.99$ for all exercises) [52].

Table 4.8 American Diabetes Association's diabetes personal health decisions: Archimedes Diabetes Model

Gender	Cardiovascular disease history
Height	Myocardial infarction
Weight	Stroke
Age	Bypass surgery
Ethnicity	Angioplasty
Family history	Heart failure
Diabetes	Renal disease history
Cardiovascular disease	Albuminuria
Systolic blood pressure	Renal dialysis
Diastolic blood pressure	Kidney transplant
Cholesterol levels	Foot disease related to DM
LDL-cholesterol	Foot sores
HDL-cholesterol	Foot ulcers
Total cholesterol	Partial foot amputation related to DM
Smoking history	Full foot amputation related to DM
Visit physician 2×/ year	Aspirin use
Activity level per week	Year started using aspirin
Have been diagnosed with T1DM?	Type 1 DM: Year when diagnosed
Current medications:	Most recent A1C
Lipitor (atorvastatin)	Do you take insulin?
Niaspan (niacin)	Foot examination at each visit
Insulin	Dilated eye exam each year
Aspirin	

Data from Eddy DM, Schlessinger L. Archimedes: A trial-validated model of diabetes. Diabetes Care 2003;26:3093–101.

Special Considerations – Asymptomatic Patients

Silent myocardial ischemia in patients with diabetes mellitus manifests as an abnormal test (exercise test, imaging test or angiography) in someone with no clinical symptoms. In a Danish study the prevalence of silent ischemia in patients with diabetes was 13.5% and this was not different from matched controls [55].

Furthermore, Nesto et al. studied 100 patients (50 with diabetes and 50 without diabetes) and found that angina pectoris symptoms were not a reliable index of myocardial ischemia [56]. In contrast, Froelicher's group found that the accuracy of an abnormal exercise test was actually *better* than myocardial imaging studies for detecting asymptomatic coronary disease in patients with diabetes. They found that myocardial perfusion imaging had an increased false-positive rate in patients with diabetes [57].

The DIAD study looked at patients with type 2 diabetes aged 50–75 years for asymptomatic heart disease [58]. The control group was randomized to clinical follow-up while the study group underwent adenosine stress perfusion imaging. The average A1C of the enrolled population was 7.1 ± 1.5%. Twenty-two percent of patients had the evidence of silent myocardial ischemia.

Performing the Test

Some authorities recommend special exercise testing preparation of persons with diabetes. Riley et al. have recommended testing patients receiving insulin in a fasting state. This group found that intravenous glucose infusion increased the incidence of ST-segment depression [59]. However, Ellestad recommends that patients who are receiving insulin be studied approximately 2 hours following breakfast or lunch with no change in the meal plan or insulin administration. With this study practice they found neither complications due to blood glucose levels nor any false-positive tests [60]. For the purposes of this chapter it is recommended that blood glucose testing be done prior to and following the exercise stress test.

Interpretation of the Test

Most physicians perform exercise tests in those with diabetes and recommend interventional therapy in those with severe ischemia. This decision is often based on those factors that are correlated with a poor prognosis (see Chapter 6). Since diabetes is considered to be a coronary artery disease equivalent, a negative exercise test result does not alter the patient's assumed increased risk for the presence of future cardiac disease. In contrast, if the results indicate severe ischemic changes, then urgent consultation and intervention would be warranted. While screening with stress imaging does detect more patients with coronary artery disease, exercise testing alone is less expensive and has a good negative predictive value (97%) for future cardiac events [61].

Duke Treadmill Score for Diabetes

Lakkireddy et al. evaluated 100 patients with diabetes who were classified into low, intermediate and high-risk groups based on the Duke Treadmill Score [62]. The study confirmed the predictive value of the score in patients with diabetes and predicted the survival free period from major adverse cardiac events. However, the prognosis was not as good in diabetic patients compared to nondiabetic patients in the intermediate risk group. Since nondiabetic patients in this intermediate group are often treated in conservative fashion, the authors felt that more studies are needed to delineate the appropriate treatment for diabetic patients in this mid-risk group.

Other Factors

Exercise capacity or cardiorespiratory fitness correlates with future all-cause mortality in patients with diabetes mellitus [63]. In this prospective observational study 1,263 men with type 2 diabetes were selected and upon entry into the study underwent a maximal stress test utilizing a modified Balke–Ware protocol. The maximal metabolic units (METs) were calculated. The men were then followed for 12 years. Men with low cardiorespiratory fitness upon entry into the study had a 2.1 fold higher risk for death than those men who were fit at baseline.

A second study by Seyoum et al. investigated exercise capacity as a predictor of future cardiovascular events in patients with type 2 diabetes [64]. In this study were 468 total patients with 307 males and 161 females. These patients underwent VO_2 testing to determine peak exercise oxygen consumption ($VO_{2\,max}$). During a 5-year follow-up period all patients (both male and female cohorts) with a lower peak VO_2 at baseline experienced a higher rate of subsequent cardiovascular events. Finally, in one study of 6,213 men the authors found that peak exercise capacity or metabolic equivalents (METs) was the strongest predictor of overall mortality [65]. In fact, with each 1-MET increase in exercise capacity, there was a 12% increase in survival in both healthy men and those with cardiovascular disease.

Coronary autonomic neuropathy is a second factor. Autonomic dysfunction is associated with increased mortality. Attenuated heart rate recovery following exercise, chronotropic incompetence and reduced heart rate variability are indicators of autonomic dysfunction [66–68].

Cole et al. described heart rate recovery at 1 min post exercise as a predictor of future overall mortality [18]. Heart rate recovery was defined as the heart rate at maximum exercise less the heart rate at 1 min into recovery. An abnormal heart rate recovery was defined as a reduction of 12 beats or less:

$$\text{Heart rate recovery (HRR)} = \text{Heart rate}_{\text{maximum exercise}} - \text{Heart rate}_{1\,\text{min in recovery}}$$

$$\text{Abnormal HRR} = \leq 12 \text{ beats}$$

Cheng et al. studied 2,333 men whose average age was 49.4 years with diabetes mellitus at the Cooper Clinic in Dallas, Texas [69]. The heart rate recovery was calculated by subtracting the heart rate at 5 min into recovery from the heart rate (peak) obtained with maximum exercise. There was a correlation between the attenuation of the heart rate recovery and subsequent cardiovascular disease and all-cause mortality (Table 4.9):

Table 4.9 Correlation between the attenuation of the heart rate recovery and subsequent cardiovascular disease and all-cause mortality

Quartile	Heart rate recovery	Cardiovascular death
1st	< 55	2.0
2nd	56–66	1.5
3rd	67–75	1.5
4th	> 75	1.0

Copyright © 2003 American Diabetes Association. From Diabetes Care Vol. 26, 2003;2052–7. Reprinted with permission from The American Diabetes Association.

$$\text{Heart rate recovery} = \text{Heart rate}_{peak} - \text{Heart rate}_{5 \text{ min of recovery}}$$

Finally, at the Cleveland Clinic, Seshadri studied 1,818 patients of which 51 patients were diagnosed with diabetes mellitus. In this small study, diabetes mellitus was associated with an abnormal heart rate recovery following maximal exercise testing in a cohort of healthy patients with no known coronary artery disease [67]:

A second factor was the chronotropic response described as the percentage of the heart rate reserve used at peak exercise. Lauer et al. defined impaired chronotropic response or chronotropic index as failure to achieve at least 80% of the heart rate reserve and chronotropic incompetence as failure to achieve 85% of age-predicted maximum heart rate. Impaired chronotropic response is known to be an independent predictor of mortality [70].

$$\text{Chronotropic response (chronotropic index)} = \text{Percentage of the heart rate reserve used at peak exercise}$$

$$\text{Heart rate reserve} = \text{Maximum achievable heart rate } (220 - \text{age}_{years}) + \text{resting heart rate}$$

$$\text{Impaired chronotropic response (impaired chronotropic index)} = < 80\% \text{ of heart rate reserve}$$

$$\text{Chronotropic incompetence} = < 85\%(220 - \text{age}_{years})$$

Reduced heart rate variability is the third indicator of autonomic dysfunction. Heart rate variability and the autonomic nervous system have been associated with cardiovascular mortality [71]. Low heart rate variability has been a predictor of coronary artery disease from many causes including diabetes [72]. The heart rate variability depends on many physiological and pathological factors (Table 4.10). This indicator is based on the variability of the RR interval and correlates with cardiac autonomic function. This variability can be calculated from tracings or via designed computer programs [73]. The normal heart rate variability is due to the interplay of the sympathetic and parasympathetic systems where a low variability

Table 4.10 Factors decreasing heart rate variability

1. Age
2. Atherosclerosis
3. Depression
4. Diabetic autonomic neuropathy
5. Elevated serum insulin level
6. Obstructive sleep apnea
7. Physical inactivity
8. Rapid, shallow breathing
9. Reduced baroreflex sensitivity
10. Smoking

of the RR interval is associated with disease states including cardiac autonomic dysfunction found in persons with diabetes [66, 74, 75].

Summary

Patients with diabetes mellitus have a high incidence of cardiovascular disease. Risk stratification of these patients is somewhat difficult since the pretest likelihood of heart disease is great. The American Diabetes Association and the American Heart Association have delineated risk factors or markers for patients with diabetes for evaluation. By utilizing these specific risk factors or markers along with specific risk scoring systems, one can further define the likelihood for cardiovascular disease in individual patients over the subsequent 10–30 years. Those patients considering exercise at a vigorous level or those in the highest risk group can be immediately submitted to exercise testing and then referred for further evaluation as indicated (Table 4.11). Those patients with a normal exercise test should be re-evaluated every 2 years.

Table 4.11 Recommendations for exercise stress testing in persons with diabetes

	Class	Level of evidence	Reference
EST (with or without imaging) is recommended in patients with diabetes prior to initiating a vigorous exercise program	IIa	C	2, 46
Routine EST is not recommended in patients with diabetes who are asymptomatic	III	C	2, 48

Conclusion

The amount of evidence is increasing regarding ECG stress testing in special populations. Coronary artery disease is no longer considered to be a disease found only in middle-aged men. Still, it is not completely clear how to apply principles of stress testing to women, diabetic patients and the elderly. Special consideration must be given to identify patients at risk, because selection of patients with the appropriate risk factors and symptoms is the key to accurately recognize the value of stress testing. Alterations in procedure and interpretation are required to gain maximal information from the test so that appropriate referral can be made for coronary angiography or imaging studies.

Acknowledgments We extend our appreciation to Gwen Sprague, MLS, for her assistance in the preparation of this manuscript.

References

1. Heart Disease and Stroke Statistics: 2007 Update. American Heart Association. *http://www.americanheart.org*
2. ACC/AHA 2002 Guideline Update for Exercise Testing: Summary Article. A Report of the American College of Cardiology/American Heart Association Task Force on Practice Guidelines (Committee to Update the 1997 Exercise Testing Guidelines) *http://www.americanheart.org*
3. Gulati M, Pandey DK, Arnsdorf MF, et al. Exercise capacity and the risk of death in women: the St James Women Take Heart Project. Circulation. 2003;108:1554–9.
4. Shaw LJ, Mieres JH. The role of noninvasive testing in the diagnosis and prognosis of women with suspected CAD. J Fam Pract. 2005;Suppl:4–5.
5. Lee WL, Cheung AM, Cape D, et al. Impact of diabetes on coronary artery disease in women and men: a meta-analysis of prospective studies. Diabetes Care. 2000;23:962–8.
6. Rosenfeld JA. Heart disease in women. Postgraduate Medicine 2000;107:111–6
7. Vittinghoff E, Shlipak MG, Varosy PD, et al. Risk factors and secondary prevention in women with heart disease: the Heart and Estrogen/progestin Replacement Study. Ann Intern Med. 2003;138:81–9.
8. Rossouw JE, Anderson GL, Prentice RL, et al. Risks and benefits of estrogen plus progestin in healthy postmenopausal women: principal results From the Women's Health Initiative randomized controlled trial. JAMA. 2002;288:321–33.
9. Kwok Y, Kim C, Grady D, et al. Meta-analysis of exercise testing to detect coronary artery disease in women. Am J Cardiol. 1999;83:660–6.
10. Michaelides AP, Psomadaki ZD, Dilaveris PE, et al. Improved detection of coronary artery disease by exercise electrocardiography with the use of right precordial leads. N Engl J Med. 1999;340:340–5.
11. Alexander KP, Shaw LJ, Shaw LK, et al. Value of exercise treadmill testing in women. J Am Coll Cardiol. 1998;32:1657–64.
12. DeCara, JM. Noninvasive cardiac testing in women. J Am Med Womens Assoc. 2003;58:254–63.
13. Pratt CM, Francis MJ, Divine GW, et al. Exercise testing in women with chest pain. Chest. 1989;95:139–144.
14. American Heart Association. Role of noninvasive testing in the clinical evaluation of women with suspected coronary artery disease: Consensus statement from the Cardiac Imaging Committee, Council on Clinical Cardiology, and the Cardiovascular Imaging and Intervention Committee, Council on Cardiovascular Radiology and Intervention. Circulation. 2005;111:682–96.
15. Fleg, J. Stress Testing in the Elderly. Am J Geriatr Cardiol. 2001;10:308–13.
16. Goraya TY, Jacobsen SJ, Pellikka PK,et al. Prognostic value of treadmill exercise testing in elderly persons. Ann Intern Med. 2000;132:862–70.
17. Messinger-Rapport B, Pothier Snader CE, Blackstone EH, et al. Value of exercise capacity and heart rate recovery in older people. J Am Geriatr Soc. 2003;51:63–8.
18. Cole CR, Blackstone EH, Pashkow FJ, et al. Heart-rate recovery immediately after exercise as a predictor of mortality. N Engl J Med 1999;341:1351–7.
19. Lai S, Kaykha A, Yamazaki T, et al. Treadmill scores in elderly men. J Am Coll Cardiol. 2004;43:606–15.
20. *www.cdc.gov/diabetes/pubs/pdf/ndfs_2005.pdf*
21. Laing SP, Swerdlow AJ, Slater SD, et al. Mortality from heart disease in a cohort of 23,000 patients with insulin-treated diabetes. Diabetologia. 2003;46:760–765.
22. *www.diabetes.org/about-diabetes.jsp*
23. *www.diabetes.org/diabetes-prevention.jsp*
24. Fox CS, Pencina MJ, Meigs JB, et al. Trends in the incidence of type 2 diabetes mellitus from the 1970s to the 1990s: the Framingham Heart Study. Circulation. 2006;113:2914–8

25. Conway DG, O'Keefe JH, Reid KJ, et al. Frequency of undiagnosed diabetes mellitus in patients with acute coronary syndrome. Am J Cardiol 2005;96:363–5.
26. Lee WL, Cheung AM, Cape D, et al. Impact of diabetes on coronary artery disease in women and men: a meta-analysis of prospective studies. Diabetes Care. 2000;23:962–8.
27. Hu FB, Stampfer MJ, Solomon CG, et al. The impact of diabetes mellitus on mortality from all causes and coronary heart disease in women: 20 years of follow-up. Arch Intern Med. 2001;161:1717–23.
28. Fox CS, Coady S, Sorlie PD, et al. Trends in cardiovascular complications of diabetes. JAMA 2004;292: 2495–9.
29. Juutilainen A, Lehto S, Ronnemaa T, et al. Similarity of the impact of type 1 and type 2 diabetes on cardiovascular mortality in middle-aged subjects. Diabetes Care 2008;31: 714–9.
30. Jemal A, Ward E, Hoa Y, et al. Trends in the leading causes of death in the United States, 1970–2002. JAMA 2005;294;1255–9.
31. Berry C, Tardif JC, Bourassa MG. Coronary heart disease in patients with diabetes: part I: recent advances in prevention and noninvasive management. J Am Coll Cardiol. 2007;49: 631–42.
32. Hammond T, Tanguay JF, Bourassa MG. Management of coronary artery disease: therapeutic options in patients with diabetes. J Am Coll Cardiol. 2000;36:355–65.
33. Shorr RI, Franse LV, Resnick HE, et al. Glycemic control of older adults with type 2 diabetes: findings from the Third National Health and Nutrition Examination Survey, 1988–1994. J Am Geriatri Soc. 2000;48:264–7.
34. www.nhlbi.nih.gov/about/ncep.index.htm
35. Buse JB, Ginsberg HN, Bakris GL, et al. Primary prevention of cardiovascular diseases in people with diabetes mellitus: A scientific statement from the American Heart Association and the American Diabetes Association. Circulation 2007;115:114–26.
36. Hogan P, Dall T, Nikolov P. American Diabetes Association. Economic costs of diabetes in the US in 2002. Diabetes Care. 2003;26:917–32.
37. Janand-DelenneB, Savin B, Habib G, et al. Silent myocardial ischemia in patients with diabetes. Diabetes Care. 1999;22:1396–400.
38. Miettinen H, Lehto S, Veikko S, et al. Impact of diabetes on mortality after the first myocardial infarction. Diabetes Care. 1998;21:69–75.
39. The BARI Investigators. Influence of diabetes on 5-year mortality and morbidity in a randomized trial comparing CABG and PTCA in patients with multivessel disease: The Bypass Angioplasty Revascularization Investigation (BARI). Circulation. 1997;96:1761–9.
40. Gu K, Cowie CC, Harris MI. Diabetes and decline in heart disease mortality in US adults. JAMA. 1999;281:1291–7.
41. Milicevic Z, Raz I, Beattie SC, et al. Natural history of cardiovascular disease in patients with diabetes. Diabetes Care. 2008;31 (Suppl 2):S155–S160.
42. Alexander CM, Landsman PB, Teutsch SM. Diabetes mellitus, impaired fasting glucose, atherosclerotic risk factors, and prevalence of coronary artery disease. Am J Cardiol. 2000:86:897–902.
43. American Diabetes Association. Consensus development conference on the diagnosis of coronary heart disease in people with diabetes: Miami, Florida. Diabetes Care. 1998;21: 1551–9.
44. Sigal, RJ, Kenny GP, Wasserman DH, et al. Physical activity/ exercise and type 2 diabetes. A Consensus Statement from the American Diabetes Association. Diabetes Care. 2006;29: 1433–8.
45. Grundy SM, Garber A, Goldberg R, et al. Prevention Conference VI: Diabetes and Cardiovascular Disease: Writing Group IV: Lifestyle and medical management of risk factors. Circulation. 2002;105;e153–8.
46. Redberg RF, Greenland P, Fuster V, et al. Prevention Conference VI: Diabetes and Cardiovascular Disease: Writing Group III: Risk assessment in persons with diabetes. Circulation 2002;105:144–52.

47. Rubler S, Arvan SB. Exercise testing in young asymptomatic diabetic patients. Angiology 1976;27:539–48.
48. Gibbons RJ, Balady GJ, Beasley JW, et al. ACC/AHA guidelines for exercise testing: executive summary. A report of the American College of Cardiology/ American Heart Association Task Force on Practice Guidelines (Committee on Exercise Testing). Circulation 1997;96: 345–54.
49. www.dtu.ox.ac.uk/riskengine/download.htm
50. Stevens RJ, Kothari V, Adler AI, et al. The UKDPS risk engine: A model for the risk of coronary artery disease in Type II diabetes (UKDPS 56). Clinical Sci 2001;101:671–9.
51. Eddy DM, Schlessinger L. Archimedes: A trial-validated model of diabetes. Diabetes Care. 2003;26:3093–101.
52. Eddy DM, Schlessinger L. Validation of the Archimedes Diabetes Model. Diabetes Care. 2003;26:3102–10.
53. Wilson PW, D'Agostino RB, Levy D, et al. Prediction of coronary heart disease using risk factor categories. Circulation. 1998;97:1837–47.
54. Fox CS, Coady S, Sorlie PD, et al. Increasing cardiovascular disease burden due to diabetes mellitus: the Framingham Heart Study. Circulation. 2007;115:1544–50.
55. May O, Arildsen H, Damsgaard EM, et al. Prevalence and prediction of silent ischaemia in diabetes mellitus: a population-based study. Cardiovasc Res. 1997;34:241–7.
56. Nesto RW, Phillips RT, Kett KG, et al. Angina and exertional myocardial ischemia in diabetic and nondiabetic patients: assessment by exercise thallium scintigraphy. Ann Intern Med. 1988;108:170–5.
57. Lee DP, Fearon WF, Froelicher VF. Clinical utility of the exercise ECG in patients with diabetes and chest pain. Chest. 2001;119:1576–81.
58. Wacker FJ, Young LH, Inzucchi SE, et al. Detection of silent myocardial ischemia in asymptomatic diabetic subjects: The DIAD study. Diabetes Care. 2004;1954–61.
59. Riley GP, Oberman A, Scheffield LT. Electrocardiographic effects of glucose ingestion. Arch Intern Med. 1972;130:703–7.
60. Ellestad MH. Stress Testing: Principles and Practice, 5th ed. New York, Oxford University Press, 2003, 485.
61. Cosson E, Paycha F, Paries J, et al. Detecting silent coronary stenosis and stratifying cardiac risk in patients with diabetes: ECG stress test or exercise myocardial scintigraphy? Diabet Med. 2004;21:342–8.
62. Lakkireddy DR, Bhakkad J, Korlakunta HL, et al. Prognostic value of the Duke Treadmill Score in diabetic patients. Am Heart J. 2005;150:516–21.
63. Wei M, Gibbons L, Kampert JB, et al. Low cardiorespiratory fitness and physical inactivity as predictors of mortality in men with type 2 diabetes. Ann Intern Med. 2000;132:605–11.
64. Seyoum B, Estacio RO, Berhanu B, et al. Exercise capacity is a predictor of cardiovascular events in patients with type 2 diabetes mellitus. Diab Vasc Dis Res. 2006;3:197–201.
65. Myers J, Prakash M, Froelicher V, et al. Exercise capacity and mortality among men referred for exercise testing. N Engl J Med. 2002;346:793–801.
66. Singh JP, Larson MG, O'Donnell CJ, et al. Association of hyperglycemia with reduced heart rate variability (The Framingham Study). Am J Cardiol. 2000;86:309–12.
67. Seshadri N, Acharya N, Lauer MS. Association of diabetes mellitus with abnormal heart rate recovery in patients without known coronary artery disease. Am J Cardiol. 2003;91: 108–11.
68. Valensi P, Sachs RN, Harfouche B, et al. Predictive value of cardiac autonomic neuropathy in diabetic patients with or without silent myocardial ischemia. Diabetes Care. 2001;24: 339–43.
69. Cheng YJ, Lauer MS, Earnest CP, et al. Heart rate recovery following maximal exercise testing as a predictor of cardiovascular disease and all-cause mortality in men with diabetes. Diabetes Care. 2003;26:2052–7.
70. Lauer MS, Francis GS, Okin PM, et al. Impaired chronotropic response to exercise stress testing as a predictor of mortality. JAMA 1999;281:524–9.

71. Task Force of the European Society of Cardiology and the North American Society of Pacing and Electrophysiology. Heart Rate Variability. Circulation. 1996;93:1043–65

72. Dekker JM, Crow RS, Folsom AR, et al. Low heart rate variability in a 2-minute rhythm strip predicts risk of coronary artery disease and mortality from several causes. The ARIC Study. Circulation. 2000;102:1239–44.

73. Risk Mj, Bril V, Broadbridge C. et al. Heart rate variability measurement in diabetic neuropathy: Review of methods. Diabetes Technol Ther. 2001;3(1):63–74.

74. Malpas SC, Maling TJ. Heart-rate variability and cardiac autonomic function in diabetes. Diabetes 1990;39:1177–81.

75. Spallone V, Menzinger G. Diagnosis of cardiovascular autonomic neuropathy in diabetes. Diabetes 1997;46(Suppl 2): S67–76.

Part II
Interpretation and Application of the Exercise Test

Chapter 5
Interpreting the Exercise Test

Corey H. Evans and Myrvin H. Ellestad

This chapter focuses on the interpretation of the exercise test. The first half discusses the important parameters of the test to be evaluated. The second half discusses how the information from the test can be used to estimate the probability of coronary disease and likelihood of future cardiac events. This important area of risk stratification allows the physician to place the patient in low-, moderate-, or high-risk groups and to identify which patients benefit from referral to cardiology for consideration of revascularization.

When the physician looks at the results of the exercise test, there are several important parameters to be evaluated. Each parameter adds essential information to the test and also should be mentioned in the final report. The following areas need to be evaluated:

1. The heart rate and blood pressure response
2. The presence or absence of symptoms
3. The presence or absence of arrhythmias
4. The aerobic capacity
5. The presence of myocardial ischemia
6. A statement about the patient's risk for coronary disease or future coronary events

Each of these areas is discussed separately and then the information is used to make probability and risk stratification statements.

Heart Rate and Blood Pressure Response

Heart Rate Response

As one exercises, the heart rate increases gradually and linearly with the increasing workload, reaching a peak at maximum exertion. One of the signs the patient is

C.H. Evans (✉)
St. Anthony's Hospital, St. Petersburg, FL; Private Practice Family Physician, Florida Institute of Family Medicine, St. Petersburg, FL, USA
e-mail: email@coreyevansmd.com

C.H. Evans, R.D. White (eds.), *Exercise Testing for Primary Care and Sports Medicine Physicians,* DOI 10.1007/978-0-387-76597-6_5
© Springer Science+Business Media, LLC 2009

reaching maximum exertion is that the heart rate plateaus, as further increases in workload fail to increase the heart rate. In the past, physicians described the maximum heart rate achieved as a percent of the patient's predicted maximum heart rate. Most of the devices on the market now continuously calculate the percent of maximal heart rate based on the formula Max HR = 220 − age. On the other hand this standard is being re-evaluated. Due to the difficulty in predicting the maximal heart rate in patients, using the predicted maximal heart rate for this purpose or for a target for exercise prescriptions should be avoided.

The maximal heart rate with dynamic exercise is affected by several factors: age, gender, level of fitness, cardiovascular disease, altitude, type of exercise, prior bed rest, and maximal effort. Age has the greatest effect on the maximal heart rate, and studies have consistently shown a gradual decrease in maximal heart rate with increasing age. Each of these other factors has a small effect on the maximal heart rate achieved.

Londeree and Moeschberger [1] performed a comprehensive review of the literature on maximal heart rate, analyzing more than 23,000 subjects. In their analysis, age accounted for 75% of the variability in the maximal heart rate, and other factors accounted for no more than 5% of the variability. Numerous authors have published formulas for using age to predict maximal heart rates, but all are imperfect, with standard deviations from 10 to 15 beats per minute. A few of these formulas are shown in Table 5.1 [2]:

Another formula widely used is maximal heart rate = 220 − age. It is important to realize that none of these formulas accurately predict the maximum heart rate in individual patients, with the usual range being about 25 beats above or below the predicted maximum. Figure 5.1, from Froelicher's [3] study of United States Air Force pilots, illustrates the age-related decline in maximal heart rate as well as the large individual variation. Although Sheffield [4] in testing 100 women found that maximal heart rates were about five beats less than men of the same age, most authors feel gender differences are minimal. Cooper [5] testing 2500 men found that those with lower fitness had lower maximal heart rates and the fitter men had a smaller decline in maximal heart rates with age. Testing at altitude, swimming, or cycle ergometry results in lower maximal heart rates compared to treadmill testing at sea level. Men with coronary artery disease or hypertension also have lower maximal heart rates than do healthy men [6]. There has been a trend to use a new formula called the heart rate reserve [7], which is calculated as follows:

$$(\text{Peak HR} - \text{Resting HR})/(220 - \text{Age} - \text{Resting HR}) \times 100$$

Table 5.1 Formulas for using age to predict maximal heart rates

Author	No. of subjects	Regression formula
Cooper	2535 men	$y = 217 - 0.845(\text{age})$
Ellestad	2583 men	$y = 197 - 0.556(\text{age})$
Froelicher	1317 men	$y = 207 - 0.64(\text{age})$

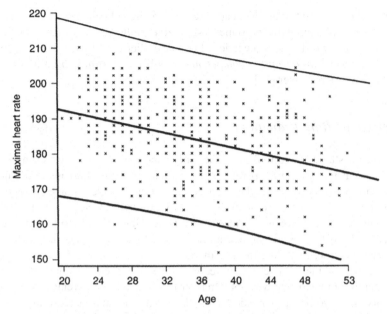

Fig. 5.1 Study of healthy air force pilots showing the relationship between maximal heart rate and age, along with the normal scatter (from Froelicher VF and Myers J [2], with permission from Elsevier.)

This includes the difference between resting HR and maximal exercise HR, which was demonstrated by Sandvik to be an important issue in predicting patients' outcome [8]. Values below 80% are a powerful predictor of adverse events.

Chronotropic Incompetence

When the maximum heart rate achieved during the exercise test is abnormally low, this is an important response called chronotropic incompetence (CI). Regardless of how it is defined, when patients show chronotropic incompetence in the absence of negative chronotropic drugs, they are at increased risk of future cardiac events and death. Ellestad initially defined CI as a maximal heart rate that was less than the fifth percentile of his published normal distribution of heart rates based on age [9]. It is currently recommended to define CI as a heart rate reserve value of less than 80% (see above discussion of heart rate reserve). Patients without ST-segment depression on an ET, but with CI, had a fourfold greater incidence of CAD, and a higher rate of death, or myocardial infarction.

Other authors have used a maximal heart rate less than 120 as a definition of CI. Using this definition, in patients with known CAD, McNeer [10] showed patients with CI had a 60% survival at 4 years versus 90% in patients with CAD but no CI on the exercise test. So whether patients have CAD or are asymptomatic, the finding of CI is important. The factors responsible for chronotropic incompetence include patients who stop the test at low heart rates due to anginal pain, severe myocardial dysfunction, and impaired autonomic dysfunction. In the last few years, Lauer has introduced the term chronotropic index [11]. The earlier work by Ellestad [12], who coined the term *chronotropic incompetence*, has been confirmed by a number of excellent studies by Lauer [11].

Other Heart Rate Indicators

More recent studies have looked at the early increase in heart rate during exercise, the total increase in heart rate, and the rapidity of the decrease in the heart rate during recovery. Falcone [13], using semi-supine bicycle ergometry, reported that an initial rapid HR increase at the onset of exercise (an increase in HR of 12 or greater at 1 min) predicted increased adverse cardiac events and CV mortality. Leeper et al. [14] using a ramp treadmill protocol looked at numerous markers of heart rate increase, including the HR increase at 15 sec, 1 min, 2 METS, the total HR increase, and the HR decrease in recovery in 1959 patients. They found that an early increase in heart rate was not a marker for increased CV events or increased mortality. The two best prognostic HR markers were the total increase in HR over resting HR (the heart rate increase or heart rate reserve) and the heart rate recovery at 2 min. The greater the heart rate increase (or heart rate reserve), the better the prognosis.

Heart Rate Recovery

A rapid recovery of the heart rate following exercise has long been associated with higher levels of fitness. This recovery is felt to be due to the reactivation of vagal tone after exercise. A failure of this normal recovery, that is, a persistently high heart rate after exercise also has been associated with increased mortality. Cole [15] studied 2428 patients and found that patients whose heart rate at 1 min recovery was 12 beats or less than the maximum had a fourfold increase in mortality over 6 years. Shelter, Marcus and Froelicher [16] attempted to address the optimum time in recovery and the cutoff value to best define patients at risk by looking at 2193 patients followed over 13 years. They reported that a heart rate decrease of 22 or less at 2 min best predicted increased mortality. When this abnormal response was also seen with a maximal MET level of less than 5, the survival was even worse. Whether one uses the 1 min heart rate recovery figure of 12 or less, or the 2 min recovery value of 22 or less, either finding is quite significant.

Blood Pressure Response to Exercise

In normal individuals undergoing exercise testing, the systolic blood pressure (BP) increases steadily with the workload reaching a maximum value at peak exercise.

In recovery the systolic BP decreases and is usually at baseline by about 6 min into recovery. The diastolic BP usually remains the same or decreases as exercise increases. Ellestad has a nice discussion of the difficulties taking BP measurements at rest and during exercise testing [17]. Even though there are difficulties in measuring BP during exercise testing, it is essential to monitor the BP throughout the test and into recovery, since abnormalities, both hypertensive and especially hypotensive responses, have strong clinical and prognostic implications.

The "double product" is a term used to describe the amount of cardiac work performed during the exercise test. This term means the systolic BP measurement multiplied by the heart rate. A normal double product at the end of a test is usually greater than 25,000. The double product correlates well with measured coronary blood flow, better than the heart rate or blood pressure alone. With stable angina, the angina will usually occur at a similar double product value on different tests. The lower the double product when ischemia occurs, in general, the worse the ischemia.

Hypertensive BP responses can be due to either unusually high systolic measurements or elevation of the diastolic readings. Although it is less clear what defines an abnormal systolic response to exercise, most agree that a rise of 10 mm in the diastolic BP is abnormal and is called a hypertensive diastolic response to exercise. In subjects free of heart disease, a hypertensive systolic response (most studies use values from 210 to 230 mm to define a hypertensive systolic response) to exercise indicates an increased risk of developing hypertension in the future [18].

It is also important to monitor the blood pressure response in recovery. In normal subjects, the systolic BP quickly returns toward normal and is close to the baseline reading by 6 min in recovery. When the systolic BP stays abnormally high in recovery, it has important prognostic implications. Taylor [19] looked at the "three-minute blood pressure ratio," the ratio of the systolic BP at 3 min in recovery divided by the maximum systolic BP. When this ratio was >0.91, the finding carried the same accuracy for the diagnosis of CAD as ST-segment depression.

Exercise-Induced Hypotension

As stated previously, the normal blood pressure response during the exercise test is a gradual increase in systolic blood pressure as the work increases. Rarely, the systolic blood pressure may start increasing, and then stop increasing and decrease. When the systolic blood pressure decreases during the test, this response is called exercise-induced hypotension (EIH). As Ellestad discusses [20], there are numerous causes for EIH, some physiologic and neurally mediated, and some are pathologic due to ischemia and left ventricular failure. When strict criteria are used to define this response, a drop in systolic blood pressure to or below the baseline [21], the response correlates with severe coronary disease and an increased mortality. When

Table 5.2 Heart rate and blood pressure responses recommendations and levels of evidence

Recommendations	Class	Level of evidence	References
1. Chronotropic incompetence predicts increased mortality	I	B	9, 10
2. Heart rate recovery indexes should be calculated and, if abnormal, indicate increased mortality	I	B	15, 16
3. Exercise-induced hypotension requires termination of the test and careful evaluation of the patient	I	B	

EIH is seen, especially when there is also evidence of myocardial ischemia, this is a worrisome response and the test should be terminated [22]. A summary of some of the important points from evaluation of the heart rate and blood pressure response and the levels of evidence are in Table 5.2.

Symptoms

The reasons for termination of the exercise test should be stated in the report and any unusual symptoms should be described. It is also helpful to describe the rate of perceived exertion experienced by the patient during the test or at termination. This is easily done using the 1–10 or 6–20 scales of perceived exertion. Although fatigue is the most common symptom, other symptoms may include chest pain characteristic of angina, atypical chest pain, leg pain suggesting claudication, unusual dyspnea or bronchospasm, and wheezing. The exercise test is especially valuable to help investigate exertion-related symptoms. It is not unusual to test a patient complaining of exertional dyspnea but denying chest pain, and to see significant myocardial ischemia with exercise causing the dyspnea (see case 2, Chapter 20). In fact, when the test is terminated exclusively for impaired breathing, those patients have a twofold increase in death from cardiac causes and a 3.5-fold increase in death from pulmonary causes [23].

When angina develops during an exercise test, the time of onset and severity should be mentioned. In most patients, angina usually develops after ECG evidence of myocardial ischemia and subsides before the ECG normalizes. The presence of angina with ECG ischemia usually suggests more severe ischemia, worse underlying CAD, and a poorer prognosis [24]. Thus, angina is an important component of most exercise scores as will be discussed later in this chapter. Exercise-induced chest pain suggestive of angina is so significant a finding, that even when it occurs without ECG evidence of ischemia, the test is interpreted as suggestive of myocardial ischemia.

Rhythm and Conduction Disturbances

Arrhythmias are commonly seen during exercise testing. Unifocal premature ventricular contractions (PVCs) and premature atrial contractions (PACs) are common and seen in 60% of exercise tests. Frequent PVCs, PACs, PVC couplets, multifocal PVCs, and rarely ventricular tachycardia (V-tach) may also be seen. Arrhythmias during exercise testing are usually divided into simple arrhythmias such as unifocal PVCs or PACs and complex arrhythmia such as multifocal PVCs, PVC couplets, and ventricular tachycardia.

Simple arrhythmias are not worrisome during the test and are common. Patients may have frequent PVCs or PACs at rest prior to testing, even bigeminy. Usually as the test begins and the heart rate elevates, these disappear. These arrhythmias are common and for years were not felt to be of any significance. Although Udall, in an analysis of 6,500 patients who were followed for 5 years in 1977, reported that when PVCs occurred with exercise the risk of a cardiac event increased by fourfold and when combined with ST-segment depression by sixfold [25]. In 2000 Jouven et al. [26] published the results of follow-up, after 23 years, of asymptomatic men who had frequent PVCs. If men had 10% or more of the QRS complexes as PVCs on any tracing during exercise, these men had an increased mortality. In fact, those asymptomatic men with frequent PVCs had the same increased mortality as those with an ischemic ST-segment response (RR = 2.3).

Other arrhythmias may occasionally be seen during the exercise test such as paroxysmal atrial tachycardia, atrial flutter, or atrial fibrillation. When a tachyarrhythmia is seen, the test is usually stopped. Patients with these atrial arrhythmias with exercise are treated in the same way as patients experiencing these arrhythmias at rest. In general these atrial arrhythmias do not suggest underlying coronary disease.

When complex arrhythmias are seen, there is more concern about underlying coronary disease. If the complex arrhythmias are increasing in frequency or severity, or if V-tach is seen, the test is usually terminated. Patients with complex arrhythmias, especially when coupled with an ischemic ST-segment response, often have significant coronary disease. Even when there is no ischemic response, patients with complex arrhythmias should undergo further testing to look for structural heart disease. This usually entails an echocardiogram and an exercise nuclear test. Arrhythmic responses are further discussed in Chapter 6.

Aerobic Capacity

When a maximal exercise test is performed, i.e., when individuals exercise until they feel they cannot go further due to maximal fatigue, and the heart rate has plateaued, the peak work load at that point defines the individual's maximal aerobic capacity. This can be expressed in METs or VO_2 max (ml of O_2/kg/min). These are related since 1 MET equals 3.5 ml O_2/kg/min. It is helpful to do maximum exercise tests since determination of the individual's maximum aerobic capacity has strong predictive power. The gold standard for determining VO_2 max is by using gas analysis (see Chapter), but the VO_2 max can be estimated from the time of termination of the test and the protocol. These estimates are usually within 10–15% of the measured VO_2 by gas analysis. Most stress systems print out an estimated maximum MET level at the end of the test. Table 5.3 shows estimations of the maximal MET level and VO_2 based on the treadmill times in the Bruce protocol.

Table 5.3 VO_2 max estimation from treadmill test from length of time on treadmill until exhaustion

VO_2 max	METS	Bruce (min:sec)
14.0	4.0	2 : 30
15.7	4.5	4 : 00
20.2	5.8	6 : 00
24.2	6.9	7 : 20
27.7	7.9	8 : 20
31.1	8.9	9 : 15
34.8	9.9	10 : 10
38.2	10.9	11 : 00
42.5	12.1	12 : 00
45.7	13.1	12 : 45
49.6	14.2	13 : 40
53.0	15.2	14 : 30
56.1	16.0	15 : 15
59.7	17.1	16 : 10
62.7	17.9	17 : 00
66.1	18.9	18 : 00
70.0	20.0	19 : 20
73.6	21.0	21 : 00
75.4	21.5	22 : 30

Modified from Nieman DC: Fitness and Your Health. Palo Alto, CA, Bull Publishing, 1993, p. 503, with permission from Bull Publishing Company.

Table 5.4 VO_2 max norms based on age and sex

Group (age, yrs)	Low	Fair	Average	Good	High	Athletic	Olympic
Women							
20–29	<28	29–34	35–43	44–48	49–53	54–59	60+
30–39	<27	28–33	34–41	42–47	48–52	53–58	59+
40–49	<25	26–31	32–40	41–45	46–50	51–56	57+
50–65	<21	22–28	29–36	37–41	42–45	46–49	50+
Men							
20–29	<38	39–43	44–51	52–56	57–62	63–69	70+
30–39	<34	35–39	40–47	48–51	52–57	58–64	65+
40–49	<30	31–35	36–43	44–47	48–53	54–60	61+
50–59	<25	26–31	32–39	40–43	44–48	49–55	56+
60–69	<21	22–26	27–35	36–39	40–44	45–49	50+

Adapted from Astrand I. Aerobic work capacity in men and women with special reference to age. ACTA Physiol Scand 49(Suppl 169):1–92, 1960, with permission.

It is helpful to use the maximal VO_2 (aerobic capacity) to determine the fitness category of the patient. This allows identification of those with low aerobic capacity, since many studies have shown a two- to threefold difference in cardiovascular mortality and all-cause mortality when one compares the lowest fitness quartile with the highest quartile [27]. In addition, when patients increase their exercise capacity by 1 MET they experience a 10–20% increase in survival and decrease in health care costs [28]. Table 5.4 shows fitness categories based on VO_2 max, age, and sex. In Chapter 15, page 280, VO_2 max values are expressed as percentile values based on VO_2 max and age.

ECG Changes with Exercise Testing

Normal ECG Changes with Exercise

With exercise, the normal response of the ECG includes the following changes: shortening of the PR segment, the P-wave becomes taller, and the repolarization wave of the atria (the Ta-wave) increases and causes downsloping of the PR segment and depression of the PQ junction. In addition, there is depression of the end of the QRS (the J point), rapid upsloping of the ST-segment, and shortening of the QT interval. Figure 5.2 shows a normal QRS complex at rest and during exercise [29].

At rest, the iso-electric PR segment can be used as a baseline to measure the amount of ST-segment elevation or depression. However with exercise, this segment is usually downsloping so it is standard practice to use the PQ junction (the end of the PR segment and beginning of the QRS) as the baseline for measurement of the ST-segment. In addition, the J point is used as a reference point to measure the ST-segment. For example, most ST-segment measurements are taken at 60 or 80 msec after the J point (J +60, J +80).

Mechanism of Myocardial Ischemia and the Ischemic Cascade

Ellestad [30] has a nice review of the mechanism of myocardial ischemia when seen with exercise testing. Basically myocardial ischemia results when there is an imbalance between supply and demand. This imbalance may be global, but usually is localized in certain areas. At least in the dog model, when coronary perfusion pressure drops to below 55 mmHg, there is a decrease in myocardial function. There are many determinants of myocardial perfusion pressure, including coronary obstructions, coronary artery spasm, the presence of collaterals, heart rate, resting wall tension, the tension of pre-capillary sphincters and velocity of blood flow in the coronary arteries. Figure 5.3 illustrates the various resistances to blood flow.

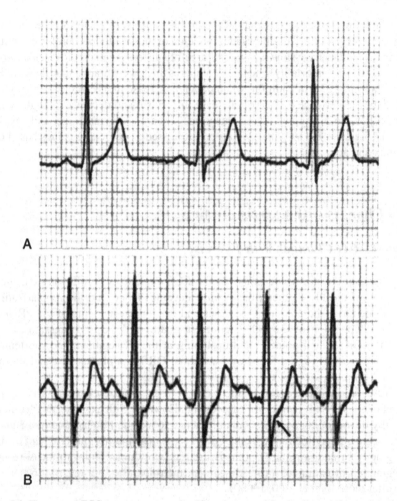

Fig. 5.2 The normal ECG response to exercise. Note the normal J point (arrow) depression and the rapid upsloping ST-segment. By agreement, the baseline is the PQ junction. A, resting tracing. B, exercise tracing (from Evans CH, Harris G, Menold V, et al. [29], with permission from Elsevier.)

Once the myocardial cells become ischemic, there is loss of contractility. This initiates what some have called the ischemic cascade. Localized myocardial ischemia is followed by localized abnormalities on thallium scanning, then wall motion abnormalities, ECG changes, then chest pain, and if the imbalance is not corrected, global dysfunction and myocardial necrosis. Figure 5.4 illustrates this ischemic cascade.

Ellestad discusses the mechanism behind ST-segment changes in his chapter on myocardial ischemia [30]. When the myocardial cells become ischemic, potassium leaves the cells creating a diastolic current of injury that flows toward the epicardium. This current of injury elevates the baseline, the P-wave, and the QRS, but

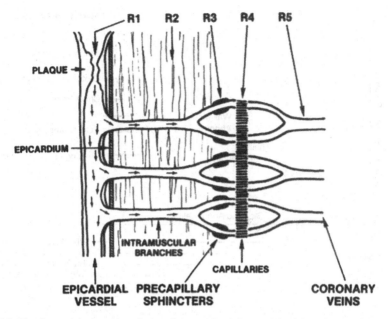

Fig. 5.3 The diagram depicts the various resistances that influence blood flow, from a plaque at R1 to the effect of coronary venous pressure at R5. When the heart is at basal state, the pre-capillary sphincters at R3 probably play the most important role (Ellestad MH [30]. With permission from Oxford University Press, Inc.)

this elevation is not recognized on the tracing. After depolarization of the ventricle, all the myocardial cells, including the ischemic cells, are depolarized and the ECG tracing returns to the original baseline, which is seen as ST-segment depression. As repolarization begins, the current of injury begins and the T-wave and baseline elevates again. When there is endocardial ischemia, the endocardium tends to develop relatively evenly distributed ischemia throughout the ventricle. The vector of this subendocardial ischemia is fairly constant in direction and points away from V_5, causing ST-segment depression in that lead. Thus, most ischemia seen on exercise testing is subendocardial ischemia and most often seen in V_5. This subendocardial ischemia tends to have the same vector regardless of which coronary vessel is the culprit vessel, and so subendocardial ischemia manifested by ST-segment depression does not identify the culprit artery.

On the other hand, when ischemia is more severe it can become transmural and is seen as ST-segment elevation. This ST-segment elevation (including J point elevation) does identify the culprit artery. So ST-segment elevation in the precordial anterior leads generally indicates disease of the left anterior descending artery (LAD), and inferior ST-segment elevation usually connotes right coronary artery disease. For further discussion of ST-segment elevation, see Chapter 6.

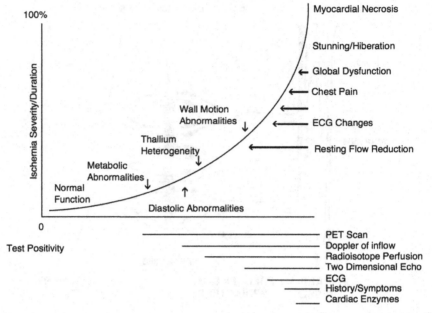

Fig. 5.4 Representation of the ischemic cascade. After reduction in myocardial blood flow sufficient to result in physiologic abnormalities, a predictable sequence of events occurs, beginning with subclinical diastolic dysfunction and progressing to electrocardiographic abnormalities and the clinical syndrome of angina. Of note, wall motion abnormalities as detected by stress echocardiography precede the development of diagnostic electrocardiographic changes and angina. The time points in the ischemic cascade at which different diagnostic tests are presumed to become positive are noted by the bars below the graph (from Ellestad MH, Stress Testing; Principles and Practice, 5th Ed. Oxford University Press, 2003, p. 128. With permission from Oxford University Press, Inc.)

Abnormal ECG Changes with Exercise

There are many abnormal ECG changes with exercise that can correlate with CAD and/or poorer outcomes. First the conventional abnormal ECG changes will be discussed. This is primarily abnormal types of ST-segment depression and elevation. Next, less common abnormal ECG changes will be discussed.

Conventional Abnormal ECG Changes with Exercise

As discussed above, during exercise the normal ST-segment starts with J point depression and a rapidly upsloping ST-segment that crosses the baseline around 80 msec past the J point. The first abnormality of the ST-segment is a slow upsloping ST-segment that is still depressed 80 msec past the J point (J + 80) (Fig. 5.5A). This response is the least specific for CAD and is also seen in some normal individuals. There is some disagreement about specific criteria to diagnose abnormal

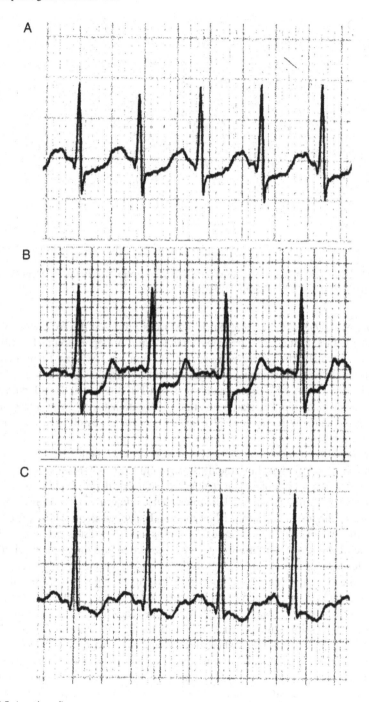

Fig. 5.5 (continued)

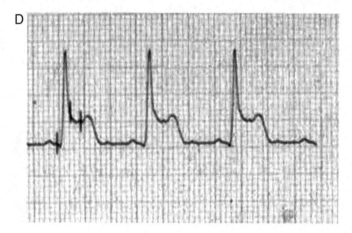

Fig. 5.5 Types of abnormal ST-segment depression indicating myocardial ischemia. A, abnormal upsloping ST-segment depression. B, horizontal ST-segment depression. C, downsloping ST-segment depression. D, ST-segment elevation. (A–C from Evans CH, Harris G, Menold V, and Ellestad MH [29], with permission from Elsevier.)

upsloping ST-segment depression, but Ellestad has proposed the following: When the ST-segment is at the baseline or less than 0.7 mm of depression at J = 80, the response is normal; when there is more than 0.7 mm but less than 1.5 mm of ST-segment depression, the response is suggestive of myocardial ischemia, and when there is 1.5 mm or more ST-segment depression at J + 80, the test is called positive for myocardial ischemia. Ellestad found that of 70 patients with 1.5 mm or more of upsloping ST-segment depression, 57% had two- or three-vessel disease at cardiac catheterization [31].

Horizontal ST-segment depression (Fig. 5.5B) occurs when there is J point depression followed by a flat (horizontal) ST-segment for 60–80 msec or more. Most clinicians use 1 mm or more of horizontal ST-segment depression as the criteria to diagnose myocardial ischemia. The criterion used determines the sensitivity and specificity of the test; if 0.5 mm of horizontal ST-segment depression is used, the test is more sensitive but less specific; if 2 mm is used, the test is not sensitive but quite specific for CAD. One millimeter of ST-segment horizontal depression is a reasonable compromise.

When the J point is depressed and the ST-segment slopes downward, this response is called *downsloping ST-segment depression*. Because the ST-segment is downsloping, the further away from the J point one reads the ST-segment, the more ST-segment depression is measured. In this case, the ST-segment is measured closer to the J point, either at J + 20 or where the ST-segment changes slope (Fig. 5.5C).

There has been considerable discussion about the relationship between types of abnormal ST-segment changes, the amount of ST-segment depression, and the severity of CAD. One often sees an evolution of ST-segment depression, starting with upsloping, then horizontal, and finally downsloping ST-segment depression as the ischemia worsens. In general upsloping ST-segment depression suggests milder disease, and downsloping ST-segment depression suggests more severe disease. Goldschlager [32] reported that less than 1% of patients with downsloping ST-segment depression had normal coronaries, and 56% had three-vessel disease. For years it has been accepted that the greater the amount of ST-segment depression, the more severe the CAD. Recently this concept has been challenged. Ellestad and others [33] have not been able to correlate the amount of maximal ST-segment depression with the number of diseased vessels.

The least common but most ominous type of ST-segment change is *ST-segment elevation* (Fig. 5.5D). This occurs when there is elevation of the J point and ST-segment. When it occurs in leads without the presence of Q-waves, it usually means significant transmural ischemia due to proximal high-grade stenosis of either the LAD or right coronary artery. Unlike ST-segment depression, ST-segment elevation does help localize the involved artery. This response can also be seen with severe coronary artery spasm, so called Prinzmetal's angina. When ST-segment elevation is seen in leads with existing Q-waves, it was thought that this phenomenon was due to an akinetic segment or area of scar, but recent reports using thallium scintigrams show there is usually an area of ischemic muscle adjacent to the scar [34].

Less Common Abnormal ECG Changes

QRS Changes

With exercise the total amplitude of the QRS complex might increase initially but usually decreases at peak exercise or early in recovery. This decrease, seen best in the lateral precordial leads, is probably due to a decrease in stroke volume at peak exercise. When there is a significant increase in R-wave height in the lateral precordial leads at high heart rates, this finding is quite specific for myocardial ischemia but not sensitive. The mechanism is probably due to increased left ventricular volume as ischemia develops. See the discussion in Ellestad [35].

Precordial T-Wave Changes

When exercise results in peaking of the T-wave in V_2 and V_3, this frequently indicates anterior wall ischemia. This may be a precursor of ST elevation in these leads (Fig. 5.6). In our experience this has been due to a high-grade narrowing in the LAD [36].

ST-Segment Depression in Ventricular Premature Complexes

PVCs are not unusual when doing an exercise test. The significance of ventricular ectopy has been previously discussed. Occasionally, however, PVCs at rest, or at low levels of exercise, will evolve into PVCs with increasing ST-segment depression. When this occurs, ischemia can be predicted with a high degree of accuracy [37].

V$_1$ V$_2$V$_3$ 0mm/mV   10mm/mV

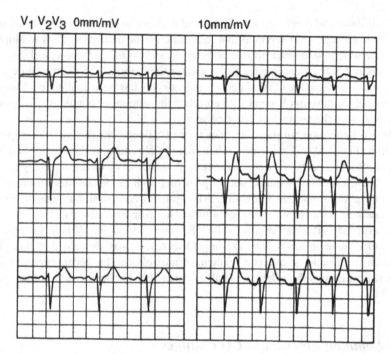

Fig. 5.6 Leads V$_1$, V$_2$, and V$_3$ on left at rest and on right immediately after exercise. The increase in amplitude of the T-wave is associated with proximal LAD disease (from Ellestad MH, Stress Testing; Principles and Practice, 5th Ed. Oxford University Press, 2003, p. 128. With permission from Oxford University Press, Inc.)

Lead Strength

It has long been known that when the R-wave amplitude is less than 10 mm and depression of 1 mm is used as a sign of ischemia there are many false-negative results, and when the R-waves are very tall ST-segment depression may represent a false-positive result. Ronald Selvester has found that ST-segment depression of 10% or less of R-wave amplitude is in the normal range, but when it exceeds this threshold, ischemia is very likely (sensitivity 95% and specificity 67%) [38]. If this is so, why not correct the magnitude of ST-segment depression for R-wave amplitude? When this is done it improves the sensitivity and has been termed lead strength analysis. Correcting ST-segment depression by calculating the ratio of ST to R amplitude, with a ratio of 0.1 as the threshold for ischemia, the sensitivity in patients with R-waves less than 10 mm was increased from 31 to 82% (Fig. 5.7) [39].

Criteria to Diagnose Myocardial Ischemia

As one can see from the previous discussion, there are numerous abnormal responses seen from the exercise test that suggest the presence of myocardial ischemia.

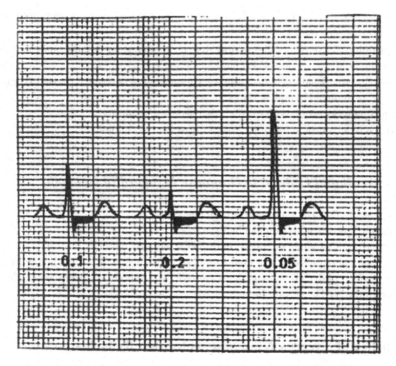

Fig. 5.7 Lead strength. The complex with a 10 mm R-wave illustrates the calculation of the ST/R ratio (1/10 = 0.10). If the R-wave is only 5 mm, an ST-segment depression of 1 mm results in a ratio of 0.2. This is equivalent to 2 mm of ST-segment depression in a patient with a 10 mm R-wave. When the R-wave is 20 mm and the ST-segment depression is 1 mm, the ratio is 0.05, which is not significant for ischemia (from Ellestad MH, Crump R, Surber M, The significance of lead strength on ST changes during treadmill stress tests. J Electrocardiol 1992;25 Suppl:31–4, with permission from Elsevier.)

Each response has its own sensitivity and specificity for the diagnosis of ischemia. Understanding this, the following criteria are generally accepted as being *diagnostic of myocardial ischemia*:

- Horizontal or downsloping ST-segment depression that is equal to or greater than 1 mm at 60 msec past the J point
- Upsloping ST-segment depression that is equal to or greater than 1.5 mm at 80 msec past the J point
- ST-segment elevation (and J point elevation) of 1 mm or more at 80 msec past the J point
- ST-segment elevation in AVR. This finding is as reliable as horizontal ST-segment depression.

It is also important to recognize when an exercise test is mildly abnormal or when some of the less commonly abnormal responses are seen. When the following responses are seen, the test is said to be *suggestive of myocardial ischemia*:

- Horizontal or downsloping ST-segment depression that is between 0.5 and 1.0 mm at 60 msec past the J point
- Upsloping ST-segment depression that is greater than 0.7 mm and less than 1.5 mm at 80 msec past the J point
- ST-segment elevation (with J point elevation) that is between 0.5 and 1.0 mm
- Exercise-induced hypotension
- Chest pain occurring with exercise that seems like angina
- High-grade ventricular ectopy especially at low work loads

Unconventional Criteria to Diagnose Myocardial Ischemia

- Increase in R-wave amplitude at high heart rates
- Peaked T-waves with exercise in V_2 and V_3
- Increasing ST-segment depression in PVCs with exercise
- ST-segment depression less than 1 mm but with a value of >0.1 when corrected for lead strength (ST-segment depression /R-wave height) or positive by calculation of the ST Heart Rate Index.

Accuracy of Exercise ST-segments to Identify Ischemia

For many years, the accuracy of ST-segment depression has been estimated by comparing it with a narrowing on the coronary angiogram of 50% or more. In the last few years, the significance of coronary narrowing has been evaluated by fractional flow reserve (FFR), which is now recognized to be a more accurate measure of narrowing that is severe enough to produce ischemia [40]. It has long been recognized that the visual analysis of the coronary angiogram, when it is believed to be moderate (40–60%) is inaccurate. When fractional flow reserve, measured with a Doppler flow wire during angiography, is compared with exercise-induced ST-segment depression it turns out that ST-segment depression is more accurate than previously reported. Wilson reports when testing single vessel disease that ST-segment depression is 84% sensitive and 87% specific [41]. This compares with a 65% sensitivity and 70% specificity previously commonly accepted. Ellestad writes [42] that noninvasive tests such as exercise tests should no longer be evaluated against coronary angiography as the gold standard, but instead should be evaluated by intra-coronary evaluation of fractional flow reserve. When this is done, the exercise test is a better predictor of significant coronary ischemia than previously thought.

Criteria to Define a Normal Exercise Test

A test is considered normal when there are no abnormal responses and the patient exercised for an adequate length of time. The usual criterion is reaching 85% of the maximal predicted heart rate. Due to the wide variability in the maximum heart rate, this criterion should not be strictly applied. In other words, if a patient reaches 80% of the maximal predicted heart rate and stops due to fatigue and describes a high rate of perceived exertion, the test is adequate. The patient probably has a lower than average maximal heart rate.

When no abnormal responses are seen, but the patient achieves less than 85% of the maximal predicted heart rate and a low level of perceived exertion, the test should be called inadequate. The test may either be repeated or, if the low heart rate was due to drugs such as beta blockers that cannot be discontinued, a stress imaging study can be done.

Significance of a Negative or Positive Exercise Test Result

The results of the exercise test can be used to help with the diagnosis of coronary artery disease or for prognostic information. In either case, the diagnostic accuracy or predictive value of the test is determined by the characteristics of the patient or population being tested. For example, in a population at low risk for CAD, a positive exercise test would have a low predictive value for CAD. The sensitivity and specificity of the exercise test depend not only on the characteristics of the population being tested, but also on the cutoff limits used to define a normal and abnormal test. For instance, if one calls only horizontal or downsloping ST-segment depression abnormal, the test will be less sensitive but more specific for the diagnosis of CAD than if one also considers upsloping ST-segment depression as abnormal. Likewise, using 2 mm of ST-segment depression as the cutoff instead of 1 mm will again make the test less sensitive but more specific for the diagnosis of CAD.

One way to consider the exercise test is that a positive test increases one's chance for having CAD, while a negative test decreases the chance. This concept is explained in greater detail in the next section. A positive exercise test can be considered an additional risk factor for CAD, and a positive test increases one's probability of having future coronary events. The reverse is true for a negative exercise test.

Practical Approaches to Analyzing the Results of the Exercise Test

When using the exercise test to evaluate and manage patients with suspected or known heart disease, there are three important considerations. First, the results of the test can be used to confirm that the patient does or does not have significant CAD. This diagnostic use of the test is best considered as using the test to generate a probability statement that the patient does or does not have CAD. Secondly, the test can be used to decide the severity of the disease. Finally, the test results can be used to develop a prognostic statement about the likelihood of future cardiac events or mortality. Each of these important concepts will be discussed.

As primary care physicians, we want to use the test to help us decide the likelihood that our patients have CAD, but even more importantly which patients we can safely follow and which need to be referred to cardiologists for consideration of revascularization to improve survival. The following discussion shows several tools useful for this important stratification of patients.

Using the Exercise Test to Develop a Probability Statement for CAD

When using the exercise test results to diagnose CAD, one needs to take into consideration not only the test results but also the risk for CAD in the patient being evaluated. The best way to do this is to determine the pretest probability for CAD in the patient and then apply the test results to determine a posttest probability for CAD in each given patient. Diamond and Forrester [43] developed this approach by applying Bayes Theorem to the data from exercise testing. They developed data on the prevalence of CAD based on the age, sex, and symptom classification of patients expressed as a probability (Fig. 5.8). One can then use the results of the exercise test to develop a posttest probability, depending upon the pretest probability and the amount of ST-segment depression seen [44] (Fig. 5.9).

This key concept means that one should develop a pretest and posttest probability of CAD in each patient tested. For example, if an asymptomatic 35-year-old male is tested, his pretest probability is about 2% of having significant CAD. If he has a positive test with 1 mm of ST-segment depression, the posttest probability is still only about 5% that he actually has significant CAD. The positive test is most likely a false-positive. However, if the same individual has more than 2.5 mm ST-segment depression, the posttest probability would increase to around 30–40%.

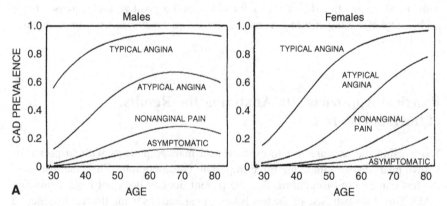

Fig. 5.8 Prevalence of CAD according to age, sex, and symptom classification (data from Diamond GA, Forrester JS [43], with permission.)

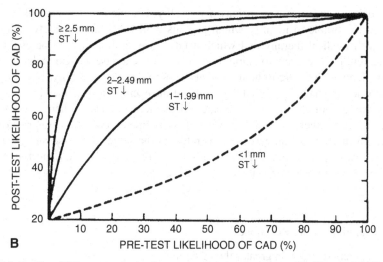

Fig. 5.9 Family of ST-segment depression curves showing the posttest likelihood of CAD (from Epstein SE [44], with permission from Elsevier.)

As another example, suppose a 70-year-old woman with typical angina is tested and has 1.5 mm of ST-segment depression. Her pretest probability of CAD is about 92% and the posttest probability is about 96%. The test did not add much to the diagnostic probability of CAD. Even if she has a negative test, the posttest probability is still about 75% that she has significant CAD. In those with high pretest probability, the test does not help much diagnostically, but can be very helpful for prognosis and determination of severity of disease.

It can be seen from this discussion that the exercise test is most helpful as a diagnostic tool in those with a pretest probability of between 20 and 80%. This is why the ACC/AHA Committee on Exercise recommends exercise testing for diagnosis in those with intermediate probability of CAD [22]. This generally includes younger men and women with typical angina, most patients with atypical angina and non-anginal pain, and asymptomatic older men with multiple risk factors such as diabetes.

This concept of posttest probability is important and should be understood by those doing exercise testing. The limitation of this approach is that the amount of ST-segment depression is the only modifying factor used, when we know there are many other conventional and unconventional markers of ischemia that can determine one's probability of CAD. Unfortunately there is no large database comparing all the factors. Exercise scores try to use multiple factors as discussed below.

Using the Exercise Test to Predict Severe CAD and for Prognosis

Using the exercise test as an aid to diagnose CAD is important, but even more important is the use of the exercise test to determine which patients with CAD have severe disease and a risk of increased mortality. For the primary care physician, we want to be able to identify which patients with CAD can be safely followed by us with medical therapy and which need to see cardiologists to be evaluated for interventional revascularization. Fortunately, the exercise test can help identify those patients with severe ischemia and at risk for increased mortality.

Many authors have compared the results of the exercise test with catheterization results. Nora Goldschlager [31] evaluated 410 patients referred to her clinic by exercise test and catheterization. The type of ST-segment depression was related to severity of disease as Fig. 5.10 demonstrates. In the same study, she analyzed the exercise test responses that correlate with severe three-vessel CAD and found the following factors correlated with severe disease:

Electrocardiographic Responses

1. ST-segment depression greater than 2.5 mm
2. ST-segment depression beginning at 5 METs or less effort
3. Downsloping ST-segment depression or ST-segment elevation
4. ST-segment depression lasting more than 8 min in recovery
5. Serious dysrhythmias at low heart rates (<120 beats per minute)
6. ST-segment depression in five or more leads

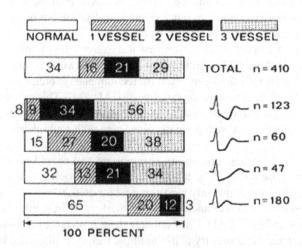

Fig. 5.10 The relation between ST response type and extent of coronary disease. The study population is represented at the top. Downsloping ST-segments are highly specific for coronary disease, with only one false-positive response encountered; most patients have double- and triple-vessel disease. Neither the horizontal nor slowly upsloping ST-segments aid in identifying severe disease. A very small percentage of patients with entirely normal treadmill tests will have double- and triple-vessel disease (from Goldschlager N, Selzer A, Cohn K [32], with permission.)

Nonelectrocardiographic Responses

1. Chronotropic incompetence (peak HR < 120 beats per minute)
2. Exercise-induced hypotension
3. Inability to exercise past a level of 5 METs (3 min on the Bruce protocol)

It is important to keep these criteria for severe disease in mind as they help physicians identify which patients are at higher risk and need consideration for cardiology consultation and cardiac catheterization.

Exercise Treadmill Scores to Develop a Prognostic Statement in Patients Undergoing Exercise Testing

In addition to identifying patients with severe disease, the exercise test can predict which patients have a poor prognosis. Several authors, after multivariate analysis of the exercise parameters and patient survival, have developed prognostic tools using the exercise parameters. One of the best known is the Exercise Treadmill Score, also known as the Duke Treadmill Score. First published by Mark et al. [45] the study compared various exercise parameters in the Duke database on 2,842 patients when followed for 5 years. The following three factors from the exercise test correlated best with prognosis: the exercise time, the degree of maximal ST-segment depression, and the presence of angina. Using regression analysis, they developed a weighted formula using these factors:

$$\text{Exercise Treadmill Score} = \text{Minutes of exercise} - (5 \times \text{Maximal ST-segment depression}) - (4 \times \text{Anginal index})$$

The exercise time was on the Bruce protocol, and the anginal index was 0 if no angina, 1 if typical angina during the test, and 2 if the test was terminated due to angina.

Based on the final score, the patients were divided into three classifications: + 5 or greater = good prognosis (5-year survival = 97%); −10 to + 4 = intermediate prognosis; and −11 or lower = poor prognosis (5-year survival = 72%).

In a later article Mark published a nomogram that enabled one to use the METs from any exercise test, the amount of ST-segment depression, and the anginal index to determine the 1- and 5-year survival of the patient [46] (Fig. 5.11).

Using the Exercise Treadmill Score in patients allows calculation of the 1- and 5-year survival of patients. When patients are at high risk, their mortality can be compared to their mortality from coronary bypass surgery and appropriate decisions can be made.

Other scores have been developed. Morrow et al. [47] developed a predictive scoring equation from an analysis of male patients in the Long Beach Veterans Administration Medical Center. This score, called the Veterans' Administration Score, uses the amount of ST-segment depression, presence of CHF or digoxin use, maximum MET level, and the systolic BP response to divide patients into low-,

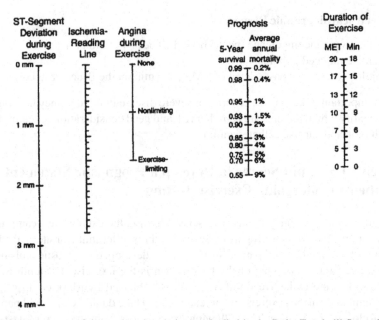

Fig. 5.11 Nomogram of the prognostic relations embodied in the Duke Treadmill Score. Determination of prognosis proceeds in five steps. First the observed amount of exercise-induced ST-segment deviation (the largest elevation or depression after resting changes have been subtracted) is marked on the line for ST-segment deviation during exercise. Second, the observed degree of angina during exercise is marked on the line for angina. Third, the marks for ST-segment deviation and degree of angina are connected with a straightedge. The point where this line intersects the ischemia-reading line is noted. Fourth, the total number of minutes of exercise in treadmill testing according to the standard Bruce protocol (or the equivalent in multiples of resting oxygen consumption (METS) from an alternative protocol) is marked on the exercise-duration line. Fifth, the mark for ischemia is connected with that for exercise duration. The point at which this line intersects the line for prognosis indicates the 5-year survival rate and average annual mortality for patients with these characteristics (From Mark DB, Shaw L Harrell FE, et al. [46], with permission.)

intermediate-, or high-risk groups. Because of its reproducibility and application to men and women, the Duke Score is recommended and should be calculated in each patient with CAD undergoing exercise testing. For further discussion of exercise testing scores see Chapter 9 by White and Goldschlager.

Clinical Management of Patients with the Exercise Test

As stated earlier, the exercise test has multiple uses in our patients at risk for CAD or with known disease. First, the test can be used to help with the diagnosis of CAD in our patients by providing a posttest probability of CAD based upon the patient's characteristics and the test results. In most patients with an intermediate probability of CAD based upon age, gender, and symptoms and a normal exercise test, the probability of significant CAD is low enough that further testing is not indicated. This is certainly true when the posttest probability of CAD is less than 10%. This will definitely be the case when asymptomatic at-risk patients are evaluated and have a normal exercise test (see Chapter). When the posttest probability of CAD after a normal exercise test will be higher, one can perform an exercise test with perfusion imaging since a normal exercise perfusion imaging test has a greater negative predictive value.

The exercise test is even more useful to help stratify our patients with known CAD. All patients with known or suspected CAD should have an exercise test for this stratification, to decide which can be managed medically and which are at high risk for severe disease and poor prognosis. Testing physicians should use both the factors correlated with severe disease mentioned previously, and also the Exercise Treadmill Score for this determination. Patients at high risk by either criterion should be further evaluated by cardiology as revascularization might improve survival.

Finally the exercise test can be used by primary care physicians to promote a healthy lifestyle and prevent CAD. The exercise test provides an important evaluation of fitness and can be used to provide an exercise prescription and encourage a higher level of fitness.

The Exercise Test Report

Each of the five main responses—the presence of myocardial ischemia, the heart rate and blood pressure response, symptoms, any dysrhythmias, and the maximal aerobic capacity—should be mentioned in the report. In addition, there should be a statement about the patients risk for CAD or future cardiac events. A suggested format for the exercise report is shown in Table 5.5.

Table 5.5 Suggested format for the exercise test report

Paragraph 1: General summary of testing
1. Patient's age, indication for testing, cardiac medicines, protocol used.
2. Baseline heart rate, blood pressure, and resting ECG findings.
3. Peak exercise data; blood pressure, heart rate, peak MET level, perceived exertion score, and reason for stopping.
4. Description of any abnormalities in the ECG response, hemodynamics, dysrhythmias, or symptoms.

Paragraph 2: Assessment
1. Presence or absence of ECG ischemia.
2. Normal or abnormal heart rate and blood pressure response to exercise.
3. Presence of dysrhythmias.
4. Presence of symptoms.
5. The maximal aerobic capacity (if a maximal test was done).
6. A statement about the patients risk of CAD or mortality, based upon the test results.

From Evans CH, Harris G, Menold V, and Ellestad MH [29], with permission from Elsevier.

References

1. Londeree BR, Moeschberger ML. Influence of age and other factors on maximal heart rate. J Cardiopulm Rehabil 1984;4: 44–49.
2. Froelicher VF, Myers J. Exercise and the Heart, 5th ed. Elsevier, 2006, 110.
3. Froelicher VF, Brammel H. Davis G, et al. A comparison of three maximal treadmill exercise protocols. J Appl Physiol 1974; 36: 720–725.
4. Sheffield LT, Malouf JA, Sawyer JA, et al. Maximal heart rate and treadmill performance of healthy women in relation to age. Circulation 1979; 57:79–84.
5. Cooper KH, Purdy JG, White SR et al. Age-fitness adjusted maximal heart rates. Med Sport 1977;10:78–88.
6. Bruce RA, Gey GO Jr., Cooper MN, et al. Seattle Heart Watch: Initial clinical, circulatory and electrocardiographic responses to maximal exercise. Am J Cardiol 1974; 33:459–469.
7. Azarbal B, Hayes SW, Lewin HC, Hachamovitch R, Cohen I, Berman DS. The incremental prognostic value of percentage of Heart Rate Reserve achieved over myocardial perfusion single-photon emission computed tomography in the prediction of cardiac death and all-cause mortality. JACC 2004;44:425–430.
8. Sandvik L, Eriksson J, Ellestad MH, Eriksson G, Thaulow E, Mundal R, Rodahl K. Heart rate increase and maximal heart rate during exercise as predictors of cardiovascular mortality: A 16 year follow-up study of 1960 healthy men. Coronary Artery Disease 1995;6: 667–679.
9. Ellestad MH. Stress Testing: Principles and Practice, 4th ed. Philadelphia, FA Davis, 1996, 346.
10. McNeer JF, Margolis JR, Le KL, et al. The role of the exercise test in the evaluation of patients for ischemic heart disease. Circulation 1978; 57:64–70.
11. Lauer MS, Okin PM, Larson MG Evans JC, Levy D. Impaired heart rate response to graded exercise: Prognostic implications of chronotropic incompetence in the Framingham Heart Study. Circulation 1996;93: 1520–1526.
12. Ellestad MH, Wan MKC. Predictive implications of stress testing follow-up of 2700 subjects after maximum treadmill stress testing. Circulation 1975;51:363.
13. Falcone C, Buzzi MP, Klersy C, Schwartz PJ. Rapid heart rate increase at onset of exercise predicts adverse cardiac events in patients with coronary artery disease. Circulation 2005; 112:1959–1964.
14. Leeper NJ, Dewey FE, Ashley EA, et al. Prognostic value of heart rate increase at onset of exercise testing. Circulation 2007; 115:468–474.
15. Cole CR, Blackstone EH, Pashkow FJ, et al. Heart-rate recovery immediately after exercise as a predictor of mortality. N Engl J Med 1999; 341:1351–1357.
16. Shetler K, Marcus R, Froelicher VF, et al. Heart rate recovery: Validation and methodologic issues. J Am Coll Cardiol 2001; 38;1980–1987.
17. Ellestad MH. Stress Testing; Principles and Practice, 5th ed. Oxford University Press, 2003, 335.
18. Froelicher VF, Myers J. Exercise and the Heart, 5th ed. Elsevier, 2006, 120.
19. Taylor AJ, Beller GA. Postexercise systolic blood pressure response: Clinical Application to the assessment of ischemic heart disease. Amer Fam Physician 58; 1126–1130, 1998.
20. Ellestad MH. Stress Testing; Principles and Practice, 5th ed. Oxford University Press, 2003, 344–345.
21. Dubach P, Froelicher VF, Klein J et al. Exercise-induced hypotension in a male population-Criteria, causes, and prognosis. Circulation 1988;78: 1380–1387.
22. Gibbons RJ, Balady GJ, Bricker JT et al. ACC/AHA 2002 Guideline update for exercise testing: a report of the ACC/AHA Task Force on Practice Guidelines 2002. Am Coll Cardiol Web Site.
23. Bodegard J, Erikssen G, Bjornholt JV, et al. Reasons for terminating an exercise test provide independent prognostic information. 2014 apparently healthy men followed for 26 years. Eur Heart J doi: 10.1093/eurheartj/ehi278.

24. Ellestad MH. Stress Testing; Principles and Practice, 5th ed. Oxford University Press, 2003, 296–297.
25. Udall JA, Ellestad MH. Predictive implications of ventricular premature contractions associated with treadmill stress testing. Circulation 1977;56:985–989.
26. Jouven X, Zurick M, Desnos M, et al. Long-term outcome in asymptomatic men with exercise-induced premature ventricular depolarizations. N Eng J Med 2000;343: 826–833.
27. ACSM's resource manual for Guidelines for exercise testing and prescription. American College of Sports Medicine; 5th ed. Lippincott Williams and Wilkins, Baltimore, 2006, 122–126.
28. Myers J, Kaykha A, George S et al. Fitness versus physical activity patterns in predicting mortality in men. Am J Med 2004;117:912–918.
29. Evans CH, Harris G, Menold V, Ellestad MH. A Basic Approach to the interpretation of the exercise test. Primary Care 2001;28: 80–81.
30. Ellestad MH. Stress Testing; Principles and Practice, 5th ed. Oxford University Press, 2003, 43–75.
31. Stuart R, Ellestad MH. Upsloping ST-segments in exercise testing. Am J Cardiol 1976;37:19.
32. Goldschlager N, Selzer A, Cohn K. Treadmill stress test as indicators of presence and severity of coronary artery disease. Ann Intern Med 1976; 85:277–286.
33. Taylor AJ, Beller GA. Patients with greater than 2 mm of ST depression do not have a greater ischemic burden by thallium-201 scintigraphy. Circulation 86(suppl II):138, 1992.
34. Dunn RF, et al. Exercise-induced ST elevation. Circulation 1980;61:889.
35. Ellestad MH. Stress Testing; Principles and Practice, 5th ed. Oxford University Press, 2003, 216–218.
36. Lee JH, Crump R, Ellestad MH. Significance of precordial T-wave increase during treadmill stress testing. Am J Cardiol 1995;76:1297–1299.
37. Rasouli ML, Ellestad MH. Usefulness of ST depression in ventricular premature complexes to predict myocardial ischemia. Am J Cardiol 2001;87: 891–894.
38. Selvester RH, Gillespie TL. Simulated ECG surface map's sensitivity to local segments of myocardium. In Lepeschkin E, Rush S. Eds. Proceeding, Vermont Conference Body Surface Mapping of Cardiac Fields. Advances in Cardiology. Vol. 10. Basel, Switzerland: S. Karger, Basel, 1974:120.
39. Ellstad MH, Crump R, Surber M. The significance of lead strength on ST changes during treadmill stress tests. J Electrocardiol 1993;25 (supp): 31.
40. Heller IH, Cates C, Popma J et al. Intracoronary Doppler assessment of moderate Coronary Artery Disease; Comparison with 201 TI imaging and coronary angiography. Circulation 1997; 96:484–490.
41. Wilson RF, Marcus ML, Christensen BV, et al. Accuracy of exercise electrocardiography in detecting physiologically significant coronary arterial lesions. Circulation 1991;83: 412–420.
42. Ellestad MH. The time has come to reexamine the gold standard when evaluating noninvasive testing. Am J Cardiol 2001;87: 100–101.
43. Diamond GA, Forrester JS. Analysis of probability as an aid in the clinical diagnosis of coronary artery disease. N Engl J Med 1979;300: 1350–1358.
44. Epstein, SE: Implications of probability analysis on the strategy used for non-invasive detection of coronary artery disease. Am J Cardiol 46:491–499, 1980.
45. Mark DB, Hlathy MA, Harrell FE Jr., et al. Exercise treadmill score for predicting prognosis in coronary artery disease. Ann Intern Med 1987;106: 793–800.
46. Mark DB, Shaw L, Harrell FE, et al. Prognostic value of a treadmill exercise score in outpatients with suspected coronary artery disease. N Engl J Med 1991; 325:849–853.
47. Morrow K, Morris CK, Froelicher VF, Hideg A. Prediction of cardiovascular death in men undergoing noninvasive evaluation for CAD. Ann Intern Med 1993;118: 689–695.

Chapter 6
Common Abnormal Responses Seen with Exercise Testing and How to Manage Them

Corey H. Evans and Victor F. Froelicher

As clinicians become more experienced with exercise testing (ET), they will experience common and less common abnormal responses. This chapter discusses several abnormal responses to ET and the management of these responses. The following abnormal responses are discussed: exercise-induced arrhythmias including complex arrhythmias and ventricular tachycardia, exercise-induced bundle branch blocks, ST-segment elevation, isolated inferior ST-segment depression and exercise-induced hypotension.

Exercise Test-Induced Arrhythmias

Pathophysiology of Exercise Test-Induced Arrhythmias

With exercise one sees a number of important physiological changes that interact with three important arrhythmogenic mechanisms; enhanced automaticity, triggered automaticity and re-entry. These physiologic changes include an increase in both the activity of the sympathetic nervous system and the circulating catecholamines. With vigorous exercise, the arterial blood circulating catecholamines can raise more than 10-fold, pH drops, and the plasma potassium increases [1]. Any of these changes can initiate arrhythmias at rest, and in some, at exercise.

It is not completely clear why these changes do not create more arrhythmias during exercise. Somehow these arrhythmogenic forces balance each other out or are suppressed by other anti-arrhythmogenic forces. What is clear is that the balance seems to be less protective in the presence of myocardial ischemia and even in recovery after vigorous exercise. Most dangerous exercise test-induced arrhythmias (ETIA) occur in recovery, especially when exercise is abruptly stopped. Tuininga [2] reported on 194 episodes of exercise test-induced ventricular tachycardia (ETIVT)

C.H. Evans (✉)
St. Anthony's Hospital, St. Petersburg, FL; Private Practice Family Physician, Florida Institute of Family Medicine, St. Petersburg, FL, USA
e-mail: email@coreyevansmd.com

C.H. Evans, R.D. White (eds.), *Exercise Testing for Primary Care and Sports Medicine Physicians*, DOI 10.1007/978-0-387-76597-6_6
© Springer Science+Business Media, LLC 2009

and found 58% occurred in recovery vs. 42% during exercise. The relative arrhythmic danger of the recovery period can be lessened by a cooldown walk during recovery [1].

A rare group of patients have genetic predispositions to exercise-induced arrhythmias. These syndromes, which include a predisposition for sudden death, are being investigated, and the molecular and genetic bases are being revealed. These include the long QT syndrome and familial catecholaminergic polymorphic VT syndrome [3,4].

Exercise Test-Induced Arrhythmias

As was discussed in Chapter 5, exercise test-induced arrhythmias (ETIA) are commonly seen with exercise testing. These are usually unifocal PVCs and PACs and have little significance. These simple arrhythmias may be seen at rest or during testing. It is not unusual for patients to have frequent unifocal PVCs at rest, but as the heart rate (HR) increases with the ET, the PVCs disappear. Although Jouven [5] did show a long-term (23-year follow-up) increased mortality in males with frequent unifocal PVCs (six or more on a 30 second tracing), we do not recommend further evaluation of patients with frequent unifocal PVCs during exercise if the rest of the ET response is normal and there are no complex arrhythmias. PVCs in recovery need more attention. Dewey [6] recently reported on PVCs during the ET and in recovery in 1847 patients followed for 5.4 years after testing. Whereas PVCs during exercise had little affect on prognosis, patients with either frequent or infrequent PVCs in recovery had a significantly increased mortality (11.6 and 12.2%, respectively) when compared to those with no recovery PVCs (4.9% mortality at 5.4 years). Thus, patients with recovery only PVCs should be considered for further evaluation or more aggressive therapy.

Complex Ventricular Arrhythmias During Exercise Testing

When one tries to look at the significance and prognostic implications of ETIA and especially exercise test-induced ventricular arrhythmias (ETIVA), it is difficult to draw conclusions. The studies are hampered by a lack of consensus on the amount of arrhythmias considered abnormal, the population tested and the study design. In spite of these limitations, it is generally felt that the incidence of ETIVA increases with age and is seen more in the presence of myocardial ischemia. The following case illustrates these concepts.

Case 1

An asymptomatic 62-year-old man without heart disease underwent ET to screen for CAD. The test was terminated at 8 minutes due to fatigue. The

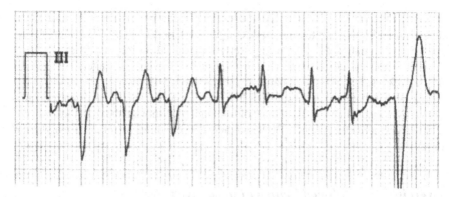

Fig. 6.1 Lead III showing a premature ventricular contraction and three beats of ventricular tachycardia at 7:16 minutes of exercise. There is also a suggestion of upsloping ST-segment depression. (From Evans CH, Froelicher VF [7], with permission from Elsevier.)

hemodynamic response was normal and he achieved 7.5 METS of work. In the last minute of exercise the patient developed complex ectopy and brief V-TACH (Fig. 6.1). There was inferior horizontal ST-segment depression of 1 mm and upsloping ST-segment depression laterally. Because of the ectopy, an Echocardiogram and a Holter monitor were performed, both normal. The patient refused recommended Beta blocker therapy and further workup. Three months later the patient presented with an acute anterior myocardial infarction, and in the ER had two episodes of sustained ventricular tachycardia, both requiring defibrillation. He was treated successfully with tPa. At cardiac catheterization he had a single high-grade proximal LAD lesion and underwent successful stenting. He has done well in follow-up without further arrhythmias. Certainly in this case, the ischemic myocardium during the ET and later with the MI contributed to the complex arrhythmias seen.

Complex or ominous ventricular arrhythmias can be defined as frequent or multifocal PVCs, couplets, ventricular tachycardia (VT) or ventricular fibrillation (VF). These responses occur somewhere between 1 and 3% of tests and also increase in frequency as the age of the patients increases. When one tries to decipher the significance of ETIVA, analysis of complex ventricular arrhythmias is more meaningful than including populations with rare PVCs. This is illustrated in the study by Califf [8] who reported on the prognostic value of ETIVA, both simple (any PVCs) and complex (paired or VT). Patients with complex ETIVA had more significant CAD, compared to those with simple ETIVA or none (75% vs. 57% vs. 44%, respectively), and a worsened survival (75% vs. 83% vs. 90%). Partington [9] at the VA Medical Center showed that patients with complex ectopy (PVCs greater than 10% of all complexes or three consecutive PVCs) had a worsened prognosis, even in the absence of myocardial ischemia. They concluded that this ETIVA was an independent predictor of cardiovascular mortality and that complex ETIVA combined with resting PVCs carried the highest risk [10].

Frolkis [11] et al. at the Cleveland Clinic reported on complex ETIVA (defined as 7 or more PVCs/minute, bigeminy, couplets, VT or VF) in 29,244 patients. The presence of complex ETIVA during exercise predicted an increased risk of death (9% vs. 5%), and complex ETIVA in recovery was even a stronger predictor of death (11% vs. 5%) when compared to those without ETIVA.

It is also apparent that complex ETIVA is especially meaningful when it occurs at low workloads. In an early study, Goldschlager [12] showed that complex ETIVA at low workloads (less than 5 METS) predicted severe three vessel disease and poor prognosis.

Exercise Test-Induced Ventricular Tachycardia

Rarely during the ET the patient will suddenly develop widening of the QRS complex. This can be the occurrence of VT or is the appearance of a Bundle Branch Block (discussed below). If the widened rhythm is sustained, and the practitioner cannot exclude the presence of VT, the test should be terminated.

Exercise test-induced ventricular tachycardia (ETIVT) is rarely seen during exercise, occurring in approximately 1 in 200 tests. The prevalence is determined by the number of consecutive PVCs one uses to determine VT. Fortunately it is usually brief and rarely needs treatment. Tamakoshi [13] et al. reported on the frequency of ETIVT (defined as 8 or more consecutive beats) among 25,075 consecutive patients. EVIVT occurred in 0.08% of the tests. Most large studies report a frequency of around 0.6% of tests when VT is considered three or more consecutive PVCs and VF is included [14].

Most patients with ETIVT will have structural heart disease and many will have ST-segment depression during the same test. Yang, Wesley and Froelicher [15] analyzed 55 cases of ETIVT among 3351 veterans. Of those with ETIVT, 45 had clinical evidence of CAD, 2 had cardiomyopathies, 3 had valvular heart disease and 5 were free of heart disease. Due to the high incidence of heart disease in these patients, when ETIVT or VF is seen the patients should undergo a careful evaluation for underlying heart disease, even if no ST-segment depression is seen. This will usually include an echocardiogram and an exercise test with perfusion imaging. Yang and associates also reported that the reoccurrence of ETIVT was low on retesting (6.9%) and the occurrence of ETIVT seemed not to increase mortality over that of the underlying heart disease.

Exercise-Induced Bundle Branch Blocks

Exercise test-related bundle branch blocks have been well described. Left bundle branch blocks (LBBB) may occur in healthy individuals, but most occur in patients with CAD. The presumed mechanism is ischemia of the conductive tissue causing delayed depolarization in the left bundle tissues. Vasey [16] described 28 patients (1.1%) with exercise-induced LBBB out of 2584 patients tested. All 10 patients who developed LBBB at a rate of 125 beats per minute or higher were free of CAD, whereas 9 of 18 patients with LBBB seen at a heart rate of less than 125 had significant CAD. Grady [17] reported on the experience of 70 patients at Mayo Clinic with exercise-induced LBBB. This response was seen in 0.5% of their patients. When they analyzed these patients against matched controls, those with exercise-induced LBBB had a three times higher risk of death and major cardiac events.

Once a LBBB develops during exercise one cannot evaluate the ECG for the presence of myocardial ischemia. Due to the underlying prevalence of CAD and the worsened prognosis, patients who develop LBBB during exercise, certainly at rates under 125, should have further evaluation for ischemia and structural heart disease.

Some patients will develop exercise-induced RBBBs. When the RBBB can be identified with certainly, the test need not be terminated, and these patients have a good prognosis. With a RBBB ST-segment depression may be seen in the anterior leads (V_1–V_3) and does not indicate myocardial ischemia. However, if the ST-segment ischemia is seen in the lateral precordial leads (V_{4-6}), ischemia is usually present since these leads are usually not affected by the RBBB [18].

ST-Segment Elevation with Exercise

ST-segment elevation is another rare response to the ET, but one that needs prompt recognition and management. As stated in Chapter 5, most myocardial ischemia during the ET is subendocardial. When the ischemia is more severe it can become transmural and cause ST-segment elevation. This ST-segment elevation can also occur in areas of old infarction, due either to peri-infarction ischemia or wall motion abnormalities. Case 2 shows a typical example of ST-segment elevation:

Case 2

A 65-year-old man presented to his family physician asking for something stronger for his "neck arthritis". He had no known heart disease but his neck arthritis occurred with exertion, most recently after running down his driveway to catch friends. An exercise test was done and in Stage I of the Bruce protocol he developed marked ST-segment elevation in the anterior leads that resolved in recovery (Fig. 6.2A and B). At catheterization he had a high-grade proximal LAD lesion and a RCA stenosis. He underwent successful bypass surgery.

ST-segment elevation can also be seen when the ischemia is due to severe coronary artery spasm. When this ST-segment elevation accompanies angina, occurs at rest and not with exercise, and is relieved with nitroglycerine, it is labeled variant angina. When Prinzmetal [20] first reported on a series of 32 patients with variant angina it was felt they had normal coronaries and severe spasm. It is now felt that many have mild CAD and spasm, and some will have ST-segment depression when tested with the ET.

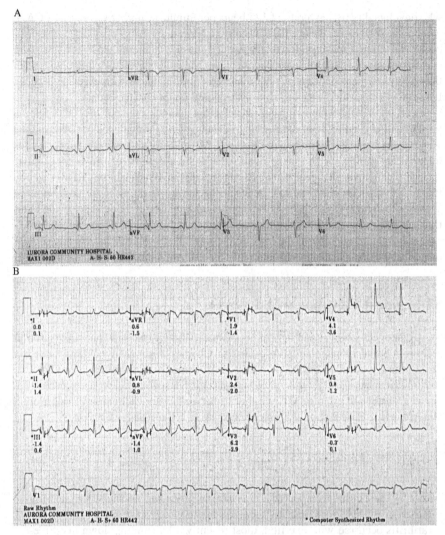

Fig. 6.2 (**A**) Resting ECG before exercise. (From Evans CH, Harris G, Menold V, et al. [19], with permission from Elsevier.) (**B**) Exercise ECG at 2:50 minutes in Stage I showing marked ST elevation in the precordial leads. The test was immediately terminated and the elevation resolved

The finding of ST-segment elevation during the exercise test is important for several reasons. First, unlike ST-segment depression, ST-segment elevation can localize the diseased artery. Anterior ST-segment elevation usually means a proximal LAD lesion and inferior ST-segment elevation is usually due to a right coronary lesion. Second, the amount of ischemia is usually considerable. Third, these patients have a high incidence of developing VT and VF and increased mortality *during the test.*

For these reasons, when ST-segment elevation is seen, the test should be terminated and the patient referred for cardiac catheterization.

Isolated ST-Segment Depression in the Inferior Leads

ST-segment depression in the anterior and lateral precordial leads is the most specific for myocardial ischemia. When this occurs, there may also be inferior ST-segment depression, usually also due to myocardial ischemia. Occasionally patients will have isolated inferior ST-segment depression without any precordial ST-segment changes. This isolated inferior ST-segment depression is usually a false-positive finding.

Case 3

A 28-year-old healthy female athlete underwent exercise testing as part of a demonstration. She exercised for 16 minutes on the Bruce protocol, and the test was terminated due to fatigue. Maximum heart rate was 178, she was asymptomatic and had a normal BP response. At 12 minutes of exercise she showed 3 mm of horizontal ST-segment depression in the inferior leads II and III, which resolved by maximal exercise at 16 minutes (Fig. 6.3).

Riff and Carleton [21] demonstrated that the duration of the atrial repolarization (the atrial T wave) may play a role in an increase in the normal rate-related depression of the J point, the amplitude of the S wave and depression of the ST-segment during exercise. This effect is greater in the inferior leads than in lateral leads. Sabin [22] evaluated 69 patients with exercise-induced ST-segment depression suggesting myocardial ischemia. Twenty-five patients had no evidence of CAD either on catheterization or by normal nuclear studies and 44 patients had at least one significant coronary lesion. Analysis of the 25 false-positive patients showed (1) markedly downsloping PR segments at peak exercise, (2) longer exercise time, (3) higher peak heart rates with exercise and (4) greater amplitude of the P waves with amplification during exercise in those leads with false-positive ST-segment depression. The two best independent predictors of a false-positive test were long exercise duration and markedly downsloping PR segments in the inferior ECG leads. Myrianthefs [23] evaluated 86 individuals with ST-segment depression during exercise and normal or near normal coronary arteries. These ST-segment responses were felt to be a false positive. When looking at the PR segment during exercise, those with short PR intervals (120 ms or less) had more false-positive ST-segment depression than those with normal PR intervals.

V_5 is the most sensitive lead for detecting myocardial ischemia. Blackburn and Katigbak [24] found that lead V_5 alone detected 89% of ischemic ST-segment responses in 100 consecutive patients. Many other authors concur. Miller et al., [25] analyzing 44 consecutive patients with abnormal ETs and thallium-201 perfusion

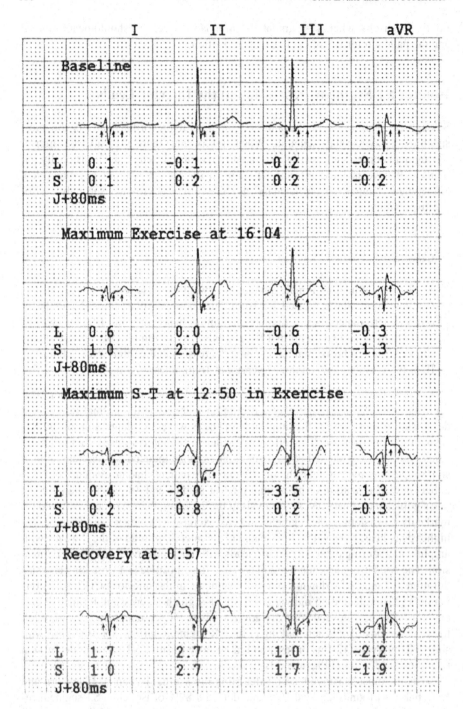

Fig. 6.3 The average complexes in leads I, II and III at baseline, maximum exercise at 16:04 minutes and at 12:50 minutes when there was 3 mm of horizontal ST-segment depression. (From Evans CH, Froelicher VF [7], with permission from Elsevier.)

imaging, found that 68% had inferior ST-segment depression but all had corresponding depression in V_4 and/or V_5. They concluded that the inferior leads added little additional diagnostic information. Studying 203 men with ETs and coronary angiography, Sketch et al. [26] found that lead II only had a sensitivity of 34%. Finally Miranda et al. [27] showed precordial lead V_5 consistently outperformed the inferior lead II, and the combination of V_5 and II was not any better than V_5 alone. Of seven patients with isolated lead II ST-segment depression with exercise, only three had a true-positive response.

In summary, when one sees exercise-induced ST-segment depression in the inferior leads and in the lateral precordial leads, this finding is usually a true-positive response indicating myocardial ischemia. When there is only isolated inferior ST-segment depression, this is usually a false-positive response. By looking for tall P waves augmented with exercise, marked downsloping PR segments and long exercise duration, one can further confirm the isolated inferior ST-segment depression is a false positive.

Exercise-Induced Hypotension

As discussed in Chapter 5, the normal systolic response to exercise is a steady increase in systolic blood pressure (SBP) as workload increases with a return to baseline SBP in recovery. Some patients experience a fall in SBP as work load increases. This response, labeled Exercise-Induced Hypotension (EIH), is usually associated with severe coronary disease or other heart disease and a poor prognosis. The following case is illustrative.

Case 4

A 65-year-old woman without known prior heart disease developed new onset atrial fibrillation. An outpatient evaluation consisted of normal blood chemistries and thyroid studies, and an echocardiogram reported as normal. She was treated with digoxin and coumadin. Two weeks later she was admitted for possible cardioversion and an ET was done to evaluate atypical chest pain. The resting ECG showed atrial fibrillation with a rate of 80, otherwise normal. At 4 minutes into the exercise test, she became lightheaded, had near-syncope and the BP became undetectable. This was associated with brief syncope and bradycardia, both of which quickly resolved in the supine position. Cardiac catheterization performed the following day showed mild LAD disease and severe constrictive calcific pericarditis, which had been missed on the earlier ECHO. She underwent pericardial stripping and did well.

EIH may be due to numerous factors in addition to severe myocardial ischemia. Other cardiac factors include severe outflow obstruction, LV failure, arrhythmias, isolated right ventricular ischemia and in some normal individuals, an excessive vagal response to exercise.

The studies on EIH are hampered by lack of consensus on the criteria for EIH. Some use a drop of 20 mmHg and some require the SBP to drop below the standing baseline. Dubach et al. [28] reported upon patients with EIH among 2036 patients at the Long Beach VA Medical Center. They compared two definitions of EIH, a drop of 20 mmHg of SBP after an initial rise, against a drop to below resting standing SBP. The "drop below rest" criterion was clearly better than a drop of 20 mmHg at predicting increased risk for death and myocardial infarctions. Forty-five percent of the patients with "drop below baseline" EIH had severe three vessel disease or left main disease, and the risk of death was two times greater than in those without EIH. Hammermeister et al. [29] in the Seattle Heart Watch study also reported that EIH (again using a drop to below baseline) had a high predictive value for three vessel or left main disease of 50%.

Because a large number of patients with EIH defined as "drop below baseline" have severe CAD or other heart disease, these patients need further evaluation to determine the exact nature of the underlying disease and consideration for revascularization. This is especially important since several authors have shown patients with EIH who receive revascularization either by CABG or by angioplasty have a lower mortality than those treated medically, and often the finding of EIH is reversed [30, 31].

This finding is very striking in the above study by Dubach [17]. There were 12 deaths in patients with EIH who were medically treated and no deaths in 22 patients who had revascularization.

Summary

In this article some of the common and less common abnormal responses to exercise testing were reviewed. Most importantly, practitioners need to recognize those abnormal responses identifying patients with severe ischemia and at high risk for poor outcomes. These abnormal high-risk responses include exercise-induced hypotension, complex arrhythmias at low workloads, ST-segment elevation and in some circumstances, exercise-induced LBBBs. Hopefully the above discussions on each of these abnormal responses will guide the practitioner as patients are evaluated with exercise testing.

References

1. Froelicher VF, Myers J; Exercise and the Heart, 5th Ed. Saunders Elsevier, Philadelphia, 2006, p. 164.
2. Tuininga YS, Crijns HJ, Wiesfeld AC, et al.; Electrocardiographic patterns relative to initiating mechanism of exercise-induced ventricular tachycardia. Am Heart J 1993; 126: 359–367.
3. Paavonen KJ, Swan H, Piippo K, et al.; Response of the QT interval to mental and physical stress in types LQT1 and LQT2 of the long QT syndrome. Heart 2001; 86: 39–44.

4. Laitinen PJ, Swan H, Piippo K, et al.; Genes, exercise and sudden death: Molecular basis for familial catecholaminergic polymorphic ventricular tachycardia. Ann Med 2004;36(suppl 1): 81–86.

5. Jouven X, Zureik M, Desnos M, et al.; Long-term outcome in asymptomatic men with exercise-induced premature ventricular depolarizations. N Engl J Med 2000; 343: 826–833.

6. Dewey FE, Kapoor JR, Williams RS, et al.; Ventricular Arrhythmias during Clinical Treadmill Testing and Prognosis. Arch Int Med 2008;168(2): 1–10.

7. Evans CH, Froelicher VF; Some common abnormal responses to exercise testing. Primary Care 2001; 28: 222.

8. Califf RM, McKinnis RA, McNeer M, et al.; Prognostic value of ventricular arrhythmias associated with treadmill exercise testing in patients studied with cardiac catheterization for suspected ischemic heart disease. J Am Coll Cardiol 1983;2: 1060–1065.

9. Partington S, Myers J, Cho S, et al.; Prevalence and prognostic value of exercise-induced ventricular arrhythmias. Am Heart J 2003; 145:139–146.

10. Beckerman J, Mathur A, Stahr S, et al.; Exercise-induced ventricular arrhythmias and cardiovascular death. Ann Noninvasive Electrocardiol 2005;10:47–52.

11. Frolkis JP, Pothier CE, Blackstone EH, Lauer MS; Frequent ventricular ectopy after exercise as a predictor of death. N Engl J Med 2003; 348: 781–790

12. Goldschlager N, Selzer A. Cohn K; Treadmill stress tests as indicators of presence and severity of coronary artery disease. Ann Intern Med 1976;85: 277–286.

13. Tamakoshi K, Fukuda E, Tajima A, et al; Prevalence and clinical background of exercise-induced ventricular tachycardia during exercise testing. J Cardiol 2002; 39: 205–212.

14. Detry JM, Abouantoun S, Wyns W; Incidence and prognostic implications of severe ventricular arrhythmias during maximal exercise testing. Cardiology 1981; 68 (suppl 2): 35–43.

15. Wang JC, Wesley RC, Froelicher VF; Ventricular tachycardia during routine treadmill testing. Risk and prognosis. Arch Int Med 1991; 151: 349–353.

16. Vasey CG, O'Donnell J, Morris SN et al.; Exercise-induced left bundle branch block and its relation to coronary artery disease. Am J Cardiol 1985; 56: 892–895.

17. Grady TA, Chiu AC, Snader CE, et al.; Prognostic significance of exercise-induced left bundle-branch block. JAMA 1998;279: 153–156.

18. Froelicher VF, Myers J; Exercise and the Heart, 5th Ed. Saunders Elsevier, Philadelphia, 2006, p. 150–151.

19. Evans CH, Harris G, Menold V, Ellestad MH; A basic approach to the interpretation of the exercise test. Primary Care 2001; 28, 84–85.

20. Prinzmetal M, Kennamer R, Merliss R, et al.; Angina pectoris. A variant form of angina pectoris; preliminary report. Am J Med 1959; 27: 375–388.

21. Riff DP, Carleton RA; Effect of exercise on the atrial recovery wave. Am Heart J 1971;82: 759–763.

22. Sapin PM, Koch G, Blauwet MB, et al.; Identification of false positive exercise tests with use of Electrocardiographic criteria: A possible role for atrial repolarization waves. J Am Coll Cardiol 1991; 18:127–135.

23. Myrianthefs MM, Nicolaides EP, Pitiris D, et al.; False positive ST-segment depression during exercise in subjects with short PR segment and angiographically normal coronaries: Correlation with exercise-induced ST depression in subjects with normal PR and normal coronaries. J Electrocardiol 1998; 31: 203–208.

24. Blackburn H, Katigbak R; What Electrocardiographic leads to take after exercise. Am Heart J 1964; 67: 184–188.

25. Miller TD, Desser KB, Lawson M; How many electrocardiographic leads are required for exercise treadmill tests? J Electrocardiol 1987; 20: 131–137.

26. Sketch MH, Nair CK, Esterbrooks DJ, et al.; Reliability of single-lead and multiple-lead electrocardiography during and after exercise. Chest 1978; 74: 394–401.

27. Miranda CP, Liu J, Kadar A, et al.; Usefulness of exercise-induced ST-segment depression in the inferior leads during exercise testing as a marker for coronary artery disease. Am J Cardiol 1992; 69:303–308.

28. Dubach P, Froelicher VF, Klein J, et al.; Exercise-induced hypotension in a male population-Criteria, causes, and prognosis. Circulation 1988; 78: 1380–1387.
29. Hammermeister KE, DeRouen TA, Dodge HT, et al.; Prognostic and predictive value of exertional hypotension in suspected coronary heart disease. Am J Cardiol 1983; 51: 1261–1265.
30. Weiner DA, McCabe CH, Cutler SS, et al.; Decrease in systolic blood pressure during exercise testing: Reproducibility, response to coronary bypass surgery and prognostic significance. Am J Cardiol 1982; 49: 1627–1631.
31. Thompson PD, Kelemen MH; Hypotension accompanying the onset of exertional angina. Circulation 1975; 52: 28–32.

Chapter 7
Nuclear Imaging with Exercise Testing

Patricia Nguyen

Advances in nuclear imaging have helped establish its role in the diagnosis and management of coronary artery disease. Recent innovations, including the advent of new radiotracers, attenuation techniques and cardiac gating, have improved the accuracy of SPECT and PET. There are extensive data demonstrating the independent diagnostic and prognostic utility of nuclear imaging for stress testing.

Nuclear Imaging Techniques

Cardiovascular nuclear imaging uses radiopharmaceuticals to provide a quantitative assessment of myocardial perfusion, metabolism, viability, left ventricular wall motion and ejection fraction. The two main technologies in nuclear imaging are single positron emission computed tomography (SPECT) and positron emission tomography (PET). Both use similar reconstruction techniques to create tomographic images of the heart but differ in the type of radiopharmaceutical and instrumentation required to create the images [1].

Radiopharmaceuticals used in SPECT, including thallium (Tl-201) and technetium (Tc-99m) [2,3], have relatively long physical half-lives and emit gamma rays (single photons) at varying energies. Gamma rays emitted by the radiotracers are localized by a gamma camera which converts the gamma rays into photons of light which are detected and then used to form an image. Although the spatial resolution of SPECT is only 12–15 mm [1], this is adequate for the evaluation of myocardial perfusion, viability and left ventricular function.

The positron-emitting radioisotopes used in PET, in contrast, are radiolabelled physiological compounds (e.g., oxygen, carbon, nitrogen). Available physiological PET radiotracers used in clinical imaging can be divided into two broad categories: (1) radiotracers which evaluate myocardial blood flow (i.e., ^{13}N-ammonia, ^{15}O-water, -rubidium-82); (2) radiotracers which evaluate myocardial metabolism (i.e., ^{13}C-palmitate, ^{11}C-acetate and ^{18}F-fluorodeoxyglucose) [3]. PET radiotracers

P. Nguyen (✉)
Department of Cardiology, Stanford University School of Medicine, Palo Alto, CA, USA
e-mail: pknguyen1@yahoo.com

C.H. Evans, R.D. White (eds.), *Exercise Testing for Primary Care and Sports Medicine Physicians*, DOI 10.1007/978-0-387-76597-6_7

have short physical half-lives and emit two gamma rays. When a high-energy positron leaves the nucleus, it collides with an electron, resulting in their complete annihilation and production of two gamma rays which travel in opposite directions that are registered by PET detectors to create an image. Because the gamma rays are perfectly collinear and more advanced methods of attenuation correction, PET has an improved spatial (4–6 mm) [1] and temporal resolution over SPECT. The higher count rate also increases its sensitivity relative to SPECT [1].

The Principle Behind Stress Myocardial Perfusion Imaging and Myocardial Viability

Myocardial Perfusion

Myocardial perfusion abnormalities are the earliest manifestation of ischemia followed by abnormalities in diastolic and systolic function [4]. Both SPECT and PET can detect abnormalities in myocardial perfusion. Detection of myocardial perfusion defects is based upon the principle that radiotracers are taken up by the myocardium in proportion to regional blood flow [2, 5] (Fig. 7.1). At rest, regional blood flow is similar in stenotic ($\geq 70\%$) and nonstenotic arteries. During stress by either exercise or vasodilators (i.e., adenosine, dipyridamole) in the presence of coronary stenosis, regional blood does not increase significantly and there is heterogeneous uptake of tracer in myocardial perfusion images. Specifically, the myocardial region supplied by the stenotic artery receives less coronary blood flow, resulting in less tracer uptake and a perfusion defect.

Ideally, tracer uptake would show a perfectly linear relationship with blood flow which exists during rest when myocardial blood flow is 1 mL/g/min; however, the relationship deviates more and more as flow rates increase. With exercise, flow rates increase to 2 mL/g/min and with pharmacologic stress, flow rate exceeds 2.5 mL/g/min. At high flow rates, relative myocardial uptake of these radiotracers may underestimate regional blood flow deficits. This "roll-off" does not significantly affect the detection of significant coronary artery stenosis ($\geq 70\%$); however, mild to moderate CAD (50–70%) may not be detected [1]. The "roll-off" at high flow rates is most notable using SPECT radiotracers [1, 6].

Myocardial Viability

An evaluation of myocardial viability allows identification of patients with potentially reversible left ventricular dysfunction who may benefit from coronary artery revascularization. Despite the absence of myocardial function (i.e., absence of wall motion) due to chronic ischemia related to significant coronary stenosis, myocardial cells may still be viable and contractile function may be restored with revascularization (Fig. 7.2) [1].

Both SPECT and PET are used for the evaluation of myocardial viability. In SPECT, myocardial viability is assessed by a TI-201 redistribution phase which follows the stress perfusion scanning. Myocardial extraction of TI-201 is dependent

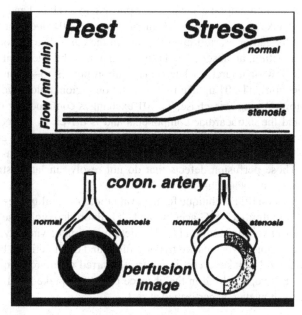

Fig. 7.1 The relationship between myocardial blood flow in normal and stenotic arteries at rest and stress. (**a**) At rest, myocardial blood flow is comparable in normal and stenotic arteries. During stress myocardial blood flow increases 2–2.5 times in the normal branch but not to the same degree in the stenosed branch. (**b**) This heterogenous blood flow results in reduced myocardial uptake in the region supplied by the stenotic artery (From Wackers FJ [5], with permission.)

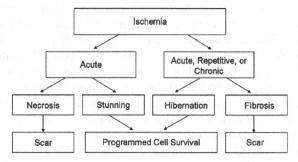

Fig. 7.2 Schematic of effects of ischemia on myocardium. An imbalance between myocardial oxygen demand and supply, usually due to myocardial perfusion abnormalities, results in ischemia. If ischemia is prolonged, necrosis occurs with the formation of fibrosis/scar. If ischemia is acute and short lived, namely, followed by revascularization or return of adequate myocardial blood flow, stunning may occur which results in temporary myocardial dysfunction. If ischemia is repetitive but short in duration, this can result in hibernation. If the myocardium is hibernating, myocytes are viable with preserved metabolic activity but function is often impaired. With revascularization, these myocytes have the potential to regain contractile function (From Dilsizian V and Narula J [1], with permission.)

on energy utilization, membrane adenosine triphosphate (ATPase) and active transport. Because uptake requires intact cell membranes, TI-201 does not concentrate in regions of infarcted or scarred myocardium. In the early distribution phase following tracer injection, an absence of TI-201 uptake may be due to either reduced regional blood flow or infarct. In late redistribution phases (3–4 hours or 24–48 hours after injection), TI-201 uptake is dependent on regional blood volume and is unrelated to flow. During this phase, TI-201 exchanges continuously between the myocardium and the extracardiac components and is driven by the concentration gradient of tracer and myocardial viability. Thus, perfusion defects appearing in the early redistribution phase but resolving in the late distribution phase are viable myocardium. Those perfusion defects that do not resolve in late distribution are infarcted or fibrotic myocardium.

The most common PET technique for the evaluation of viability uses a metabolic tracer (i.e., ^{13}C-palmitate, ^{11}C-acetate and ^{18}F-fluorodeoxyglucose) to detect metabolically inactive myocardium [7]. The determination of viability is based on the premise that viable myocytes are hypoperfused and dysfunctional but metabolically active and will uptake tracer; in contrast, scarred or infarcted myocytes are metabolically inactive, resulting in the absence of tracer uptake [8]. Imaging with PET for viability, however, is performed at rest.

Methodology

Exercise as a Stressor for Nuclear Imaging

Dynamic exercise is the stress test of choice for the evaluation of coronary artery disease if the patient is able to exercise to an acceptable workload (i.e., 85% of target heart rate [220 − age]) [9, 10]. Exercise protocols are similar to standard exercise testing. Patients should be assessed for their ability to exercise adequately prior to referral for exercise stress testing. In preparation for an exercise nuclear test, patients should withhold B adrenergic agonists and rate-limiting calcium channel blockers for at least five half-lives (approximately 48 hours) prior to testing unless contraindicated or required for evaluating the efficacy of current treatment regimens. These drugs may interfere with the physiological exercise response. Patients should avoid caffeine-containing foods, beverages and drugs (i.e., methylxanthines) for a minimum of 12 hours prior to testing to allow for use of vasodilators (adenosine and dipyridamole) in cases where exercise is terminated early (i.e., due to insufficient workload) and a pharmacological stress is undertaken. Caffeine and methylxanthines interfere with the pharmacological actions of adenosine and dipyridamole. Fasting 12 hours prior to testing is encouraged as it may improve image quality. Patients should also be instructed to wear proper attire for exercise.

Patients are continuously monitored with a 12-lead ECG, and heart rate and blood pressure are recorded frequently throughout the examination. Exercise should be symptom limited and patients should be encouraged to reach target heart rate (85% of maximum age-predicted heart rate). The radiopharmaceutical should be injected close to peak exercise. The patient should continue exercising for 1 min after TI-201 and 2 min after Tc-99m injection. Exercise should be stopped if patients show any symptoms or signs of inadequate perfusion (please refer to Chapter– Procedure: Terminating the Test) [9]. Horizontal or downsloping ST-segment depression (≥ 0.2 mV) is not necessarily an indication for termination of exercise unless it is progressive or associated with other symptoms [9]. Please refer to Chapter – Performance of Exercise Testing: Contraindications [9].

Imaging Protocols, Acquisition and Display

Different imaging protocols are utilized in exercise SPECT imaging, most commonly, one- or two-day exercise stress protocols [2, 11]. Early redistribution images are acquired 30–60 min after injection to allow for hepatobiliary clearance but may be acquired as early as 5–7 min post-injection for TI-201 and 15 min for Tc-99m [2]. Late redistribution images are acquired 3–4 hours and/or 24–48 hours post-injection in the supine position using a gamma camera (Fig. 7.3) [11]. Images are then processed and tomographic images are reconstructed. An attenuation correction is performed to reduce artifact. Although exercise can be used as a stressor in PET myocardial perfusion protocols, vasodilator stress is more com-

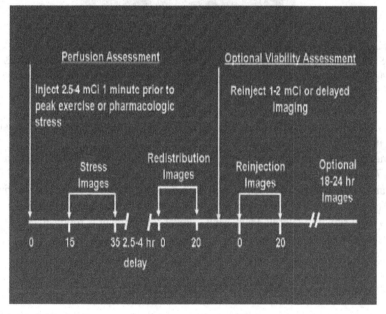

Fig. 7.3 Example of a stress/rest reinjection/18–24 hour TI-201 imaging protocol. In the stress/rest reinjection/late redistribution protocol using TI-201, patients are injected prior to peak stress. Stress images are obtained as early as 15 min post-injection. Redistribution images are then obtained 2.5–4 hours later. A reinjection of TI-201 is given at 50% dose and late redistribution images are taken 18–24 hours later. Alternatively (not shown), redistribution images can be taken 24–48 hours after the first injection (From Henzlova MJ, Cerqueira MD, Mahmarian JJ, Yao SS [11], with permission from Elsevier.)

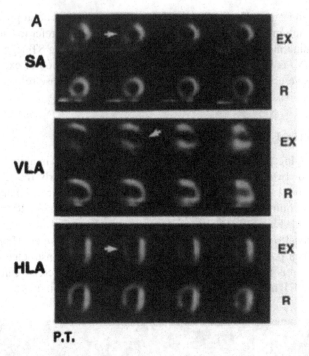

Fig. 7.4 Exercise and stress SPECT Tc-99m-sestamibi images. Exercise rest (*bottom*) and stress (*top*) SPECT Tc-99m-sestamibi images are shown in the standard three axes: short axis (SAX), vertical long axis (VLA) and horizontal long axis (HLA). Reversible anteroapical and septal perfusion defects are present (arrows) (From Wackers FJ [5], with permission.)

monly used because of the short physical half-lives of radiopharmaceutical agents used in PET [12].

Images are displayed horizontally generally with stress images above rest images (Fig. 7.4) [9, 13]. Images are displayed along three axes: short axis, horizontal long axis and vertical axis. Short axis images are displayed from apex to base; horizontal long axis views are displayed from anterior to inferior and vertical long axis views from septal to lateral. Thus, each myocardial segment is represented in three different views.

Assessment of Myocardial Perfusion Studies

Hemodynamic and ECG Findings

Hemodynamic and ECG findings provide important prognostic information. For details on the prognostic value of hemodynamic response and ECG findings during and after exercise testing, please refer to Chapter II – Interpreting the Exercise Test. Briefly, the four most important exercise variables include chest pain at maximal exertion, exercise duration less than 6 METs, heart rate impairment and ST-segment depression [14].

17-Segment Model

Radionuclide images are analyzed based on the 17-segment model [15], which divides the left ventricle into 17 segments. For each segment, an assessment of the tracer uptake is performed which reflects the severity of the perfusion defect. Tracer uptake is assessed semi-qualitatively as normal (70–100% maximum uptake), mildly reduced (50–69%), moderately reduced (30–49%), severely reduced (10–29%) and absent (0–9%). Rest and stress images are compared relative to each other. Artifacts must also be taken into consideration in image interpretation. In addition to severity, an estimate of the extent of the perfusion defect is also performed. The extent of the defect can be small (5–10% of the left ventricle), moderate (15–20%) or large (>20%) (Fig. 7.4).

Perfusion defects are then assigned to coronary artery territories based on their segment location. In the 17-segment model, segments are assigned to the three major coronary artery territories [13], recognizing that there is anatomical variability, especially in the assignment of segment 17, the apical cap. In general, the anterior wall (segments 1, 7, 13), anterior septum (segments 2, 8, 14) and apical cap are assigned to the left anterior descending artery. The anterior-lateral (segments 6, 12, 16) and inferior-lateral (segments 5, 11) walls are assigned to the left circumflex. The inferior wall (segments 4, 11, 15) and inferior septal wall (segments 3, 9) are assigned to the right coronary artery. Thus, perfusion defects can be localized to the site of ischemia and/or infarct to a culprit vessel.

Summed Stress Score and Summed Difference Score

Although not commonly performed in routine clinical evaluation, studies have demonstrated the prognostic value of a summed stress score (SSS) and summed difference score (SDS) for MPI [16, 17]. Both scores use the 17-segment model and similar grades for the severity of tracer uptake. The summed rest score is the sum of all severity scores in each segment on the rest scan and estimates the amount of resting or hibernating myocardium. A summed stress score is the sum of all severity scores in each segment on the stress scan and estimates the amount of infracted, ischemic or jeopardized myocardium. The summed difference score is the difference between the SSS and SRS, estimating the amount of ischemic or jeopardized myocardium. The SSS and SDS scores have been shown to have prognostic value.

Other Prognostic Markers

The presence of other prognostic markers should also be determined. The presence of transient post-stress ischemic dilation (TID) is determined by performing a qualitative assessment of left ventricular cavity size at rest and stress [1]. Dilation that is worse on stress than rest images indicates TID. Because of delayed imaging, this is not commonly seen with Tc-99m. Another important marker of poor prognosis is abnormal lung uptake represented by increased lung/heart ratio [18].

Assessment of Left Ventricular Volumes and Function

ECG-gated SPECT and PET images can provide an estimate of wall motion, left ventricular volumes and left ventricular function. There is good correlation between left ventricular function determined by post-stress-gated SPECT and rest echocardiography [19]. However, some studies have demonstrated that gated SPECT performed immediately after exercise may manifest post-stress stunning [20] and is not representative of rest EF in some patients [21].

Assessment of Myocardial Viability

The severity and extent of the perfusion defect is evaluated similarly for myocardial perfusion and viability images. Although there are several techniques described for assessing viability using SPECT images [10], the most commonly used is the comparison of rest, early redistribution (15–20 min after stress) and redistribution images 3–4 hours after stress imaging. Perfusion defects that resolve in redistribution images obtained 3–4 hours after injection are viable. The absence of uptake on redistribution images, however, is not a sufficient sign of the absence of viability [10]. In the case of an inconclusive result, either a TI-201 reinjection or a late redistribution image can be performed. In the former, 50% of the initial dose is reinjected after redistribution images are complete and a third set of images is performed. About 50% of reinjection images will show significant tracer uptake which has been shown to predict improvement of LV function post-revascularization. A severe defect indicates low probability of functional recovery. In the late redistribution protocol, a third set of images is acquired 24–48 hours after initial tracer injection, which allows more time for redistribution to occur. Although it has a high positive predictive value, the negative predictive value is limited by image quality [22]. Although data are more limited using Tc-99m, previous studies [23, 24] have demonstrated that redistribution images after 3–4 hours of technetium provide similar information about viability as TI-201, although some studies have suggested technetium may underestimate viability [25].

For PET viability images, tracer uptake (or the number of counts) is interpreted using the same scoring system as used in myocardial perfusion imaging ranging from normal to absent and reflects the amount of preserved metabolic activity [13] (Fig. 7.5). To determine if patients may benefit from revascularization, images acquired with a tracer used to detect metabolic activity (e.g., ^{18}F-fluorodeoxyglucose) are compared to images acquired with a tracer used to measure myocardial blood flow (e.g., ^{13}N-ammonia) performed at rest. Four distinct perfusion–metabolism have been observed [26–29]: normal perfusion–metabolism, perfusion–metabolism

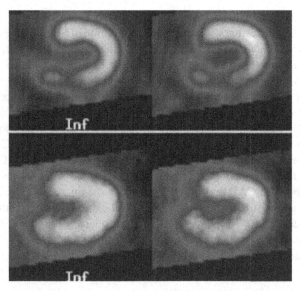

Fig. 7.5 The perfusion images show a defect in the inferior, posterior and lateral walls (*top row*); FDG uptake was preserved in these segments. Thus, a perfusion–FDG mismatch was present in the inferior, posterior and lateral walls. The anterior, septal and apical walls had preserved perfusion and FDG uptake (matched perfusion–FDG) (From Vitola JV, Delbeke D, Nuclear Cardiology and Correlative Imaging: A Teaching File, New York, Springer, 2004, with permission of Springer Science + Business Media.)

match, perfusion–metabolism mismatch and reverse perfusion mismatch. A normal pattern indicates normal metabolic activity (viable myocardium) with normal blood flow. A matched pattern showing no uptake for both tracers indicates nonviable myocardium with severely reduced blood flow consistent with scarred myocardium. A mismatch pattern indicates that metabolic activity is preserved despite severely reduced blood flow. A reverse perfusion–metabolism mismatch [30–32] indicates normal or near-normal blood flow with reduced metabolism. This pattern is often due to technical limitations but if a true reverse perfusion mismatch occurs, the myocardium is considered viable [13].

The potential for contractile recovery post-revascularization is low for perfusion–metabolism matches even if perfusion and metabolism defects are mild or moderate. In contrast, the potential for functional recovery is high if perfusion is normal, if perfusion and FDG are normal and if FDG uptake is significantly greater than perfusion (mismatch). If the mismatch affects >20% of the myocardium, the potential for recovery of at least 5% of left ventricular ejection fraction is high [26, 27].

Clinical Indications

Although an exercise ECG stress test remains the most reasonable initial test in patients who are able to exercise and who have a resting and interpretable ECG [33], patients with an ECG pattern that interferes with the interpretation of ST segments should have exercise testing with imaging. The addition of SPECT imaging provides significant incremental benefit only in those patients with an abnormal baseline ECG [10, 34]. Patients with the following resting ECG abnormalities should have stress testing with an imaging modality: ST abnormalities (≥ 0.10 mV), intraventricular conduction defects, right bundle branch blocks, LV hypertrophy, pre-excitation or digoxin effect [10]. Patients with left bundle branch block and paced rhythm should undergo an adenosine stress test. Because ECG stress evaluation is considered less accurate than imaging studies in women for the diagnosis of CAD [33, 35], the optimal initial testing strategy in women is not clearly defined. Compared to men, women may have a higher rate of false positives [36, 37] because of a lower pretest probability of CAD and a higher prevalence of microvascular disease rather than large vessel obstructive disease [36]. Initial exercise testing with imaging is also recommended [10] for patients who are considered at high risk for coronary artery disease, namely patients with diabetes or those having >20% 10-year risk of coronary artery disease event. For details of clinical indications for imaging, please refer to the ACC/AHA/ASNC guidelines for clinical use of radionuclide imaging [10].

Patients who can exercise and who require additional imaging should have an initial exercise stress because determining exercise capacity can provide valuable functional and prognostic data. Exercise stress testing is indicated in diagnosis and risk stratification in patients with acute coronary syndrome (Table 7.1) and chronic ischemic heart disease (Tables 7.2 and 7.3). Patients who cannot exercise adequately, however, should be referred for pharmacologic stress testing [10]. The choice of imaging modality, either nuclear imaging or echocardiography, however, is largely based upon patient preference, availability and local expertise.

Table 7.1 Indications for exercise MPI in acute coronary syndrome

	Patient group	Indication	Class
1	Possible ACS with nondiagnostic ECG and negative markers or normal rest scan	Diagnosis of CAD	I
2	STEMI patients after thrombolytic therapy without catheterization	Assessment of therapy: detection of inducible ischemia and myocardium at risk	I
3	Acute STEMI	Assessment of infarct size and residual viable myocardium	I
4	Non-STEMI	Identification of inducible ischemia	I
5	Non-STEMI after coronary angiography	Identification of hemodynamic significance of coronary stenosis	I

Table 7.2 Indications for exercise MPI in patients with chronic coronary artery disease

	Patient group	Indication	Class
1	Patients with intermediate likelihood of CAD who are able to exercise and do not have baseline ECG abnormalities	Diagnosis of CAD	I
2	Intermediate risk patients after catheterization	Identification of hemodynamic significance of intermediate lesions (25–75%)	I
3	Patients with a change in symptoms who have had previous stress imaging	Risk assessment	I
4	High-risk asymptomatic patients post-revascularization (3–5 years)	Risk assessment	IIa
5	High-risk asymptomatic patients (diabetes or greater than 20% 10-year risk of coronary event)	Initial diagnostic assessment	IIa

Table 7.3 Indications for radionuclide techniques for myocardial viability

	Indication	Test	Class
1	Predicting improvement in regional and global LV function after revascularization	Stress/redistribution TI-201	I
		Rest–redistribution imaging	I
		Perfusion plus PET FDG imaging	I
		Gated-SPECT sestamibi imaging	IIa
2	Predicting improvement in heart failure symptoms after revascularization	Perfusion plus PET FDG imaging	IIa
3	Predicting improvement in natural history after revascularization	TI-201 imaging (rest–redistribution and stress/redistribution/reinjection)	I
		Perfusion plus PET FDG imaging	I

Acute Coronary Syndrome

Diagnosis

There is no role for exercise nuclear testing in the initial diagnosis in patients who present with acute coronary syndrome. However, in patients who present with suspected or possible acute coronary syndrome (ACS) whose follow-up (after 6–8 hours) 12-lead ECG and cardiac biomarkers are normal, early exercise stress testing can be considered [10]. Alternatively, they can be discharged and can return for an outpatient stress test within 72 hours. Patients who are capable of exercise and who have an uninterpretable ECG should be evaluated with an exercise imaging study.

Risk Assessment and Prognosis

Radionuclide imaging with exercise can also be used for prognosis and assessment of therapy in patients after ST elevation myocardial infarction. The prognosis after STEMI is primarily dependent on ejection fraction, infarct size and residual myocardium at risk, information which is provided by radionuclide imaging [38]. Radionuclide imaging can also identify patients who may benefit from revascularization by detecting the presence of viable myocardium.

Previous studies [39, 40] have shown that submaximal exercise testing with myocardial perfusion imaging is more effective in predicting patient outcomes than exercise ECG testing alone. Myocardial perfusion images also provide incremental data over clinical data and left ventricular function. Moreover, the addition of coronary angiography data to clinical data, left ventricular function and myocardial perfusion images may not provide incremental prognostic value [40]. Submaximal exercise stress imaging, however, cannot be performed until 4 days after ST elevation MI [10]. If earlier assessment is necessary, radionuclide imaging with vasodilator stress can be performed safely as early as 2 days post-myocardial infarction.

In patients presenting with unstable angina and non-ST elevation MI, radionuclide imaging has been useful in predischarge risk stratification [41–43]. Radionuclide imaging can identify areas of inducible ischemia in the distribution of the culprit lesion or in remote areas. The presence and extent of reversible defects [41–43] and, in some studies [44] a fixed defect, were predictive of future events. Radionuclide imaging can also help determine the significance of moderate lesions noted on angiography in patients who are referred for early invasive strategy [10]. Depending on clinical risk assessment, submaximal exercise testing can be performed 24–72 hours after chest pain once the patient is stabilized.

Chronic Coronary Artery Disease

Diagnosis

Similar to other diagnostic testing, exercise nuclear testing is most useful in patients with an intermediate likelihood of angiographically significant CAD based on age, sex, symptoms, risk factors and results of prior stress testing (i.e., intermediate Duke treadmill score). Repeat exercise MPI after initial perfusion imaging is most useful in patients whose symptoms have changed to redefine the risk for cardiac event [10]. Exercise nuclear testing is sensitive and specific for the diagnosis and assessment of patients with coronary artery disease [10, 45–60]. The average sensitivity and

Table 7.4 Sensitivity and specificity of exercise nuclear MPI for detecting CAD ($\geq$50% stenosis by angiography)

Author/Ref	Year	Radiopharmaceutical	Prior MI (%)	Sensitivity	Specificity
SPECT					
Van Train [60]	1994	Sestamibi	19	89	36
Sylven [57]	1994	Sestamibi	37	72	50
Rubello [54]	1995	Sestamibi	57	93	61
Palmas [53]	1995	Sestamibi	30	91	75
Hambye [50]	1996	Sestamibi	0	82	75
Van Eck-Smit [59]	1997	Tetrofosmin	NR	87	86
Taillefer [58]	1997	Sestamibi	17	72	81
Ho [52]	1997	Tl-201	33	76	77
Heiba [93]	1997	Sestamibi	31	93	50
Yao [94]	1997	Sestamibi	55	94	93
Candell-Riera [48]	1997	Sestamibi	0	93	94
Iskandrian [95]	1997	Tl-201	21	87	69
Ho [51]	1998	Tl-201	22	79	75
Acampa [45]	1998	Sestamibi	47	96	86
Acampa [45]	1998	Tetrofosmin	47	92	71
Santana-Boado [56]	1998	Sestamibi	0	91	90
Budoff [47]	1998	Sestamibi	0	75	71
San Roman [55]	1998	Sestamibi	0	87	70
Azzarelli [46]	1999	Tetrofosmin	66	95	77
Elhendy [49]	2001	Sestamibi/tetrofosmin	0	76	73
PET					
Tamaki [62]	1988	^{13}N-ammonia	75	98	100
Steward [61]	1991	Rubidium-82*	42	83	86

The use of dipyridamole included in sensitivity and specificity calculations. No adjustment for referral bias.
Adapted from Klocke FJ, Baird MG, Lorell BH, et al. [10], with permission of J Am Coll Cardiol, with permission from Elsevier.

specificity for SPECT MPI using angiography as the gold standard are 87 and 73% (Table 7.4) [45–60], respectively, which is significantly higher than ECG testing alone. Although exercise PET imaging has been performed (Table 7.5) [61,62], PET perfusion imaging is more commonly performed with vasodilator stress. In a study of 48 patients with CAD and 3 without [62], PET demonstrated 98% sensitivity and 100% specificity. Although PET provides improved resolution, the few head-to-head comparisons between SPECT and PET have not conclusively improved sensitivity and specificity [10].

It should be noted that normal perfusion patterns have been observed in some patients with extensive or diffuse CAD due to balanced ischemia or globally abnormal flow reserve. If patients have an intermediate or high pretest probability of disease, other markers of a poor prognosis should be carefully evaluated. Abnormal LV function as a result of hibernation and stunning, TID and increased lung uptake have been reported in these patients.

Table 7.5 Prognostic value of exercise stress myocardial perfusion

Author	Year	Agent	Mean F/U (month)	HE (%/year)	HE/abnormal SPECT (%/year)	HE/normal SPECT (%/year)
Stratmann [74]	1994	Sestamibi	13	4.2	6.7	0.5
Machecourt [73]	1994	TI-201*	33	2.0	2.9	0.5
Boyne [71]	1997	Sestamibi	19.2	2.2	5.1	0.8
Snader [96]	1997	TI-201	24	1.6	3.8	1.0
Alkeylani [70]	1998	Sestamibi*	27.6	3.4	5.0	0.6
Olmos [97]	1998	TI-201	44.4	1.8	2.7	0.9
Hachamovitch [16]	1998	Sestamibi (Dual)	19.4	2.2	4.7	0.7
Vanzetto [75]	1999	T1-201	72	1.5	2.0	0.6
Galassi [72]	2001	Tetrofosmin	37	2.5	3.0	0.9

The use of dipyridamole included in sensitivity and specificity calculations. No adjustment for referral bias.
Adapted from Klocke FJ, Baird MG, Lorell BH, et al. [10], with permission from Elsevier.

Risk Stratification and Prognosis

Similar to optimal application of diagnostic testing, nuclear tests are most useful for risk stratification in patients who have an intermediate risk of subsequent cardiac events (1–3% annual cardiac mortality) [33]. For a more detailed discussion of interpretation and risk stratification in symptomatic patients, please refer to Chapter II, Interpreting the Exercise Test, and Chapter 9, Stratifying Symptomatic Patients Using the Exercise Test and Other Tools. Patients who have an intermediate Duke treadmill score on ECG testing who are not directly referred to angiography should be referred for MPI for further risk assessment [63–65]. Previous studies have shown that referral to cardiac catheterization more closely parallels SPECT MPI than exercise testing [64, 66]. In addition, a study of 4,649 patients [67] with normal or near-normal SPECT MPI and intermediate Duke treadmill score demonstrated a 7-year mortality of 1.5% (less than 1% per year) which translated into a cumulative catheterization in these patients of only 17% over 7 years.

The major determinants of prognosis in patients with chronic CAD include the amount of infarcted myocardium, jeopardized myocardium and left ventricular function [10]. Studies [10,68] have shown that the best predictor of cardiac mortality is the extent of infarcted myocardium, TID, increased lung uptake and the extent of LV dysfunction which can be estimated by the left ventricular ejection fraction. In contrast, the best predictor of subsequent ischemic events are markers of inducible ischemia which include exertional symptoms, ECG changes, the extent of reversible defects and stress-induced wall motion abnormalities.

Myocardial perfusion data provide independent and incremental prognostic information over clinical, exercise ECG [16, 67, 68] and angiography [69] in patients with chronic CAD. A normal stress SPECT MPI is highly predictive of benign prognosis, predicting a less than 1% annual risk of cardiac death and MI [16, 70–75] (Table 7.5). In patients with abnormal SPECT MPI, the risk of adverse outcome is dependent on the extent of perfusion abnormalities. Rates of MI and cardiac death increase with worsening scan abnormalities. In a prospective study of 5,183 patients [16], the rate of adverse outcome (cardiac death or MI) with normal exercise SPECT scan was 0.7% per year compared to 6.7% in patients with SSS > 65% of the myocardium.

Other markers of worse prognosis include TID and increased lung uptake post-exercise. TID correlates with severe stenosis (>90%) in the proximal left anterior descending artery and/or two- to three-vessel CAD [76, 77]. Increased lung uptake indicates stress-induced global LV dysfunction and is associated with increased pulmonary hypertension in the presence of severe CAD [78]. In addition, it has been associated with severe and extensive CAD and is a marker of poor prognosis.

In addition to myocardial perfusion data, exercise-gated MPI can provide an evaluation of LV function which provides incremental value over myocardial perfusion data alone [79]. In a study [79] of 1,680 patients, post-stress LVEF and LV end systolic volume provided additional prognostic information over SSS in prediction of cardiac death. In another study of 2,686 patients [68], post-stress LVEF was predictive of cardiac mortality, whereas SDS was predictive of subsequent ischemia. The combined assessment was more predictive of outcome than either assessment alone. Using a threshold of 50%, resting LV function by radionuclide angiography [80] has also been shown to have prognostic value. In patients with abnormal resting EF, a decline in EF with exercise is an important predictor of CAD severity and poor prognosis [80, 81]. Data in patients with normal resting EF, however, are inconclusive [82].

Risk Assessment Before and After Revascularization

Radionuclide imaging can be used to guide referral to angiography and revascularization [10]. Previous studies [64] have shown that SPECT MPI can identify patients who have a reduction in morbidity and mortality with revascularization compared to medical therapy. In general, patients with moderate to severe perfusion abnormalities (SSS > 8) should be referred for revascularization. SDS, a measure of ischemic extent and severity, however, may be a more powerful predictor of who will benefit from revascularization. In a study [64] of 10,627 patients, patients with moderate to severe ischemia benefited most from revascularization, whereas in the setting of no to mild ischemia, medical therapy showed a greater survival advantage. The percent of myocardium with fixed defects showed no predictive benefit. Moreover, compared to direct angiography, using SPECT to guide referral to angiography has been shown to provide significant cost savings.

MPI can also be used to assess the functional significance of single or multiple stenoses. When revascularization is targeted to the culprit vessel, exercise MPI can identify compromised myocardium supplied by the culprit vessel(s) and guide revascularization. In addition, MPI can determine the functional significance of mild or moderate stenosis on angiography [83, 84]. Despite their appearance on angiography, these lesions can be functionally significant and warrant revascularization. Moreover, if no ischemia is noted on SPECT MPI, there is a low risk of cardiac events even in patients with three-vessel or left main disease [85, 86]. Unless there is a change in symptoms suggesting restenosis or new disease, radionuclide imaging is generally not recommended early (<2 months) or late after PCI or CABG [10]. However, in high-risk asymptomatic patients, exercise MPI is recommended 3–5 years after PCI or CABG [10] because these patients have a higher risk of cardiac events [87, 88].

Preoperative Risk Assessment

Initial preoperative risk assessment should rest on an assessment of clinical, demographic and surgical indicators of risk. Noninvasive testing prior to noncardiac surgery should be reserved for patients at intermediate risk who are scheduled to undergo an intermediate- or high-risk operation. In general, an assessment of functional status, either by history or exercise testing, is the major determinant of perioperative and long-term outcomes. Referral to noninvasive testing should follow similar guidelines [89] as referral in patients with chronic coronary artery disease in the nonoperative setting.

Most studies [10] using radionuclide imaging for risk stratification prior to noncardiac surgery have used vasodilator stress. Findings, however, are comparable between exercise and vasodilator stress. Based on studies using radionuclide MPI, the positive predictive value is low ranging from 4 to 20% with a high negative predictive value ranging from 96 to 100% [10]. The presence of reversible perfusion defects is associated with perioperative ischemia, whereas the presence of fixed defects may be a marker of long-term risk.

The indications for angiography or intervention are the same as for patients in the nonoperative setting. There are no randomized trials that have shown that revascularization improves outcomes. However, a number of studies have demonstrated the benefits of beta blockade in the perioperative setting [89]. For details on ECG stress testing for perioperative risk assessment, see Chapter 10, Exercise Testing as Applied to the Preoperative Patient.

Viability Assessment

The goal of the viability assessment is to determine which patients with significant regional ventricular dysfunction may improve after revascularization. In SPECT imaging, the magnitude of tracer uptake reflects the magnitude of preserved viability and consequently the probability of functional recovery after revascularization in areas with abnormal perfusion. Most studies evaluating myocardial viability have used resting images (i.e., images using thallium redistribution or PET metabolic activity) and assigned a specific threshold or cutoff for viability, often 50–60% [10]. For SPECT, sensitivity and specificity ranges are from 81 to 86% and 50 to 66%, respectively; for PET, sensitivity and specificity are 93 and 58%, respectively. The negative and positive predictive values are comparable and approximately 70 and 85%, respectively [90]. However, when values are intermediate, assessment of stress-induced ischemia may provide additional important information. The finding of stress-induced ischemia (a reversible perfusion defect) is a more powerful predictor of functional recovery than a fixed defect with similar amounts of tracer uptake.

In addition to imaging rest metabolic activity, PET viability protocols have included an evaluation of myocardial perfusion. Patients with CAD and LV dysfunction who have demonstrated viable myocardium by PET have a higher risk of cardiac death if they are treated with medical therapy compared to a much lower risk after revascularization [91]. PET protocols using this technique have slightly better overall accuracy than single photon techniques; however, a meta-analysis of outcome studies related to viability showed no differences in regard to reduction of morbidity and mortality [92].

Thus, the evaluation of patients with CAD and severe LV dysfunction should include an assessment of the potential benefit of revascularization [10]. Active angina in the setting of LV dysfunction alone would warrant revascularization. If angina is not present, an evaluation of myocardial viability is needed. If extensive viability if found associated with stenotic arteries then patients would likely benefit from revascularization. In absence of ischemia or viability, this benefit is less probable.

References

1. Dilsizian V, Narula J. Atlas of Nuclear Cardiology. Philadelphia: Current Medicine, 2003.
2. Husain SS. Myocardial perfusion imaging protocols: is there an ideal protocol? J Nucl Med Technol 2007;35(1):3–9.
3. Beller GA, Bergmann SR. Myocardial perfusion agents: SPECT and PET. J Nucl Cardiol 2004;11(1):74–86.
4. Feigenbaum H, Armstrong WF, Ryan, T. Feigenbaum's Echocardiography. 6 ed: Philadelphia, Lippincott Williams and Wilkins, 2005.
5. Wackers FJ. Exercise myocardial perfusion imaging. J Nucl Med 1994;35(4):726–9.
6. Meleca MJ, McGoron AJ, Gerson MC, et al. Flow versus uptake comparisons of thallium-201 with technetium-99m perfusion tracers in a canine model of myocardial ischemia. J Nucl Med 1997;38(12):1847–56.
7. Slart RH, Bax JJ, van Veldhuisen DJ, et al. Prediction of functional recovery after revascularization in patients with coronary artery disease and left ventricular dysfunction by gated FDG-PET. J Nucl Cardiol 2006;13(2):210–9.
8. Arrighi JA. Assessment of myocardial viability: more than measurements of radiotracer uptake alone. J Nucl Cardiol 2006;13(2):180–3.
9. Anagnostopoulos C, Harbinson M, Kelion A, et al. Procedure guidelines for radionuclide myocardial perfusion imaging. Heart 2004;90 Suppl 1:i1–10.
10. Klocke FJ, Baird MG, Lorell BH, et al. ACC/AHA/ASNC guidelines for the clinical use of cardiac radionuclide imaging – executive summary: a report of the American College of Cardiology/American Heart Association Task Force on Practice Guidelines (ACC/AHA/ASNC Committee to Revise the 1995 Guidelines for the Clinical Use of Cardiac Radionuclide Imaging). J Am Coll Cardiol 2003;42(7):1318–33.
11. Henzlova MJ, Cerqueira MD, Mahmarian JJ, Yao SS. Stress protocols and tracers. J Nucl Cardiol 2006;13(6):e80–90.
12. Bateman TM. Cardiac positron emission tomography and the role of adenosine pharmacologic stress. Am J Cardiol 2004;94(2A):19D–24D; discussion D-5D.
13. Schelbert HR, Beanlands R, Bengel F, et al. PET myocardial perfusion and glucose metabolism imaging: Part 2-Guidelines for interpretation and reporting. J Nucl Cardiol 2003;10(5):557–71.

14. McNeer JF, Margolis JR, Lee KL, et al. The role of the exercise test in the evaluation of patients for ischemic heart disease. Circulation 1978;57(1):64–70.

15. Cerqueira MD, Weissman NJ, Dilsizian V, et al. Standardized myocardial segmentation and nomenclature for tomographic imaging of the heart: a statement for healthcare professionals from the Cardiac Imaging Committee of the Council on Clinical Cardiology of the American Heart Association. Circulation 2002;105(4):539–42.

16. Hachamovitch R, Berman DS, Shaw LJ, et al. Incremental prognostic value of myocardial perfusion single photon emission computed tomography for the prediction of cardiac death: differential stratification for risk of cardiac death and myocardial infarction. Circulation 1998;97(6):535–43.

17. Hachamovitch R. Prognostic characterization of patients with mild coronary artery disease with myocardial perfusion single photon emission computed tomography: validation of an outcomes-based strategy. J Nucl Cardiol 1998;5(1):90–5.

18. Sanders GP, Pinto DS, Parker JA, Koutkia P, Aepfelbacher FC, Danias PG. Increased resting Tl-201 lung-to-heart ratio is associated with invasively determined measures of left ventricular dysfunction, extent of coronary artery disease, and resting myocardial perfusion abnormalities. J Nucl Cardiol 2003;10(2):140–7.

19. Omar WA, Reda A. Comparison between gated SPECT and echocardiography in evaluation of left ventricular ejection fraction. J Egypt Nat Canc Inst 2000;12(4):301–6.

20. Berman D, Germano G, Lewin H, et al. Comparison of post-stress ejection fraction and relative left ventricular volumes by automatic analysis of gated myocardial perfusion single-photon emission computed tomography acquired in the supine and prone positions. J Nucl Cardiol 1998;5(1):40–7.

21. Verberne HJ, Dijkgraaf MG, Somsen GA, van Eck-Smit BL. Stress-related variations in left ventricular function as assessed with gated myocardial perfusion SPECT. J Nucl Cardiol 2003;10(5):456–63.

22. Kiat H, Berman DS, Maddahi J, et al. Late reversibility of tomographic myocardial thallium-201 defects: an accurate marker of myocardial viability. J Am Coll Cardiol 1988;12(6): 1456–63.

23. Sansoy V, Glover DK, Watson DD, et al. Comparison of thallium-201 resting redistribution with technetium-99m-sestamibi uptake and functional response to dobutamine for assessment of myocardial viability. Circulation 1995;92(4):994–1004.

24. Nicolai E, Cuocolo A, Acampa W, Varrone A, Pace L, Salvatore M. Exercise-test Tc-99m tetrofosmin SPECT in patients with chronic ischemic left ventricular dysfunction: direct comparison with Ti-201 reinjection. J Nucl Cardiol 1999;6(3):270–7.

25. Matsunari I, Fujino S, Taki J, et al. Myocardial viability assessment with technetium-99m-tetrofosmin and thallium-201 reinjection in coronary artery disease. J Nucl Med 1995;36(11):1961–7.

26. Schoder H, Campisi R, Ohtake T, et al. Blood flow-metabolism imaging with positron emission tomography in patients with diabetes mellitus for the assessment of reversible left ventricular contractile dysfunction. J Am Coll Cardiol 1999;33(5):1328–37.

27. Pagano D, Townend JN, Littler WA, Horton R, Camici PG, Bonser RS. Coronary artery bypass surgery as treatment for ischemic heart failure: the predictive value of viability assessment with quantitative positron emission tomography for symptomatic and functional outcome. J Thorac Cardiovasc Surg 1998;115(4):791–9.

28. Gambhir SS, Schwaiger M, Huang SC, et al. Simple noninvasive quantification method for measuring myocardial glucose utilization in humans employing positron emission tomography and fluorine-18 deoxyglucose. J Nucl Med 1989;30(3):359–66.

29. Choi Y, Hawkins RA, Huang SC, et al. Parametric images of myocardial metabolic rate of glucose generated from dynamic cardiac PET and 2-[18F]fluoro-2-deoxy-d-glucose studies. J Nucl Med 1991;32(4):733–8.

30. Maes A, Van de Werf F, Nuyts J, Bormans G, Desmet W, Mortelmans L. Impaired myocardial tissue perfusion early after successful thrombolysis. Impact on myocardial flow, metabolism, and function at late follow-up. Circulation 1995;92(8):2072–8.

31. Maes A, Mortelmans L, Nuyts J, et al. Importance of flow/metabolism studies in predicting late recovery of function following reperfusion in patients with acute myocardial infarction. Eur Heart J 1997;18(6):954–62.
32. Yamagishi H, Akioka K, Hirata K, et al. A reverse flow-metabolism mismatch pattern on PET is related to multivessel disease in patients with acute myocardial infarction. J Nucl Med 1999;40(9):1492–8.
33. Gibbons RJ, Balady GJ, Bricker JT, et al. ACC/AHA 2002 guideline update for exercise testing: summary article. A report of the American College of Cardiology/American Heart Association Task Force on Practice Guidelines (Committee to Update the 1997 Exercise Testing Guidelines). J Am Coll Cardiol 2002;40(8):1531–40.
34. Mattera JA, Arain SA, Sinusas AJ, Finta L, Wackers FJ. Exercise testing with myocardial perfusion imaging in patients with normal baseline electrocardiograms: cost savings with a stepwise diagnostic strategy. J Nucl Cardiol 1998;5(5):498–506.
35. Douglas PS, Ginsburg GS. The evaluation of chest pain in women. N Engl J Med 1996;334(20):1311–5.
36. Wong Y, Rodwell A, Dawkins S, Livesey SA, Simpson IA. Sex differences in investigation results and treatment in subjects referred for investigation of chest pain. Heart 2001;85(2): 149–52.
37. Sketch MH, Mohiuddin SM, Lynch JD, Zencka AE, Runco V. Significant sex differences in the correlation of electrocardiographic exercise testing and coronary arteriograms. Am J Cardiol 1975;36(2):169–73.
38. Ryan TJ, Antman EM, Brooks NH, et al. 1999 update: ACC/AHA guidelines for the management of patients with acute myocardial infarction. A report of the American College of Cardiology/American Heart Association Task Force on Practice Guidelines (Committee on Management of Acute Myocardial Infarction). J Am Coll Cardiol 1999;34(3):890–911.
39. Dakik HA, Mahmarian JJ, Kimball KT, Koutelou MG, Medrano R, Verani MS. Prognostic value of exercise 201Tl tomography in patients treated with thrombolytic therapy during acute myocardial infarction. Circulation 1996;94(11):2735–42.
40. Basu S, Senior R, Dore C, Lahiri A. Value of thallium-201 imaging in detecting adverse cardiac events after myocardial infarction and thrombolysis: a follow up of 100 consecutive patients. BMJ 1996;313(7061):844–8.
41. Amanullah AM, Lindvall K. Prevalence and significance of transient – predominantly asymptomatic – myocardial ischemia on Holter monitoring in unstable angina pectoris, and correlation with exercise test and thallium-201 myocardial perfusion imaging. Am J Cardiol 1993;72(2):144–8.
42. Stratmann HG, Younis LT, Wittry MD, Amato M, Miller DD. Exercise technetium-99m myocardial tomography for the risk stratification of men with medically treated unstable angina pectoris. Am J Cardiol 1995;76(4):236–40.
43. Kroll D, Farah W, McKendall GR, Reinert SE, Johnson LL. Prognostic value of stress-gated Tc-99m sestamibi SPECT after acute myocardial infarction. Am J Cardiol 2001;87(4):381–6.
44. Stratmann HG, Tamesis BR, Younis LT, Wittry MD, Amato M, Miller DD. Prognostic value of predischarge dipyridamole technetium 99m sestamibi myocardial tomography in medically treated patients with unstable angina. Am Heart J 1995;130(4):734–40.
45. Acampa W, Cuocolo A, Sullo P, et al. Direct comparison of technetium 99m-sestamibi and technetium 99m-tetrofosmin cardiac single photon emission computed tomography in patients with coronary artery disease. J Nucl Cardiol 1998;5(3):265–74.
46. Azzarelli S, Galassi AR, Foti R, et al. Accuracy of 99mTc-tetrofosmin myocardial tomography in the evaluation of coronary artery disease. J Nucl Cardiol 1999;6(2):183–9.
47. Budoff MJ, Gillespie R, Georgiou D, et al. Comparison of exercise electron beam computed tomography and sestamibi in the evaluation of coronary artery disease. Am J Cardiol 1998;81(6):682–7.
48. Candell-Riera J, Santana-Boado C, Castell-Conesa J, et al. Simultaneous dipyridamole/maximal subjective exercise with 99mTc-MIBI SPECT: improved diagnostic yield in coronary artery disease. J Am Coll Cardiol 1997;29(3):531–6.

49. Elhendy A, van Domburg RT, Sozzi FB, Poldermans D, Bax JJ, Roelandt JR. Impact of hypertension on the accuracy of exercise stress myocardial perfusion imaging for the diagnosis of coronary artery disease. Heart 2001;85(6):655–61.

50. Hambye AS, Vervaet A, Lieber S, Ranquin R. Diagnostic value and incremental contribution of bicycle exercise, first-pass radionuclide angiography, and 99mTc-labeled sestamibi single-photon emission computed tomography in the identification of coronary artery disease in patients without infarction. J Nucl Cardiol 1996;3(6 Pt 1):464–74.

51. Ho YL, Wu CC, Huang PJ, et al. Assessment of coronary artery disease in women by dobutamine stress echocardiography: comparison with stress thallium-201 single-photon emission computed tomography and exercise electrocardiography. Am Heart J 1998;135(4): 655–62.

52. Ho YL, Wu CC, Huang PJ, et al. Dobutamine stress echocardiography compared with exercise thallium-201 single-photon emission computed tomography in detecting coronary artery disease-effect of exercise level on accuracy. Cardiology 1997;88(4):379–85.

53. Palmas W, Friedman JD, Diamond GA, Silber H, Kiat H, Berman DS. Incremental value of simultaneous assessment of myocardial function and perfusion with technetium-99m sestamibi for prediction of extent of coronary artery disease. J Am Coll Cardiol 1995;25(5):1024–31.

54. Rubello D, Zanco P, Candelpergher G, et al. Usefulness of 99mTc-MIBI stress myocardial SPECT bull's-eye quantification in coronary artery disease. Q J Nucl Med 1995;39(2): 111–5.

55. San Roman JA, Vilacosta I, Castillo JA, et al. Selection of the optimal stress test for the diagnosis of coronary artery disease. Heart 1998;80(4):370–6.

56. Santana-Boado C, Candell-Riera J, Castell-Conesa J, et al. Diagnostic accuracy of technetium-99m-MIBI myocardial SPECT in women and men. J Nucl Med 1998;39(5):751–5.

57. Sylven C, Hagerman I, Ylen M, Nyquist O, Nowak J. Variance ECG detection of coronary artery disease – a comparison with exercise stress test and myocardial scintigraphy. Clin Cardiol 1994;17(3):132–40.

58. Taillefer R, DePuey EG, Udelson JE, Beller GA, Latour Y, Reeves F. Comparative diagnostic accuracy of Tl-201 and Tc-99m sestamibi SPECT imaging (perfusion and ECG-gated SPECT) in detecting coronary artery disease in women. J Am Coll Cardiol 1997;29(1):69–77.

59. van Eck-Smit BL, Poots S, Zwinderman AH, Bruschke AV, Pauwels EK, van der Wall EE. Myocardial SPET imaging with 99Tcm-tetrofosmin in clinical practice: comparison of a 1 day and a 2 day imaging protocol. Nucl Med Commun 1997;18(1):24–30.

60. Van Train KF, Garcia EV, Maddahi J, et al. Multicenter trial validation for quantitative analysis of same-day rest-stress technetium-99m-sestamibi myocardial tomograms. J Nucl Med 1994;35(4):609–18.

61. Stewart RE, Schwaiger M, Molina E, et al. Comparison of rubidium-82 positron emission tomography and thallium-201 SPECT imaging for detection of coronary artery disease. Am J Cardiol 1991;67(16):1303–10.

62. Tamaki N, Yonekura Y, Senda M, et al. Value and limitation of stress thallium-201 single photon emission computed tomography: comparison with nitrogen-13 ammonia positron tomography. J Nucl Med 1988;29(7):1181–8.

63. Sharir T, Kang X, Germano G, et al. Prognostic value of poststress left ventricular volume and ejection fraction by gated myocardial perfusion SPECT in women and men: gender-related differences in normal limits and outcomes. J Nucl Cardiol 2006;13(4):495–506.

64. Hachamovitch R, Berman DS, Kiat H, et al. Exercise myocardial perfusion SPECT in patients without known coronary artery disease: incremental prognostic value and use in risk stratification. Circulation 1996;93(5):905–14.

65. Shaw LJ, Hachamovitch R, Peterson ED, et al. Using an outcomes-based approach to identify candidates for risk stratification after exercise treadmill testing. J Gen Intern Med 1999;14(1):1–9.

66. Hlatky MA, Pryor DB, Harrell FE, Jr., Califf RM, Mark DB, Rosati RA. Factors affecting sensitivity and specificity of exercise electrocardiography. Multivariable analysis. Am J Med 1984;77(1):64–71.

67. Gibbons RJ, Hodge DO, Berman DS, et al. Long-term outcome of patients with intermediate-risk exercise electrocardiograms who do not have myocardial perfusion defects on radionuclide imaging. Circulation 1999;100(21):2140–5.

68. Sharir T, Germano G, Kang X, et al. Prediction of myocardial infarction versus cardiac death by gated myocardial perfusion SPECT: risk stratification by the amount of stress-induced ischemia and the poststress ejection fraction. J Nucl Med 2001;42(6):831–7.

69. Iskandrian AS, Chae SC, Heo J, Stanberry CD, Wasserleben V, Cave V. Independent and incremental prognostic value of exercise single-photon emission computed tomographic (SPECT) thallium imaging in coronary artery disease. J Am Coll Cardiol 1993;22(3):665–70.

70. Alkeylani A, Miller DD, Shaw LJ, et al. Influence of race on the prediction of cardiac events with stress technetium-99m sestamibi tomographic imaging in patients with stable angina pectoris. Am J Cardiol 1998;81(3):293–7.

71. Boyne TS, Koplan BA, Parsons WJ, et al. Predicting adverse outcome with exercise SPECT technetium-99m sestamibi imaging in patients with suspected or known coronary artery disease. Am J Cardiol 1997;79(3):270–4.

72. Galassi AR, Azzarelli S, Tomaselli A, et al. Incremental prognostic value of technetium-99m-tetrofosmin exercise myocardial perfusion imaging for predicting outcomes in patients with suspected or known coronary artery disease. Am J Cardiol 2001;88(2):101–6.

73. Machecourt J, Longere P, Fagret D, et al. Prognostic value of thallium-201 single-photon emission computed tomographic myocardial perfusion imaging according to extent of myocardial defect. Study in 1,926 patients with follow-up at 33 months. J Am Coll Cardiol 1994;23(5):1096–106.

74. Stratmann HG, Williams GA, Wittry MD, Chaitman BR, Miller DD. Exercise technetium-99m sestamibi tomography for cardiac risk stratification of patients with stable chest pain. Circulation 1994;89(2):615–22.

75. Vanzetto G, Ormezzano O, Fagret D, Comet M, Denis B, Machecourt J. Long-term additive prognostic value of thallium-201 myocardial perfusion imaging over clinical and exercise stress test in low to intermediate risk patients : study in 1137 patients with 6-year follow-up. Circulation 1999;100(14):1521–7.

76. Mazzanti M, Germano G, Kiat H, et al. Identification of severe and extensive coronary artery disease by automatic measurement of transient ischemic dilation of the left ventricle in dual-isotope myocardial perfusion SPECT. J Am Coll Cardiol 1996;27(7):1612–20.

77. Weiss AT, Berman DS, Lew AS, et al. Transient ischemic dilation of the left ventricle on stress thallium-201 scintigraphy: a marker of severe and extensive coronary artery disease. J Am Coll Cardiol 1987;9(4):752–9.

78. Bacher-Stier C, Sharir T, Kavanagh PB, et al. Postexercise lung uptake of 99mTc-sestamibi determined by a new automatic technique: validation and application in detection of severe and extensive coronary artery disease and reduced left ventricular function. J Nucl Med 2000;41(7):1190–7.

79. Sharir T, Germano G, Kavanagh PB, et al. Incremental prognostic value of post-stress left ventricular ejection fraction and volume by gated myocardial perfusion single photon emission computed tomography. Circulation 1999;100(10):1035–42.

80. Lee KL, Pryor DB, Pieper KS, et al. Prognostic value of radionuclide angiography in medically treated patients with coronary artery disease. A comparison with clinical and catheterization variables. Circulation 1990;82(5):1705–17.

81. Mazzotta G, Bonow RO, Pace L, Brittain E, Epstein SE. Relation between exertional ischemia and prognosis in mildly symptomatic patients with single or double vessel coronary artery disease and left ventricular dysfunction at rest. J Am Coll Cardiol 1989;13(3):567–73.

82. Taliercio CP, Clements IP, Zinsmeister AR, Gibbons RJ. Prognostic value and limitations of exercise radionuclide angiography in medically treated coronary artery disease. Mayo Clin Proc 1988;63(6):573–82.

83. Legrand V, Mancini GB, Bates ER, Hodgson JM, Gross MD, Vogel RA. Comparative study of coronary flow reserve, coronary anatomy and results of radionuclide exercise tests in patients with coronary artery disease. J Am Coll Cardiol 1986;8(5):1022–32.

84. Miller DD, Donohue TJ, Younis LT, et al. Correlation of pharmacological 99mTc-sestamibi myocardial perfusion imaging with poststenotic coronary flow reserve in patients with angiographically intermediate coronary artery stenoses. Circulation 1994;89(5):2150–60.
85. Brown KA, Rowen M, Altland E. Prognosis of patients with an isolated fixed thallium-201 defect and no prior myocardial infarction. Am J Cardiol 1993;72(15):1199–201.
86. Abdel Fattah A, Kamal AM, Pancholy S, et al. Prognostic implications of normal exercise tomographic thallium images in patients with angiographic evidence of significant coronary artery disease. Am J Cardiol 1994;74(8):769–71.
87. Kang X, Berman DS, Lewin HC, et al. Incremental prognostic value of myocardial perfusion single photon emission computed tomography in patients with diabetes mellitus. Am Heart J 1999;138(6 Pt 1):1025–32.
88. Giri S, Shaw LJ, Murthy DR, et al. Impact of diabetes on the risk stratification using stress single-photon emission computed tomography myocardial perfusion imaging in patients with symptoms suggestive of coronary artery disease. Circulation 2002;105(1):32–40.
89. Eagle KA, Berger PB, Calkins H, et al. ACC/AHA guideline update for perioperative cardiovascular evaluation for noncardiac surgery – executive summary: a report of the American College of Cardiology/American Heart Association Task Force on Practice Guidelines (Committee to Update the 1996 Guidelines on Perioperative Cardiovascular Evaluation for Noncardiac Surgery). J Am Coll Cardiol 2002;39(3):542–53.
90. Rahimtoola SH, La Canna G, Ferrari R. Hibernating myocardium: another piece of the puzzle falls into place. J Am Coll Cardiol 2006;47(5):978–80.
91. Bax JJ, Wijns W, Cornel JH, Visser FC, Boersma E, Fioretti PM. Accuracy of currently available techniques for prediction of functional recovery after revascularization in patients with left ventricular dysfunction due to chronic coronary artery disease: comparison of pooled data. J Am Coll Cardiol 1997;30(6):1451–60.
92. Allman KC, Shaw LJ, Hachamovitch R, Udelson JE. Myocardial viability testing and impact of revascularization on prognosis in patients with coronary artery disease and left ventricular dysfunction: a meta-analysis. J Am Coll Cardiol 2002;39(7):1151–8.
93. Heiba SI, Hayat NJ, Salman HS, et al. Technetium-99m-MIBI myocardial SPECT: supine versus right lateral imaging and comparison with coronary arteriography. J Nucl Med 1997;38(10):1510–4.
94. Yao Z, Liu XJ, Shi R, et al. A comparison of 99mTc-MIBI myocardial SPET with electron beam computed tomography in the assessment of coronary artery disease. Eur J Nucl Med 1997;24(9):1115–20.
95. Iskandrian AE, Heo J, Nallamothu N. Detection of coronary artery disease in women with use of stress single-photon emission computed tomography myocardial perfusion imaging. J Nucl Cardiol 1997;4(4):329–35.
96. Snader CE, Marwick TH, Pashkow FJ, Harvey SA, Thomas JD, Lauer MS. Importance of estimated functional capacity as a predictor of all-cause mortality among patients referred for exercise thallium single-photon emission computed tomography: report of 3,400 patients from a single center. J Am Coll Cardiol 1997;30(3):641–8.
97. Olmos LI, Dakik H, Gordon R, et al. Long-term prognostic value of exercise echocardiography compared with exercise 201Tl, ECG, and clinical variables in patients evaluated for coronary artery disease. Circulation 1998;98(24):2679–86.

Chapter 8
Stress Echocardiography

Patricia Nguyen

Stress echocardiography offers an alternative to stress nuclear imaging for the evaluation of coronary artery disease. Although the choice of imaging modality often varies depending on patient characteristics, availability and local expertise [1], stress echocardiography offers several advantages [2] to nuclear techniques including (1) versatility to obtain additional diagnostic information, (2) lower cost, (3) no radiation exposure, and (4) convenience because patients do not need to return for late imaging.

Principle Behind Stress Echocardiography

Physiologic stress increases heart rate and contractility, resulting in an increase in myocardial oxygen demand. In the absence of flow-limiting stenosis, myocardial blood flow augments to meet this demand. In the presence of a coronary stenosis, the increase in myocardial blood flow is inadequate to meet demand, resulting in a demand–supply mismatch, which, if persistent, leads to the ischemia [3].

Although stress echocardiography can evaluate for earlier markers of ischemia including myocardial perfusion defects and diastolic dysfunction, the mainstay for assessment of coronary artery disease is the detection of new or worsening regional wall motion abnormalities induced by ischemia [2]. The severity of the wall motion abnormality depends on several factors including the magnitude of blood flow change, the spatial extent of defect, the presence of collateral blood flow, the left ventricular pressure and wall stress, and the duration of ischemia [4].

Elimination of the stressor decreases myocardial oxygen demand and ischemia resolves. Recovery of baseline wall motion occurs typically within 1 or 2 min. In rare cases, wall motion abnormalities may persist (stunning), lasting for days or weeks but these abnormalities eventually return to baseline.

P. Nguyen (✉)
Department of Cardiology, Stanford University School of Medicine, Palo Alto, CA, USA
e-mail: pknguyen1@yahoo.com

C.H. Evans, R.D. White (eds.), *Exercise Testing for Primary Care and Sports Medicine Physicians,* DOI 10.1007/978-0-387-76597-6_8
© Springer Science+Business Media, LLC 2009

Methodology

For stress echocardiography, images are taken at rest (baseline) while the patient is supine and during (i.e., supine bicycle, pharmacologic stress) or immediately after stress (i.e., treadmill, upright bicycle). Images are acquired in four views (Fig. 8.1): Parasternal long axis displaying the left ventricle (excluding apex) and left ventricular outflow tract/aorta (A, top); short axis view of the left ventricle at the mid-papillary level (A, bottom); apical four-chamber view, displaying the right and left chambers of the heart (B, top); and apical two-chamber view, displaying the left side of the heart (B, bottom). Patients are continuously monitored with a 12 lead ECG and heart rate and blood pressure are recorded frequently throughout the examination. Because the accuracy of echo interpretation is highly dependent on the quality of images, stress echo images should be acquired by an experienced technician who performs these examinations regularly.

Types of Stress

Stress echocardiography can be performed with exercise, a pharmacologic agent or pacing [1,2,5] (Table 8.1). Exercise echocardiography is most often performed using either treadmill or bicycle (supine or upright) exercise. With treadmill and upright bicycle exercise, only immediate post-exercise images are available, increasing the potential for false negatives, especially in patients with mild or single vessel disease.

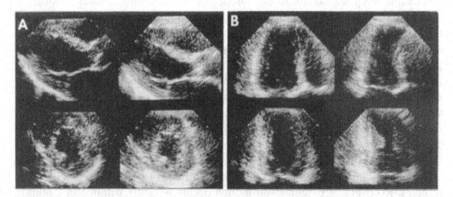

Fig. 8.1 Display of images of the left ventricle in systole in the four standard views used in echo stress testing. (**A**) Parasternal long axis (*top*) and short axis images (*bottom*), at rest (*left*) and after exercise (*right*). (**B**) Apical four-chamber (*top*) and two-chamber images (*bottom*) at rest (*left*) and after exercise (*right*). At rest the function of the left ventricle is normal and all walls demonstrate symmetrical thickening. At peak stress, the basal left ventricle became hyperdynamic, the normal stress response. The apex became dysketic (*arrows*) suggesting disease in the region supplied by the left anterior descending artery. The patient was found to have a high grade lesion of the mid-left anterior descending artery. (From Mayo Clinic Cardiovascular Working Group on Stress Testing [106], with permission of *Mayo Clin Proc.*)

Table 8.1 Types of stress

Exercise
Post-treadmill exercise
Supine bicycle
Upright bicycle
Handgrip exercise
Pharmacologic
Dobutamine
Adenosine
Dipyridamole
Other
Transesophageal atrial pacing
Transvenous pacing

Supine bicycle is preferred because imaging can be performed at peak exercise, reducing the risk that regional wall motion abnormalities resolve prior to imaging.

In addition to the type of exercise, the amount of exercise patients perform may reduce the potential of having false negatives [6]. Stress echocardiography uses standard treadmill exercise protocols, including the Bruce and modified Bruce protocols. Unless a sub-maximal stress test is required (i.e., shortly after myocardial infarction) or patients develop indications for early test termination [7] (Table 8.2), target heart rate [85% (220 – age)] should be achieved. If target heart rate is not achieved and the test is reported normal, it is possible the result is a false negative [6] and a pharmacologic stress test should be ordered. Unless stress testing is used to evaluate patients on their existing medical regimen, beta blockers and non-dihydropyridine calcium channel blockers should be withheld for 48 h [1] prior to stress testing to ensure adequate heart rate response.

Patients who cannot adequately exercise (i.e., those with claudication, deconditioning, etc.) should be referred for pharmacological stress testing [1]. Dobutamine is the most common pharmacologic stress agent in echocardiography. Dobutamine is a synthetic catecholamine that causes both inotropic (lower doses) and chronotropic (higher doses). Because of the inotropic effects of dobutamine, reaching target heart rate is not as critical as with exercise echocardiography [5]. The peripheral effects of dobutamine may be either vasoconstriction or vasodilation, so blood pressure response is less predictable. Dobutamine, thus, increases myocardial work load and indirectly coronary blood flow. In myocardial regions supplied by a coronary artery with significant stenosis, a steal phenomenon occurs and myocardial oxygen

Table 8.2 Indications for termination of stress testing

Target HR achieved: 85% (220 – age) or 70% if recent MI
Severe symptoms (chest pain, dyspnea, dizziness)
Severe ischemia (ST >2 mm or ST >1 mm)
Signs of poor perfusion (pallor, cyanosis)
Hypertension (SBP >250 mmHg, DBP >115 mmHg)
Hypotension (≥10 mmHg compared to baseline or ≥20 mmHg compared to previous stage)
Sustained VT or complex arrhythmias

Table 8.3 Relative contraindications to dobutamine stress testing

Hemodynamically unstable patients
Decompensated CHF
Acute coronary syndrome
Uncontrolled atrial fibrillation
Abdominal aortic aneurysm
Severe aortic stenosis*
Hypertrophic cardiomyopathy
Severe ventricular arrhythmia
Uncontrolled hypertension

*Exception is for the evaluation of severe aortic stenosis associated with low cardiac output.

demand exceeds supply. Ischemia develops because blood is diverted away from the stenotic artery and the subendocardium to the normal arteries and the subepicardium.

Dobutamine is administered as a continuous, stepwise infusion starting at 5 μg/kg/min. The infusion is increased every 3 min in 10 μg/kg/min increments until one of the following endpoints is reached: (a) peak dose of 40 μg/kg/min has been reached, (b) the patient develops symptoms or reaches target heart rate (Table 8.2) [7], or (c) new or worsening regional wall motion abnormalities are noted. Patients who do not achieve adequate heart rate response (i.e., those on beta blockers) may receive 0.2–1 mg intravenous atropine to increase heart rate. Images are taken at baseline, low-dose dobutamine (5 μg/kg/min), pre-peak and peak dobutamine infusion with or without atropine. If patients develop significant symptoms or persistent tachycardia occurs, esmolol can be administered to terminate the effects of dobutamine. Beta blockers which reduce the chronotropic and inotropic effects of dobutamine should also be stopped 48 h before testing [1] unless an evaluation of the patients' current medical regimen is indicated.

Although coronary vasodilators including adenosine and dipyridamole have been used in stress echocardiography, their usage has been mainly in myocardial perfusion imaging (i.e., myocardial contrast imaging). Previous studies [8] have suggested that the use of coronary vasodilators for detection of wall motion abnormalities is not as sensitive as dobutamine. Thus, if patients have contraindications to dobutamine (Table 8.3) [5] and are unable to exercise, nuclear imaging should be considered.

Another option for inducing stress is with transesophageal atrial pacing or transvenous pacing [9]. Stress is determined by a controlled increase in heart rate which is a major determinant of myocardial oxygen demand. Pacing, however, is not routinely used as a stress agent.

Choice of Stressor

The choice of the stress agent is dependent on patient's physical status and the clinical question to be addressed. In general, if patients can exercise, exercise testing is

Table 8.4 Stress testing and clinical decision making

	TME	Bike	DSE
Chest pain evaluation	+	+	±
Post-MI risk	+	+	+
Viability	−	±	+
Dypsnea/fatigue	+	+	−
Preoperative risk assessment	±	±	+
Valvular disease	−	+	−
Pulmonary hypertension	−	+	−

TME, treadmill exercise; DSE, dobutamine stress echocardiography.
Adapted from Armstrong WF, Zoghbi WA, Stress echocardiography: current methodology and clinical applications. J Am Coll Cardiol. 2005;45:1739–1747, with permission of Elsevier.

preferred over pharmacological stress testing because a possible causal relationship can be established between the amount of physical activity and provokable symptoms [5]. Moreover, exercise provides information on functional status (i.e., number of METs performed) which is useful for risk stratification and prognosis [10]. Thus, patients should be encouraged to exercise for the duration of the test and even longer if they are able to provide adequate assessment of their functional status.

Another consideration in choosing type of stress test is the clinical question to be answered (Table 8.4) [5]. Exercise testing is preferred to evaluate the association of physical activity with symptoms including chest pain, dypsnea or fatigue. Similarly, exercise testing (with supine bicycle) is required to measure pulmonary artery pressure response to exercise for early diagnosis of primary pulmonary hypertension [11]. For preoperative assessment prior to non-cardiac surgery and for evaluation of myocardial viability, dobutamine is the stressor of choice. To evaluate the severity of mitral valve stenosis, exercise testing (usually with supine bicycle) is required. Dobutamine echo is also used to evaluate the severity of aortic stenosis in patients with severe LV dysfunction and to determine contractile reserve for risk stratification and prognosis in these patients prior to cardiac surgery.

Coronary Artery Disease

Interpretation

Wall Motion Abnormalities

Analysis of stress echocardiograms is based on a subjective assessment of the regional wall motion, comparing the wall thickening and endocardial excursion of the left ventricle at rest and with stress (Table 8.5). Normally, after exercise or dobutamine infusion, the wall motion becomes hyperkinetic. Worsening of wall motion abnormalities or the development of new wall motion abnormalities indicates stress-induced ischemia. Wall motion abnormalities range from hypokinetic (graded

Table 8.5 Interpretation of regional wall motion abnormalities

Rest	Stress	Interpretation
Normal	Hyperkinetic	Normal
Normal	New or worsening WMA	Ischemia
WMA	No change	Infarct
WMA	Worsening of WMA	Peri-infarct ischemia

WMA, wall motion abnormality.

as mild, moderate and severe), to akinetic (not moving), to dyskinetic (moving the opposite direction). The lack of hyperkinetic motion may indicate ischemia but is less specific [7]. If a wall motion abnormality is present at rest, an infarct is present. If the wall motion abnormality is present at rest and worsens with stress, an infarct in addition to ischemia is present.

Assignment of Wall Motion Abnormalities to Coronary Artery Territories

Similar to nuclear myocardial perfusion images, stress echocardiograms can be analyzed using the 17-segment model [12], which divides the left ventricle into 17 segments. Segments are then assigned to the three major coronary artery territories [12], recognizing that there is anatomical variability, especially in the assignment of segment 17, the apical cap. In general, the anterior wall (segments 1, 7, 13), anterior septum (segments 2, 8, 14) and apical cap are assigned to the left anterior descending artery. The anterior-lateral (segments 6, 12, 16) and inferior-lateral (segments 5, 11) walls are assigned to the left circumflex. The inferior wall (segments 4, 11, 15) and inferior septal wall (segments 3, 9) are assigned to the right coronary artery. Alternatively, a 16 segment model is used and the apical cap is divided between segments 13–16. The 16 segment model is more accurate in the distribution of the myocardium between base, mid and apex but the 17 segment model has been advocated as the standard for all imaging modalities. Thus, regional wall motion abnormalities can be used to localize the site of ischemia and/or infarct to a culprit vessel.

Wall Motion Index: An Objective Measure of Ischemia

A wall motion index (WMI) can be calculated which can provide a more objective measure of ischemia. The WMI is the total sum of the wall motion abnormalities graded on a five-point scale (3, hyperkinesis; 2, normokinesis; 1, hypokinesis; 0, akinesis; and −1, paradoxical) for each segment divided by the number of analyzable segments. Patients with a score >1.8 have been shown to have worse prognosis [13].

Other Markers of Ischemia

In addition to changes in wall motion, other markers of ischemia include LV cavity dilatation [14], a decrease in global systolic function [7], diastolic dysfunction [15] or new or worsening mitral regurgitation [7]. These echocardiographic markers are specific but not sensitive [7]. Because the stress response produced by exercise is not identical to dobutamine, the frequency and significance of these markers differ for each type of stressor [7].

Assessment of Myocardial Viability

Dobutamine echocardiography is also used to differentiate viable from nonviable myocardium (scarred or irreversibly dysfunctional myocardium). Although a segment appears akinetic (not moving), the myocardium may still be viable because myocardial contractility ceases when ≥20% or more of the entire myocardial thickness is involved by ischemia or infarction [7]. Viable myocardium can be normal, stunned or hibernating. Stunned myocardium results from transient coronary artery occlusion and recovers spontaneously after days to weeks. Hibernating myocardium results from chronic myocardial ischemia which recovers after revascularization. During infusion of low-dose dobutamine (5–20 μg/kg/min), coronary blood flow increases and recruitment of contractile reserve improves wall motion of dysfunctional myocardium. If the dobutamine dose is increased in the presence of an obstructive lesion, coronary blood flow does not increase further and myocardial ischemia occurs, resulting in worsening of wall motion. This biphasic response to dobutamine indicates the presence of hibernating myocardium [16]. If there is continued augmentation of systolic wall thickening with higher doses of dobutamine, a critical stenosis is not present [1].

Clinical Indications: Acute Coronary Syndrome

Diagnosis of Acute Coronary Syndrome

There is no role for stress echocardiography in the initial diagnosis of suspected acute coronary syndrome or infarction [17]. Transthoracic echocardiography (without stress), however, can be performed in patients whose diagnosis is not evident by other means (e.g., ECG, cardiac enzymes, etc.). Specifically, transthoracic echocardiography can be used to identify segmental wall motion abnormalities that suggest the presence of CAD but cannot differentiate from inducible ischemia, recent myocardial infarction or scar. Preservation of normal wall thickness and normal reflectivity, however, suggests an acute event. The absence of wall motion abnormalities also has a high negative predictive value as high as 98% [18].

In patients presenting with suspected or possible acute coronary syndrome (ACS) who have normal follow-up (after 6–8 h) 12 lead ECGs and cardiac biomarkers, early exercise stress testing can be considered (Table 8.6) [1, 17, 19]. Alternatively, they can be discharged and can return for an outpatient stress test within 72 h. Patients who are capable of exercise and who have an uninterpretable ECG should be evaluated with an exercise imaging study (e.g., stress echocardiography). Patients who are unable to exercise should have a pharmacologic stress test. Patients who have definite ACS should be admitted for further evaluation [17].

Risk Stratification and Prognosis in Acute Coronary Syndrome

The management of ACS requires continuous risk stratification, from initial assessment to discharge. Risk stratification identifies high-risk patients who would benefit

Table 8.6 Indications for stress echocardiography in acute coronary syndromes

	Patient group	Indication	Class
1	Possible ACS with nondiagnostic ECG and negative markers or normal rest scan in the presence of baseline abnormalities which are expected to compromise ECG interpretation	Diagnosis and risk stratification	I
2	Assessment of myocardial viability when required to define potential efficacy of revascularization 4–10 days after myocardial infarction	Guide therapy	I
3	Possible ACS with nondiagnostic ECG and negative markers or normal rest scan *in the absence* of baseline abnormalities which are expected to compromise ECG interpretation	Diagnosis and risk stratification	IIa

from coronary angiography and revascularization. In low- to intermediate-risk patients, a noninvasive testing is recommended for risk stratification prior to discharge if patients have been free of ischemia at rest or with low-level activity and free of heart failure for a minimum of 24 h [17] (Table 8.7) [20–29]. Stress echocardiographic features that suggest high-risk warrant referral to revascularization are shown in Table 8.8 [17].

Stress echocardiography for risk stratification can also be performed safely in patients presenting with ACS early after infarction. Graded exercise testing is preferred [1, 21, 26, 30], but graded dobutamine echocardiogram can also be performed [1,31]. Although serious complications have been reported with dobutamine echocardiography [32], most agree [1] that a carefully performed pharmacological stress echocardiography using a graded protocol starting with low-dose dobutamine is feasible and safe if performed 4–10 days after infarction. Those patients with a

Table 8.7 Prognostic value of stress echocardiography early after acute myocardial infarction

		Time after			Annualized event rate	
Author	Year	MI D	Stress	Events	Ischemia (%)	No ischemia (%)
Applegate [21]	1987	13	TME	D, MI, Re	55	14
Ryan [27]	1987	11–21	TME	D, MI	59	0
Quintana [26]	1995	7	BE	D, MI	22.2	4.7
Sicari [29]	1997	12	DASE	D, MI	6.4	6.6
Greco [23]	1997	12	DASE	D, MI	7.77	1.5
Carlos [22]	1997	2–7	DASE	D, MI, VT	26.6	4.3
Minardi [24]	1997	3–5	DSE	D, MI	4.3	0
Previtali [25]	1998	9	DASE	D, MI	8.4	0
Sicari [28]	2002	10	DASE/Dipyr	D, MI	7.7	3.7
Acampa [20]	2005	3–7	DASE	D, MI	N/A	0.8

Stress: Treadmill exercise (TME), bicycle exercise (BE), dobutamine–atropine (DASE), dobutamine (DSE); events: death (D), myocardial infarction (MI), revascularization (Re).
Adapted from Cheitlin et al. [1], with permission of Elsevier.

Table 8.8 Indications for stress echocardiography in chronic ischemia

	Patient group	Indication	Class
1	Symptomatic patients with intermediate likelihood of CAD who have baseline ECG abnormalities	Diagnosis of CAD	I
2	Intermediate-risk patients after cath	Identification of hemodynamic significance of intermediate lesions (25–75%)	I
3	Patients prior to revascularization	Assessment of myocardial viability	I
4	Prognosis in patients with baseline ECG abnormalities with an intermediate pretest likelihood of CAD	Risk assessment	IIa
5	Detection of CAD by DSE in patients after cardiac transplant	Initial diagnostic assessment	IIa
6	Detection of myocardial ischemia in women with a pretest probability of CAD	Diagnosis of CAD	IIa

positive ischemic response have a higher rate of death and reinfarction and should be referred for revascularization [1, 21, 26, 30].

Assessment before and after revascularization in acute coronary syndrome:

Graded dobutamine echocardiography can also be used to assess myocardial viability early after infarction. Specifically, dobutamine echocardiography can differentiate between hypokinetic segments at rest that are infarcted (i.e., contractility deteriorates after dobutamine), stunned (i.e., contractility improves with increasing dobutamine) or hibernating (i.e., contractility improves with low dose and deteriorates with high dose, "the biphasic response") [16]. Functional recovery occurs in stunned (spontaneously) and hibernating myocardium (after revascularization).

Routine follow-up testing after successful PCI or surgery is generally not recommended because the identification of residual but asymptomatic lesions has not improved patient outcomes [1]. However, an exercise or pharmacologic stress echo is recommended in patients who present with recurrent atypical or typical symptom [1] despite recent percutaneous coronary intervention or bypass surgery to assess restenosis and the functional significance of residual lesions.

Clinical Indications: Chronic Ischemic Heart Disease

Diagnosis of Coronary Artery Disease

Stress imaging adds significant clinical value for detecting and localizing ischemia compared to standard treadmill testing [1]. Some studies [33, 34] have also suggested that it is more cost-effective than exercise testing alone in patients with intermediate risk and in women where exercise testing alone is considered less accurate. Despite an increased risk in false-positive exercise ECG test results in women [35,36], data are currently insufficient to recommend initial evaluation with stress imaging in women [1].

Stress echocardiography is sensitive and specific for the diagnosis of CAD in patients with intermediate to high pretest probability (Table 8.9) [1, 17, 18]. Using coronary angiography as the gold standard, exercise echocardiography has a weighted mean sensitivity of 86%, specificity of 81% and overall accuracy of 85% (Table 8.10) [1, 37–48]. With dobutamine stress echocardiography, the sensitivity, specificity and overall accuracy are 82, 84, 83% (Table 8.11) [1, 24, 37, 43–60], respectively. Sensitivity is higher for patients with multivessel disease, severe stenosis (≥70%) and prior infarction [24, 37–41, 45, 51–60]. Sensitivity and specificity are comparable in men and women [1]. The sensitivity can be diminished if all myocardial segments are not adequately visualized [37]. Visualization can be improved with contrast echocardiography. Alternatively, dobutamine with transesophageal echocardiography [61, 62] can be used.

Stress echocardiography should not be used to screen asymptomatic patients because in these patients who have a low likelihood for coronary artery disease, positive stress echocardiography results are often false positives [1]. However, patients who may have false-positive treadmill exercise tests could benefit from referral to stress echocardiography for further risk stratification.

Risk Stratification and Prognosis in Chronic Heart Disease

The presence and absence of inducible ischemia provide useful prognostic data, independent of clinical and exercise data in predicting cardiac events in men and women. Although data are not as extensive compared to radionuclide imaging, studies have shown that a negative stress echocardiogram denotes a low risk of adverse cardiovascular events during follow-up (Table 8.12) [55, 58, 63–70]. A re-

Table 8.9 Noninvasive risk stratification

High risk (greater than 3% mortality)
Severe resting LV dysfunction (LVEF less than 35%)
High-risk treadmill score (score −11 or less)
Severe exercise LV dysfunction (exercise LVEF less than 35%)
Wall motion abnormality (involving more than two segments) developing at low-dose dobutamine (10 mcg/kg/min or less) or at a low heart rate (less than 120 bpm)
Stress echocardiogram evidence of extensive ischemia (wall motion score index greater than 1)
Intermediate risk (1–3% annual mortality)
Mild-to-moderate resting LV dysfunction (LVEF 35–45%)
Intermediate-risk treadmill score (−11 to 5)
Limited stress echocardiographic ischemia with wall motion abnormality only at higher doses of dobutamine involving less than or equal to two segments
Low risk (less than 1% annual mortality)
Low-risk treadmill score (score 5 or greater)
Normal stress echocardiographic wall motion or no new wall motion abnormalities with stress

Table 8.10 Diagnostic accuracy of exercise echocardiography in detecting angiographically proven CAD (without correction for referral bias)

Author/Ref		Exercise	CAD (%)	Sens (%)	Spec (%)	PPV (%)	NPV (%)	Overall accuracy (%)
Marwick [37]	1994	BE	>50	91	80	89	77	85
Roger [47]	1994	TME	≥50	91	–	–	–	–
Marangelli [46]	1994	TME	≥75	89	91	93	86	90
Beleslin [44]	1994	TME	≥50	88	82	97	50	88
Williams [38]	1994	UBE	>50	88	84	83	89	86
Roger [45]	1995	TME	≥50	88	72	93	60	–
Dagianti [43]	1995	SBE	>70	76	94	90	85	87
Marwick [37]	1995	TME or UBE	≥50	80	81	71	91	81
Bjornstad [48]	1995	UBE	≥50	84	67	93	44	81
Marwick [37]	1995	TME	>50	71	91	85	81	82
Tawa [39]	1996	TME	>70	94	83	94	83	91
Luotolahti [40]	1996	UBE	≥50	94	70	97	50	92
Tian [41]	1996	TME	>50	88	93	97	76	89
Roger [42]	1997	TME	≥50	78	41	79	40	69

Exercise: bicycle (BE), treadmill exercise (TME), supine bicycle ergometry (SBE), upright bicycle ergometry (UBE); Sens: sensitivity; Spec: specificity; PPV: positive predictive value; NPV: negative predictive value.

Adapted from Cheitlin et al. [1], with permission of Elsevier.

Table 8.11 Diagnostic accuracy of dobutamine stress echocardiography in detecting angiographically proven CAD (without correction for referral bias)

Author/Ref	Year	Protocol	CAD (%)	Sens (%)	Spec (%)	PPV (%)	NPV (%)	Overall accuracy (%)
Ostojic [51]	1994	DSE	≥50	75	79	96	31	75
Marwick [37]	1994	DSE	>50	54	83	86	49	64
Beleslin [44]	1994	DSE	≥50	82	76	96	38	82
Sharp [52]	1994	DSE	≥50	83	71	89	59	80
Pellikka [45]	1995	DSE	≥50	98	65	84	94	87
Ho [50]	1995	DSE	≥50	93	73	93	73	89
Daoud [49]	1995	DSE	≥50	92	73	95	62	89
Dagianti [43]	1995	DSE	≥50	72	97	95	83	87
Pingitore [53]	1996	DSE	≥50	84	89	97	52	85
Schroder [54]	1996	DSE	≥50	76	88	97	44	78
Anthopoulos [55]	1996	DSE	≥50	87	84	94	68	86
Ling [56]	1996	DSE	≥50	93	62	95	54	90
Takeuchi [60]	1996	DSE	≥50	75	92	79	90	87
Minardi [24]	1997	DSE	≥50	75	67	97	15	74
Dionisopoulos [57]	1997	DSE	≥50	87	89	95	71	87
Elhendy [58]	1997	DSE	≥50	74	85	94	50	76
Ho [59]	1998	DSE	≥50	93	82	87	90	88

Adapted from Cheitlin et al. [1], with permission of Elsevier.

cent study [71] of 1325 patients who had normal exercise echocardiograms, the event-free survival rate was 99.2% at 1 year, 97.8% at 2 years and 97.4% at 3 years. In contrast, patients with a positive stress test have a higher risk of morbidity and mortality [66, 72, 73]. The overall event rates, however, are more variable.

Assessment Before and After Revascularization

Stress echocardiography can be used to demonstrate the functional significance of a lesion [1]. If the degree of angiographic stenosis is moderate or uncertain, stress echocardiography can help determine whether the lesion has functional significance and whether the patient would benefit from PCI [74]. Although not indicated for routine testing post-PCI, stress echocardiography could be used to assess restenosis in patients with recent PCI who present with recurrent symptoms [1].

As mentioned previously, dobutamine echocardiography can be used to identify patients with hibernating myocardium that would benefit from revascularization (Table 8.13) [16, 75–83]. The negative and positive predictive value of low-dose dobutamine is approximately 80% [1].

Preoperative Evaluation

Exercise stress testing is recommended for initial preoperative evaluation because it can provide information on functional capacity and myocardial ischemia. For patients with baseline ECG abnormalities, either echocardiography or radionuclide imaging is indicated. Although either exercise or dobutamine echocardiography is indicated for preoperative evaluation, the majority of studies [58, 84–97] have used dobutamine (Table 8.14) [58, 84–97]. The positive predictive value for MI or death ranged from 7 to 25% with negative predictive values ranging from 93 to 100%. The

Table 8.12 Prognostic value of stress echocardiography in various patient populations

Author	Year	Stress	Events	Annualized event rate		
				Ischemia (%)	No ischemia (%)	Normal
Afridi [63]	1994	DSE	D, MI	48	8.9	3
Poldermans [58]	1994	DSE	D, MI	6.6	3.4	–
Kamaran [67]	1995	DSE	D, MI	69	1	–
Williams [70]	1996	DSE	D, MI, Re	32.6	7.3	–
Anthopoulous [55]	1996	DSE	D, MI	13.6	0	–
Marcovitz [68]	1996	DSE	D, MI	12.8	8.2	1.1
Heupler [66]	1997	TME	D, MI, Re	9.2	1.3	–
McCully [69]	1998	TME	D, MI	–	–	0.5
Chuah [64]	1998	DSE	D, MI	6.9	6.3	1.9
Davar [65]	1999	DSE	D, MI	–	–	0

Stress: treadmill exercise (TME), bicycle exercise (BE), dobutamine–atropine (DASE), dobutamine (DSE);

Events: death (D), myocardial infarction (MI), revascularization (Re).

Adapted from Cheitlin et al. [1], with permission of Elsevier.

Table 8.13 Myocardial viability: detection of hibernating myocardium by DSE in patients with chronic CAD and LV dysfunction

Author/Ref	Year	Stress	Criteria	Sens. (%)	Spec. (%)	PPV (%)	NPV (%)	Overall accuracy (%)
Iliceto [79]	1996	LD-DSE	Imp Wm	71	88	73	87	83
Varga [83]	1996	LD-DSE	Imp Wm	74	94	93	78	84
Baer [75]	1996	LD-DSE	Imp Wm	92	88	92	88	90
Vanoverschelde [78]	1996	LD-DSE	Imp Wm	88	77	84	82	84
Gerber [78]	1996	LD-DSE	Imp Wm	71	87	89	65	77
Bax [76]	1996	LD-DSE	Imp Wm	85	63	49	91	70
Perrone-Filardi [81]	1996	LD-DSE	Imp Wm	79	83	92	65	81
Qureshi [82]	1997	LD-DSE	Imp Wm	86	68	51	92	73
Quershi [82]	1997	DSE	Biphasic resp	74	89	72	89	85
Naguch [80]	1997	LD-DSE	Imp Wm	91	66	61	93	75
Naguch [80]	1997	DSE	Biphasic resp	68	83	70	82	77
Furukawa [77]	1997	LD-DSE	Imp Wm	79	72	76	75	76
Cornel [16]	1997	LD-DSE	Imp Wm	89	82	74	93	85

Adapted from Cheitlin et al. [1], with permission of Elsevier.

presence of a new worsening extensive wall motion abnormalities, especially at low ischemic thresholds, is predictive of short- and long-term outcomes [1].

Valvular Disease

In addition to evaluation of coronary artery disease, stress echocardiography has prognostic utility in the evaluation of valvular stenosis in specific patient subsets.

Mitral Stenosis

A conclusive diagnosis can be obtained by resting 2D echocardiography and Doppler evaluation in the majority of patients with mitral stenosis. In patients with unexplained symptoms but mild-to-moderate mitral stenosis, a Doppler evaluation with either exercise or dobutamine should be performed for further evaluation (Class IIa) [1]. In mitral valve stenosis, the increase in heart rate associated with stress increases the transmitral gradient and pulmonary pressures (estimated from the tricuspid regurgitation jet), resulting in symptoms. The degree of symptoms correlates with the degree of pulmonary hypertension which can be measured by Doppler hemodynamics.

In a study [98] of 60 patients with mitral stenosis using Doppler echocardiography, exercise increased maximum and mean transmitral gradients and tricuspid regurgitation velocity (i.e., pulmonary artery systolic pressure), thus, providing further evaluation of the functional significance of mitral stenosis. Patients with increases in transmitral gradient and pulmonary artery pressure with exercise had worse prognosis. Similarly, dobutamine echocardiography provides valuable prognostic information. A recent study [99] has suggested that patients who develop

Table 8.14 Preoperative risk assessment using dobutamine echocardiography

Author/Ref	Year	n	Pts with ischemia (%)	Events (MI or death) (%)	Criteria for abnormal test	PPV (%)	NPV (%)
Lane [92]	1991	38	50	8	New WMA	16	100
Lalka [91]	1992	60	50	15	New or worsening WMA	23	93
Eichelberger [89]	1993	75	36	2	New or worsening WMA	7	100
Langan [93]	1993	74	24	3	New WMA or ECG changes	17	100
Poldermans [58]	1993	131	27	5	New or worsening WMA	14	100
Davila-Roman [88]	1993	88	23	2	New or worsening WMA	10	100
Poldermans [58]	1995	302	24	6	New or worsening WMA	24	100
Shafriz [96]	1997	42	0	1	New or worsening WMA	n/a	97
Plotkin [95]	1998	80	8	2	New or worsening WMA, ECG changes and/or chest pain or dypsnea	33	100
Ballal [84]	1999	233	17	7	New or worsening WMA	0	96
Bossone [86]	1999	46	9	1	New or worsening WMA	25	100
Das [87]	2000	530	40	32	New or worsening WMA or failure to develop hypodynamic function	15	100
Boersma [85]	1097	1097	20	4	New or worsening WMA	4	98
Morgan [94]	2002	78	5	0	Undefined	0	100
Torres [97]	2002	105	47	10	New or worsening WMA	18	98
Labib [90]	2004	429	7	2	New or worsening WMA	9	98

Adapted from Fleisher et al. [105], with permission of Elsevier.

a mean diastolic gradient of ≥ 18 mmHg during dobutamine stress are at increased risk for clinical events including hospitalization, intervention, arrhythmia and death. DSE, therefore, may provide additional prognostic information and identify those patients who would benefit from intervention. Consistent with these findings, in a study [100] of 44 patients with mitral stenosis, those with a mean mitral gradient ≥ 15 mmHg and pulmonary artery pressure > 60 mmHg with dobutamine stress had a rapid evolution of disease after 24 months.

Thus, patients with mild MS (MVA < 1.5 cm^2) who are symptomatic with a significant elevation of pulmonary artery pressure (> 60 mmHg), mean transmitral gradient (>15 mmHg) or mean pulmonary wedge pressure (≥25 mmHg) have significant mitral stenosis and should be referred for surgical intervention [101].

Aortic Stenosis

Like mitral stenosis, 2D and Doppler echocardiography provide complete evaluation of aortic stenosis in most patients. In patients with low gradient AS (defined as transaortic pressure <30 mmHg, reduced LV function and low cardiac output), dobutamine echocardiography may be indicated for further evaluation [101]. Dobutamine echocardiography is used to differentiate patients with true fixed, severe aortic stenosis from functional AS (pseudo-AS). Although patients with pseudo-AS have thickened valves, the effective orifice area is small because of a reduced stroke volume. Dobutamine increases cardiac output which opens the valve wider without increasing the transvalvular gradient. In contrast, in patients with true, fixed severe AS, during dobutamine infusion, the valve does not open wider and the transvalvular gradient increases. A comparison of the gradient change before and after dobutamine differentiates pseudo-AS (i.e., no gradient change) from true AS (i.e., gradient increases). Patients with pseudo-AS usually have mild-to-moderate AS and do not benefit from valvular surgery. Their symptoms are primarily due to LV dysfunction and not aortic stenosis, and they should receive management for cardiomyopathy.

Dobutamine echocardiography has been used to determine whether the LV dysfunction is due to the aortic valve stenosis (failed compensatory LV hypertrophy to an increase in afterload) or due to LV contractile dysfunction secondary to other processes. Patients whose LV dysfunction is primarily due to AS will have LV contractile reserve, defined as an increase in peak velocity (>0.6 m/s), stroke volume (>20%) or mean transvalvular pressure gradient (>10 mmHg) with DSE [101]. Previous studies have shown that patients who have LV contractile reserve have a lower perioperative mortality than those without contractile reserve (approximately 6 versus 33%) [102,103]. If the patient survives the valvular surgery, however, those with and without contractile reserve had similar symptoms postoperatively (New York Heart Association functional class I or II in 93 versus 85%, respectively), (2) 2-year survival (92 versus 90%, respectively), (3) increase in LVEF (19 versus 17%, respectively) and (4) postoperative LVEF (47 versus 48%, respectively) [104]. Because the prognosis for these patients without surgery is poor, symptomatic patients with severe, low gradient AS should be referred to surgery and DSE is not needed to determine the presence or absence of contractile reserve [104].

Choice of Stress Echo or Nuclear Perfusion

The choice of either stress or nuclear testing should be based on the expertise of the local facility and the patient. To date, there are no large, well-controlled trials comparing stress echocardiography with nuclear perfusion. Table 8.15 details the advantages and disadvantages of stress echocardiography versus nuclear

Table 8.15 Comparison of stress echo and nuclear myocardial perfusion

	Stress echo	Nuclear
Time of detection	Later than nuclear if detecting abnormal wall motion	Earliest marker of ischemia
Information additional to ischemia extent and LV size and function	Diastolic function Valvular function Filling pressures Assessment of pericardium Chamber sizes RV function	No additional information
Technical expertise	High technical expertise required for image acquisition	Moderate technical expertise required for image acquisition

myocardial perfusion. In general, the advantages of stress echocardiography are that it is less expensive, it does not expose the patient to radiation and can supply additional structural and functional information. Stress echocardiography, however, is highly dependent on the technical skills of the sonographer because images must be attained quickly once the patient achieves target heart rate. In contrast, the advantages of nuclear perfusion are that it can detect the earliest changes of ischemia and is less technically dependent. However, it does expose patients to radiation and is twice as costly. The sensitivities and specificities are similar, approximately 80–85%, respectively, depending on the study; however, a lower specificity is often reported with nuclear perfusion due to a higher rate of false positives secondary to interference from the breast or diaphragm. The choice of stressor agent is more dependent on patient characteristics than imaging modality. Both stress echocardiography and nuclear perfusion can be performed with exercise, dobutamine or vasodilators. In general, dobutamine stress is more commonly used with echocardiography and vasodilator stress is more commonly used with nuclear perfusion.

All patients who can exercise adequately should have an exercise stress echocardiogram with the exception of patients with LBBB or paced rhythms. In patients with native or ventricular pacemaker-induced LBBB, a false-positive stress test for ischemia in LAD distribution may occur irrespective of imaging technique if stress induction is performed with exercise or dobutamine. This may be avoided if a coronary vasodilator (dipyridamole or adenosine) is used for stress induction. It is generally agreed that dipyridamole or adenosine stress testing is the preferred stress test modality in patients with LBBB.

Obese patients are particularly challenging for both stress and nuclear imaging techniques. Excessive adipose tissue impairs access to adequate cardiac windows in echocardiography and may cause attenuation artifacts in nuclear scanning. In addition, patients who are morbidly obese may exceed the weight limit on the table (usually >300 lbs) and should be referred for stress echocardiography.

Patients with end-stage liver disease or bronchospastic disorders including asthma and COPD who cannot exercise should be referred for dobutamine stress testing. The ACC/AHA/ASNC guidelines [18] state that both adenosine and dipyridamole may exacerbate bronchospasm and should be used with extreme caution in these patients, if at all. Patients with end-stage liver disease often have preoperative risk assessment prior to orthotropic liver transplantation. The use of vasodilators in this group has been associated with poor positive predictive value because of decreased arteriolar resistance at baseline.

On the other hand, patients with uncontrolled systolic blood pressure at rest are at risk for severe hypertension during either exercise or dobutamine. These patients should be considered for vasodilator stress.

References

1. Cheitlin MD, Armstrong WF, Aurigemma GP, et al. ACC/AHA/ASE 2003 guideline update for the clinical application of echocardiography – summary article: a report of the American College of Cardiology/American Heart Association Task Force on Practice Guidelines (ACC/AHA/ASE Committee to Update the 1997 Guidelines for the Clinical Application of Echocardiography). J Am Coll Cardiol 2003; 42(5):954–70.
2. Gottdiener JS. Overview of stress echocardiography: uses, advantages, and limitations. Curr Probl Cardiol 2003;28(8):485–516.
3. Leong-Poi H, Rim SJ, Le DE, Fisher NG, Wei K, Kaul S. Perfusion versus function: the ischemic cascade in demand ischemia: implications of single-vessel versus multivessel stenosis. Circulation 2002;105(8):987–92.
4. Grover-McKay M, Matsuzaki M, Ross J, Jr. Dissociation between regional myocardial dysfunction and subendocardial ST segment elevation during and after exercise-induced ischemia in dogs. J Am Coll Cardiol 1987;10(5):1105–12.
5. Feigenbaum HA, W; Ryan, Thomas. Feigenbaum's Echocardiography. 6 ed: Lippincott Williams and Wilkins; 2005.
6. Higgins JP, Higgins JA. Electrocardiographic exercise stress testing: an update beyond the ST segment. Int J Cardiol 2007;116(3):285–99.
7. Oh J SJ, Tajik AJ. The Echo Manual Second ed: Lippincott, Williams and Wilkins; 1999.
8. San Roman JA, Vilacosta I, Castillo JA, et al. Selection of the optimal stress test for the diagnosis of coronary artery disease. Heart 1998;80(4):370–6.
9. Gligorova S, Agrusta M. Pacing stress echocardiography. Cardiovasc Ultrasound 2005;3:36.
10. Gibbons RJ, Balady GJ, Bricker JT, et al. ACC/AHA 2002 guideline update for exercise testing: summary article: a report of the American College of Cardiology/American Heart Association Task Force on Practice Guidelines (Committee to Update the 1997 Exercise Testing Guidelines). Circulation 2002;106(14):1883–92.
11. Grunig E, Janssen B, Mereles D, et al. Abnormal pulmonary artery pressure response in asymptomatic carriers of primary pulmonary hypertension gene. Circulation 2000;102(10):1145–50.
12. Cerqueira MD, Weissman NJ, Dilsizian V, et al. Standardized myocardial segmentation and nomenclature for tomographic imaging of the heart: a statement for healthcare professionals from the Cardiac Imaging Committee of the Council on Clinical Cardiology of the American Heart Association. Circulation 2002;105(4):539–42.
13. Moller JE, Hillis GS, Oh JK, Reeder GS, Gersh BJ, Pellikka PA. Wall motion score index and ejection fraction for risk stratification after acute myocardial infarction. Am Heart J 2006;151(2):419–25.

14. Yao SS, Shah A, Bangalore S, Chaudhry FA. Transient ischemic left ventricular cavity dilation is a significant predictor of severe and extensive coronary artery disease and adverse outcome in patients undergoing stress echocardiography. J Am Soc Echocardiogr 2007;20(4):352–8.

15. von Bibra H, Tuchnitz A, Klein A, Schneider-Eicke J, Schomig A, Schwaiger M. Regional diastolic function by pulsed Doppler myocardial mapping for the detection of left ventricular ischemia during pharmacologic stress testing: a comparison with stress echocardiography and perfusion scintigraphy. J Am Coll Cardiol 2000;36(2):444–52.

16. Bax JJ, Wijns W, Cornel JH, Visser FC, Boersma E, Fioretti PM. Accuracy of currently available techniques for prediction of functional recovery after revascularization in patients with left ventricular dysfunction due to chronic coronary artery disease: comparison of pooled data. J Am Coll Cardiol 1997;30(6):1451–60.

17. Anderson JL, Adams CD, Antman EM, et al. ACC/AHA 2007 guidelines for the management of patients with unstable angina/non-ST-Elevation myocardial infarction: a report of the American College of Cardiology/American Heart Association Task Force on Practice Guidelines (Writing Committee to Revise the 2002 Guidelines for the Management of Patients With Unstable Angina/Non-ST-Elevation Myocardial Infarction) developed in collaboration with the American College of Emergency Physicians, the Society for Cardiovascular Angiography and Interventions, and the Society of Thoracic Surgeons endorsed by the American Association of Cardiovascular and Pulmonary Rehabilitation and the Society for Academic Emergency Medicine. J Am Coll Cardiol 2007;50(7):e1–e157.

18. Sabia P, Abbott RD, Afrookteh A, Keller MW, Touchstone DA, Kaul S. Importance of two-dimensional echocardiographic assessment of left ventricular systolic function in patients presenting to the emergency room with cardiac-related symptoms. Circulation 1991;84(4):1615–24.

19. Klocke FJ, Baird MG, Lorell BH, et al. ACC/AHA/ASNC guidelines for the clinical use of cardiac radionuclide imaging – executive summary: a report of the American College of Cardiology/American Heart Association Task Force on Practice Guidelines (ACC/AHA/ASNC Committee to Revise the 1995 Guidelines for the Clinical Use of Cardiac Radionuclide Imaging). J Am Coll Cardiol 2003;42(7):1318–33.

20. Acampa W, Spinelli L, Petretta M, Salvatore M, Cuocolo A. Comparison of prognostic value of negative dobutamine stress echocardiography versus single-photon emission computed tomography after acute myocardial infarction. Am J Cardiol 2005;96(1):13–6.

21. Applegate RJ, Dell'Italia LJ, Crawford MH. Usefulness of two-dimensional echocardiography during low-level exercise testing early after uncomplicated acute myocardial infarction. Am J Cardiol 1987;60(1):10–4.

22. Carlos ME, Smart SC, Wynsen JC, Sagar KB. Dobutamine stress echocardiography for risk stratification after myocardial infarction. Circulation 1997;95(6):1402–10.

23. Greco CA, Salustri A, Seccareccia F, et al. Prognostic value of dobutamine echocardiography early after uncomplicated acute myocardial infarction: a comparison with exercise electrocardiography. J Am Coll Cardiol 1997;29(2):261–7.

24. Minardi G, Di Segni M, Manzara CC, et al. Diagnostic and prognostic value of dipyridamole and dobutamine stress echocardiography in patients with Q-wave acute myocardial infarction. Am J Cardiol 1997;80(7):847–51.

25. Previtali M, Fetiveau R, Lanzarini L, Cavalotti C, Klersy C. Prognostic value of myocardial viability and ischemia detected by dobutamine stress echocardiography early after acute myocardial infarction treated with thrombolysis. J Am Coll Cardiol 1998;32(2):380–6.

26. Quintana M, Lindvall K, Ryden L, Brolund F. Prognostic value of predischarge exercise stress echocardiography after acute myocardial infarction. Am J Cardiol 1995;76(16):1115–21.

27. Ryan T, Armstrong WF, O'Donnell JA, Feigenbaum H. Risk stratification after acute myocardial infarction by means of exercise two-dimensional echocardiography. Am Heart J 1987;114(6):1305–16.

28. Sicari R, Landi P, Picano E, et al. Exercise-electrocardiography and/or pharmacological stress echocardiography for non-invasive risk stratification early after uncomplicated

myocardial infarction. A prospective international large scale multicentre study. Eur Heart J 2002;23(13):1030–7.

29. Sicari R, Picano E, Landi P, et al. Prognostic value of dobutamine–atropine stress echocardiography early after acute myocardial infarction. Echo Dobutamine International Cooperative (EDIC) Study. J Am Coll Cardiol 1997;29(2):254–60.

30. Picano E, Pingitore A, Sicari R, et al. Stress echocardiographic results predict risk of reinfarction early after uncomplicated acute myocardial infarction: large-scale multicenter study. Echo Persantine International Cooperative (EPIC) Study Group. J Am Coll Cardiol 1995;26(4): 908–13.

31. Previtali M, Poli A, Lanzarini L, Fetiveau R, Mussini A, Ferrario M. Dobutamine stress echocardiography for assessment of myocardial viability and ischemia in acute myocardial infarction treated with thrombolysis. Am J Cardiol 1993;72(19):124G–30G.

32. Orlandini AD, Tuero EI, Diaz R, Vilamajo OA, Paolasso EA. Acute cardiac rupture during dobutamine–atropine echocardiography stress test. J Am Soc Echocardiogr 2000;13(2): 152–3.

33. Garber AM, Solomon NA. Cost-effectiveness of alternative test strategies for the diagnosis of coronary artery disease. Ann Intern Med 1999;130(9):719–28.

34. Kuntz KM, Fleischmann KE, Hunink MG, Douglas PS. Cost-effectiveness of diagnostic strategies for patients with chest pain. Ann Intern Med 1999;130(9):709–18.

35. Wong Y, Rodwell A, Dawkins S, Livesey SA, Simpson IA. Sex differences in investigation results and treatment in subjects referred for investigation of chest pain. Heart 2001;85(2): 149–52.

36. Sketch MH, Mohiuddin SM, Lynch JD, Zencka AE, Runco V. Significant sex differences in the correlation of electrocardiographic exercise testing and coronary arteriograms. Am J Cardiol 1975;36(2):169–73.

37. Snader CE, Marwick TH, Pashkow FJ, Harvey SA, Thomas JD, Lauer MS. Importance of estimated functional capacity as a predictor of all-cause mortality among patients referred for exercise thallium single-photon emission computed tomography: report of 3,400 patients from a single center. J Am Coll Cardiol 1997;30(3):641–8.

38. Stratmann HG, Williams GA, Wittry MD, Chaitman BR, Miller DD. Exercise technetium-99m sestamibi tomography for cardiac risk stratification of patients with stable chest pain. Circulation 1994;89(2):615–22.

39. Tawa CB, Baker WB, Kleiman NS, Trakhtenbroit A, Desir R, Zoghbi WA. Comparison of adenosine echocardiography, with and without isometric handgrip, to exercise echocardiography in the detection of ischemia in patients with coronary artery disease. J Am Soc Echocardiogr 1996;9(1):33–43.

40. Luotolahti M, Saraste M, Hartiala J. Exercise echocardiography in the diagnosis of coronary artery disease. Ann Med 1996;28(1):73–7.

41. Tian J, Zhang G, Wang X, Cui J, Xiao J. Exercise echocardiography: feasibility and value for detection of coronary artery disease. Chin Med J (Engl) 1996;109(5):381–4.

42. Roger VL, Pellikka PA, Bell MR, Chow CW, Bailey KR, Seward JB. Sex and test verification bias. Impact on the diagnostic value of exercise echocardiography. Circulation 1997;95(2):405–10.

43. Dagianti A, Penco M, Agati L, et al. Stress echocardiography: comparison of exercise, dipyridamole and dobutamine in detecting and predicting the extent of coronary artery disease. J Am Coll Cardiol 1995;26(1):18–25.

44. Beleslin BD, Ostojic M, Stepanovic J, et al. Stress echocardiography in the detection of myocardial ischemia. Head-to-head comparison of exercise, dobutamine, and dipyridamole tests. Circulation 1994;90(3):1168–76.

45. Roger VL, Pellikka PA, Oh JK, Miller FA, Seward JB, Tajik AJ. Stress echocardiography. Part I. Exercise echocardiography: techniques, implementation, clinical applications, and correlations. Mayo Clin Proc 1995;70(1):5–15.

46. Marangelli V, Iliceto S, Piccinni G, De Martino G, Sorgente L, Rizzon P. Detection of coronary artery disease by digital stress echocardiography: comparison of exercise, transesophageal atrial pacing and dipyridamole echocardiography. J Am Coll Cardiol 1994;24(1):117–24.

47. Roger VL, Pellikka PA, Oh JK, Bailey KR, Tajik AJ. Identification of multivessel coronary artery disease by exercise echocardiography. J Am Coll Cardiol 1994;24(1):109–14.

48. Bjornstad K, Aakhus S, Hatle L. Comparison of digital dipyridamole stress echocardiography and upright bicycle stress echocardiography for identification of coronary artery stenosis. Cardiology 1995;86(6):514–20.

49. Daoud EG, Pitt A, Armstrong WF. Electrocardiographic response during dobutamine stress echocardiography. Am Heart J 1995;129(4):672–7.

50. Ho FM, Huang PJ, Liau CS, et al. Dobutamine stress echocardiography compared with dipyridamole thallium-201 single-photon emission computed tomography in detecting coronary artery disease. Eur Heart J 1995;16(4):570–5.

51. Ostojic M, Picano E, Beleslin B, et al. Dipyridamole-dobutamine echocardiography: a novel test for the detection of milder forms of coronary artery disease. J Am Coll Cardiol 1994;23(5):1115–22.

52. Sharp SM, Sawada SG, Segar DS, et al. Dobutamine stress echocardiography: detection of coronary artery disease in patients with dilated cardiomyopathy. J Am Coll Cardiol 1994;24(4):934–9.

53. Pingitore A, Picano E, Colosso MQ, et al. The atropine factor in pharmacologic stress echocardiography. Echo Persantine (EPIC) and Echo Dobutamine International Cooperative (EDIC) Study Groups. J Am Coll Cardiol 1996;27(5):1164–70.

54. Schroder K, Voller H, Dingerkus H, et al. Comparison of the diagnostic potential of four echocardiographic stress tests shortly after acute myocardial infarction: submaximal exercise, transesophageal atrial pacing, dipyridamole, and dobutamine–atropine. Am J Cardiol 1996;77(11):909–14.

55. Anthopoulos LP, Bonou MS, Kardaras FG, et al. Stress echocardiography in elderly patients with coronary artery disease: applicability, safety and prognostic value of dobutamine and adenosine echocardiography in elderly patients. J Am Coll Cardiol 1996;28(1):52–9.

56. Bax JJ, Visser FC, van Lingen A, Visser CA, Teule GJ. Myocardial F-18 fluorodeoxyglucose imaging by SPECT. Clin Nucl Med 1995;20(6):486–90.

57. Dionisopoulos PN, Collins JD, Smart SC, Knickelbine TA, Sagar KB. The value of dobutamine stress echocardiography for the detection of coronary artery disease in women. J Am Soc Echocardiogr 1997;10(8):811–7.

58. Elhendy A, van Domburg RT, Sozzi FB, Poldermans D, Bax JJ, Roelandt JR. Impact of hypertension on the accuracy of exercise stress myocardial perfusion imaging for the diagnosis of coronary artery disease. Heart 2001;85(6):655–61.

59. Ho YL, Wu CC, Huang PJ, et al. Assessment of coronary artery disease in women by dobutamine stress echocardiography: comparison with stress thallium-201 single-photon emission computed tomography and exercise electrocardiography. Am Heart J 1998;135(4): 655–62.

60. Yamagishi H, Akioka K, Hirata K, et al. A reverse flow-metabolism mismatch pattern on PET is related to multivessel disease in patients with acute myocardial infarction. J Nucl Med 1999;40(9):1492–8.

61. Prince CR, Stoddard MF, Morris GT, et al. Dobutamine two-dimensional transesophageal echocardiographic stress testing for detection of coronary artery disease. Am Heart J 1994;128(1):36–41.

62. Laurienzo JM, Cannon RO, 3rd, Quyyumi AA, Dilsizian V, Panza JA. Improved specificity of transesophageal dobutamine stress echocardiography compared to standard tests for evaluation of coronary artery disease in women presenting with chest pain. Am J Cardiol 1997;80(11):1402–7.

63. Afridi I, Quinones MA, Zoghbi WA, Cheirif J. Dobutamine stress echocardiography: sensitivity, specificity, and predictive value for future cardiac events. Am Heart J 1994;127(6):1510–5.

64. Chuah SC, Pellikka PA, Roger VL, McCully RB, Seward JB. Role of dobutamine stress echocardiography in predicting outcome in 860 patients with known or suspected coronary artery disease. Circulation 1998;97(15):1474–80.
65. Davar JI, Brull DJ, Bulugahipitiya S, Coghlan JG, Lipkin DP, Evans TR. Prognostic value of negative dobutamine stress echo in women with intermediate probability of coronary artery disease. Am J Cardiol 1999;83(1):100–2, A8.
66. Heupler S, Mehta R, Lobo A, Leung D, Marwick TH. Prognostic implications of exercise echocardiography in women with known or suspected coronary artery disease. J Am Coll Cardiol 1997;30(2):414–20.
67. Kamaran M, Teague SM, Finkelhor RS, Dawson N, Bahler RC. Prognostic value of dobutamine stress echocardiography in patients referred because of suspected coronary artery disease. Am J Cardiol 1995;76(12):887–91.
68. Marcovitz PA, Shayna V, Horn RA, Hepner A, Armstrong WF. Value of dobutamine stress echocardiography in determining the prognosis of patients with known or suspected coronary artery disease. Am J Cardiol 1996;78(4):404–8.
69. McCully RB, Roger VL, Mahoney DW, et al. Outcome after normal exercise echocardiography and predictors of subsequent cardiac events: follow-up of 1,325 patients. J Am Coll Cardiol 1998;31(1):144–9.
70. Williams MJ, Odabashian J, Lauer MS, Thomas JD, Marwick TH. Prognostic value of dobutamine echocardiography in patients with left ventricular dysfunction. J Am Coll Cardiol 1996;27(1):132–9.
71. Chung G, Krishnamani R, Senior R. Prognostic value of normal stress echocardiogram in patients with suspected coronary artery disease – a British general hospital experience. Int J Cardiol 2004;94(2–3):181–6.
72. Gambhir SS, Schwaiger M, Huang SC, et al. Simple noninvasive quantification method for measuring myocardial glucose utilization in humans employing positron emission tomography and fluorine-18 deoxyglucose. J Nucl Med 1989;30(3):359–66.
73. Sawada SG, Ryan T, Conley MJ, Corya BC, Feigenbaum H, Armstrong WF. Prognostic value of a normal exercise echocardiogram. Am Heart J 1990;120(1):49–55.
74. McNeill AJ, Fioretti PM, el-Said SM, Salustri A, de Feyter PJ, Roelandt JR. Dobutamine stress echocardiography before and after coronary angioplasty. Am J Cardiol 1992;69(8):740–5.
75. Baer FM, Voth E, Deutsch HJ, et al. Predictive value of low dose dobutamine transesophageal echocardiography and fluorine-18 fluorodeoxyglucose positron emission tomography for recovery of regional left ventricular function after successful revascularization. J Am Coll Cardiol 1996;28(1):60–9.
76. Bax JJ, Cornel JH, Visser FC, et al. Prediction of recovery of myocardial dysfunction after revascularization. Comparison of fluorine-18 fluorodeoxyglucose/thallium-201 SPECT, thallium-201 stress-reinjection SPECT and dobutamine echocardiography. J Am Coll Cardiol 1996;28(3):558–64.
77. Furukawa T, Haque T, Takahashi M, Kinoshita M. An assessment of dobutamine echocardiography and end-diastolic wall thickness for predicting post-revascularization functional recovery in patients with chronic coronary artery disease. Eur Heart J 1997;18(5): 798–806.
78. Gerber BL, Ordoubadi FF, Wijns W, et al. Positron emission tomography using(18)F-fluoro-deoxyglucose and euglycaemic hyperinsulinaemic glucose clamp: optimal criteria for the prediction of recovery of post-ischaemic left ventricular dysfunction. Results from the European Community Concerted Action Multicenter study on use of(18)F-fluoro-deoxyglucose Positron Emission Tomography for the Detection of Myocardial Viability. Eur Heart J 2001;22(18):1691–701.
79. Iliceto S, Galiuto L, Marchese A, et al. Analysis of microvascular integrity, contractile reserve, and myocardial viability after acute myocardial infarction by dobutamine echocardiography and myocardial contrast echocardiography. Am J Cardiol 1996;77(7):441–5.

80. Nagueh SF, Vaduganathan P, Ali N, et al. Identification of hibernating myocardium: comparative accuracy of myocardial contrast echocardiography, rest-redistribution thallium-201 tomography and dobutamine echocardiography. J Am Coll Cardiol 1997;29(5):985–93.

81. Perrone-Filardi P, Pace L, Prastaro M, et al. Assessment of myocardial viability in patients with chronic coronary artery disease. Rest-4-hour-24-hour 201Tl tomography versus dobutamine echocardiography. Circulation 1996;94(11):2712–9.

82. Qureshi U, Nagueh SF, Afridi I, et al. Dobutamine echocardiography and quantitative rest-redistribution 201Tl tomography in myocardial hibernation. Relation of contractile reserve to 201Tl uptake and comparative prediction of recovery of function. Circulation 1997;95(3): 626–35.

83. Varga A, Ostojic M, Djordjevic-Dikic A, et al. Infra-low dose dipyridamole test. A novel dose regimen for selective assessment of myocardial viability by vasodilator stress echocardiography. Eur Heart J 1996;17(4):629–34.

84. Ballal RS, Kapadia S, Secknus MA, Rubin D, Arheart K, Marwick TH. Prognosis of patients with vascular disease after clinical evaluation and dobutamine stress echocardiography. Am Heart J 1999;137(3):469–75.

85. Boersma E, Poldermans D, Bax JJ, et al. Predictors of cardiac events after major vascular surgery: Role of clinical characteristics, dobutamine echocardiography, and beta-blocker therapy. JAMA 2001;285(14):1865–73.

86. Bossone E, Martinez FJ, Whyte RI, Iannettoni MD, Armstrong WF, Bach DS. Dobutamine stress echocardiography for the preoperative evaluation of patients undergoing lung volume reduction surgery. J Thorac Cardiovasc Surg 1999;118(3):542–6.

87. Das MK, Pellikka PA, Mahoney DW, et al. Assessment of cardiac risk before nonvascular surgery: dobutamine stress echocardiography in 530 patients. J Am Coll Cardiol 2000;35(6):1647–53.

88. Davila-Roman VG, Waggoner AD, Sicard GA, Geltman EM, Schechtman KB, Perez JE. Dobutamine stress echocardiography predicts surgical outcome in patients with an aortic aneurysm and peripheral vascular disease. J Am Coll Cardiol 1993;21(4):957–63.

89. Eichelberger JP SK, Black ER, Green RM, Ouriel K. Predictive value of dobutamine echocardiography just before noncardiac vascular surgery. Am J Cardiol 1993;72(7):602–7.

90. Labib SB, Goldstein M, Kinnunen PM, Schick EC. Cardiac events in patients with negative maximal versus negative submaximal dobutamine echocardiograms undergoing noncardiac surgery: importance of resting wall motion abnormalities. J Am Coll Cardiol 2004;44(1): 82–7.

91. Lalka SG SS, Dalsing MC, Cikrit DF, Sawchuk AP, Kovacs RL, Segar DS, Ryan T, Feigenbaum H. Dobutamine stress echocardiography as a predictor of cardiac events associated with aortic surgery. J Vasc Surg 1992;15(5):831–40.

92. Lane RT, Sawada SG, Segar DS, et al. Dobutamine stress echocardiography for assessment of cardiac risk before noncardiac surgery. Am J Cardiol 1991;68(9):976–7.

93. Langan EM, 3rd, Youkey JR, Franklin DP, Elmore JR, Costello JM, Nassef LA. Dobutamine stress echocardiography for cardiac risk assessment before aortic surgery. J Vasc Surg 1993;18(6):905–11; discussion 12–3.

94. Morgan PB, Panomitros GE, Nelson AC, Smith DF, Solanki DR, Zornow MH. Low utility of dobutamine stress echocardiograms in the preoperative evaluation of patients scheduled for noncardiac surgery. Anesth Analg 2002;95(3):512–6, table of contents.

95. Plotkin JS, Benitez RM, Kuo PC, et al. Dobutamine stress echocardiography for preoperative cardiac risk stratification in patients undergoing orthotopic liver transplantation. Liver Transpl Surg 1998;4(4):253–7.

96. Shafritz R, Ciocca RG, Gosin JS, Shindler DM, Doshi M, Graham AM. The utility of dobutamine echocardiography in preoperative evaluation for elective aortic surgery. Am J Surg 1997;174(2):121–5.

97. Torres MR, Short L, Baglin T, Case C, Gibbs H, Marwick TH. Usefulness of clinical risk markers and ischemic threshold to stratify risk in patients undergoing major noncardiac surgery. Am J Cardiol 2002;90(3):238–42.

98. Cheriex EC, Pieters FA, Janssen JH, de Swart H, Palmans-Meulemans A. Value of exercise Doppler-echocardiography in patients with mitral stenosis. Int J Cardiol 1994;45(3):219–26.
99. Reis G, Motta MS, Barbosa MM, Esteves WA, Souza SF, Bocchi EA. Dobutamine stress echocardiography for noninvasive assessment and risk stratification of patients with rheumatic mitral stenosis. J Am Coll Cardiol 2004;43(3):393–401.
100. Chirio C, Anselmino M, Mangiardi L, et al. Is dobutamine stress echocardiography predictive of middle and late term outcomes in mitral stenosis patients? Minerva Cardioangiol 2007;55(3):317–23.
101. Mazzotta G, Bonow RO, Pace L, Brittain E, Epstein SE. Relation between exertional ischemia and prognosis in mildly symptomatic patients with single or double vessel coronary artery disease and left ventricular dysfunction at rest. J Am Coll Cardiol 1989;13(3):567–73.
102. Quere JP, Monin JL, Levy F, et al. Influence of preoperative left ventricular contractile reserve on postoperative ejection fraction in low-gradient aortic stenosis. Circulation 2006;113(14):1738–44.
103. Monin JL, Quere JP, Monchi M, et al. Low-gradient aortic stenosis: operative risk stratification and predictors for long-term outcome: a multicenter study using dobutamine stress hemodynamics. Circulation 2003;108(3):319–24.
104. Lange RA, Hillis LD. Dobutamine stress echocardiography in patients with low-gradient aortic stenosis. Circulation 2006;113(14):1718–20.
105. Fleisher LA, Beckman JA, Brown KA, Calkins H, Chaikof E, Fleischmann KE, Freeman WK, Froehlich JB, Kasper EK, Kersten JR, Riegel B, Robb JF, Smith SC, Jacobs AK, Adams CD, Anderson JL, Antman EM, Buller CE, Creager MA, Ettinger SM, Faxon DP, Fuster V, Halperin JL, Hiratzka LF, Hunt SA, Lytle BW, Nishimura R, Ornato JP, Page RL, Riegel B, Lynn G. ACC/AHA 2007 guidelines on perioperative cardiovascular evaluation and care for noncardiac surgery: A report of the American College of Cardiology/American Heart Association Task Force on practice guidelines. J Am Coll Cardiol 2007;50(17):1707–322.
106. Mayo Clinic Cardiovascular Working Group on Stress Testing. Cardiovascular stress testing: a description of the various types of stress tests and indications for their use. Mayo Clin Proc 1996;71(1):43–52.

Chapter 9
Stratifying Symptomatic Patients Using the Exercise Test and Other Tools

Russell D. White and Nora Goldschlager

Risk stratification of patients with chest pain occurs daily by physicians in the primary care setting. When patients present in the office with recent or new-onset chest pain, the physician must determine the appropriate evaluation. Does this pain represent coronary artery disease or is the pain due to some other cause? When a patient with pre-existing risk factors for coronary artery disease presents with typical angina symptoms, the physician must recommend appropriate evaluation. Finally, how does one manage the patient in the emergency department with chest pain? All of these clinical situations presenting to the primary care physician require assessment through the performance of specific evaluations in the proper setting and time period. Some patients can be evaluated over hours or days. Other patients require immediate consultation with a cardiologist.

This chapter first reviews the concept of risk stratification, definitions of coronary disease and looks at multiple stratification tools. Second, these tools are discussed as they are applied to stratifying patients with chest pain. The final section presents multiple case studies illustrating the use of these tools in the approach to the patient with chest pain.

Risk stratification involves determining the likelihood of coronary artery disease being present (diagnosis) and the future risk of cardiac events for the patient (prognosis). This process may require careful objective testing while at other times subjective intuitive evaluation based on experience and statistical data occurs. When a 62-year-old man with multiple cardiac risk factors (positive family history of coronary artery disease, personal history of smoking, hypertension, type 2 diabetes mellitus and hyperlipidemia) presents with a pressure discomfort in the anterior chest precipitated by exertion and relieved with rest, one promptly places this patient at a high likelihood for coronary artery disease. This immediate determination from the history that coronary artery disease is probably present occurs *before* the patient is examined and with no objective test results. Other clinical presentations may require thorough evaluation and testing for subsequent risk stratification.

R.D. White (✉)
Department of Community and Family Medicine, University of Missouri—Kansas City, Truman Medical Center Lakewood, 7900 Lee's Summit Road, Kansas City, MO 64139, USA
e-mail: Russell.White@tmcmed.org

C.H. Evans, R.D. White (eds.), *Exercise Testing for Primary Care and Sports Medicine Physicians,* DOI 10.1007/978-0-387-76597-6_9

Most risk stratification systems utilize a composite of different factors for predicting the presence of coronary artery disease (CAD). These factors include patient age, sex, presenting symptoms, personal history of cardiac risk factors, family history of premature coronary artery disease (defined as infarction, angioplasty, bypass or sudden death in a first-degree relative <55 years for males and <65 years for females), baseline electrocardiogram (ECG) abnormalities (such as previous infarction), ST-segment abnormalities developing with exercise, duration of treadmill exercise time or metabolic equivalents (METs) of work and angina occurring during the exercise test [1–9]. In the primary care setting risk stratification begins with a methodical history and physical examination. Exercise stress testing is one clinical method utilized in completing the risk stratification process and delineating further treatment and management.

Defining Coronary Artery Disease

Definitions

Risk stratification is done not only for the diagnosis but also for the prognosis or severity of the underlying heart disease. Likelihood is the probability of coronary artery disease relating to diagnosis and refers to the presence or absence of significant coronary artery disease. The clinical evaluation for coronary artery disease is based on demographics, cardiovascular history, risk factors, baseline electrocardiogram, chest film and physical examination [10] (Table 9.1).

Mark has defined *significant* coronary artery disease as the presence of at least one major coronary vessel with ≥70% diameter stenosis by angiography while *severe* coronary artery disease is three-vessel disease or left main disease [11]. There are variations on the angiographic definition of coronary artery disease. Froelicher's group has defined significant angiographic coronary artery disease as 70% narrowing of the left anterior descending, left circumflex, or right coronary arteries or their major branches, or a 50% narrowing in the left main coronary artery [6]. This variation in definition may affect the statistical analysis and subsequent correlation of data.

Risk Stratification

Likelihood (Diagnosis) and Risk (Prognosis)

The term risk is reserved for the prognosis (future threat of morbidity and mortality) due to underlying coronary artery disease [11]. When risk-stratifying a patient for coronary artery disease, one determines the likelihood or probability of coronary artery disease being present and defines the prognosis or the future risk for the patient. In other words, does this patient with chest complaints have coronary artery disease? If this patient does have coronary artery disease, what is the risk that this

Table 9.1 Diagnosis versus prognosis in the initial clinical evaluation of suspected CAD

	Diagnosis	Prognosis
Demographics		
Age	+	+
Sex	+	+
Race	−	−
Anginal symptoms		
Typical angina	+	+
Anginal course	−	+
Anginal frequency	−	+
Nocturnal angina	−	+
Anginal severity	−	−
Duration of symptoms	+	−
Risk factors		
Diabetes	+	−
Hypertension	+	−
Hyperlipidemia	+	−
Smoking	+	−
Family history	−	−
Other history		
Previous MI	+	+
Congestive heart failure	−	+
Non-cardiac vascular disease	−	+
Electrocardiogram		
ST-T wave changes	+	+
Pathologic Q waves	+	+
Premature ventricular contractions	−	−
Chest film		
Cardiomegaly	−	+
Pulmonary congestion	−	+
Physical examination		
S_3 gallop	−	+
Blood pressure	−	−
S_4 gallop	−	−

+ = most useful; − = less useful.
From Mark [10], with permission from Elsevier.

patient will suffer a myocardial infarction with significant morbidity or death in the next one or more years. This stratification for the likelihood of coronary artery disease and determination of the future risk is done simultaneously with exercise stress testing.

One patient may have minimal obstructive coronary disease (<40% obstruction of the right coronary artery) and perform well with treadmill stress testing. This same patient may experience the acute rupture of a plaque and suddenly develop unstable angina and a lethal arrhythmia or possible myocardial infarction. Risk-stratifying this patient prior to acute cardiovascular compromise described above is difficult since the acute event is statistically unpredictable.

Most myocardial infarctions are now known to result from coronary arteries with less than 50% obstruction. Plaque rupture usually occurs in a non-obstructive lesion. Since most plaque formation occurs in the medial layer and is not a luminal lesion, angiography does not reveal this non-luminal pathology. Functional testing, such as exercise treadmill testing, determines ischemia from fixed disease but does not predict future myocardial infarction and cardiac events from unpredictable plaque rupture. Consequently, less obstructive lesions may be more relevant to myocardial infarction and sudden death than more obstructive, symptomatic and exercise-related ischemic lesions typically detected with current evaluation [12].

Recent studies in cardiac microvascular flow indicate that some patients may have "normal coronary arteries" on angiographic studies but experience a decrease in flow with an increase in myocardial oxygen consumption in the presence of exercise or tachycardia [13, 14]. It was previously thought that blood flow was normal or maximal beyond an identified coronary artery stenotic lesion. It is now known that coronary artery resistance paradoxically increases downstream to a coronary artery stenotic lesion and causes further ischemia [13, 15]. Thus, a patient may have a minimally stenotic lesion on angiography but perform poorly on exercise testing and have a high risk for a subsequent cardiac event such as cardiac arrhythmia or acute infarction. In this case poor performance with exercise testing (poor MET level achieved, poor maximal double product [systolic blood pressure × heart rate], ST-segment changes) may define this high-risk category.

Finally, a patient may have normal coronary arteries and yet experience angina in the presence of severe coronary artery spasm or alterations in the coronary microcirculation. In contrast, some patients may have a 90% coronary artery obstruction and not experience pain or symptoms [16]. These patients maintain an excellent vasodilator reserve defined as the ability to increase and maintain distal blood flow in response to compression or stenosis. Agents such as endogenous nitrous oxide and prostaglandins may act to modify the inherent ischemic response in some individuals. Thus, a functional test (exercise stress testing) and an anatomical test (angiography) may complement each other in completing the risk stratification process.

Defining Diagnosis and Prognosis by Analysis, Test Scores and Criteria

Several test scores have been developed for the evaluation of symptomatic patients. Included are the (1) multivariate analysis scores, (2) Duke treadmill score and the (3) Veterans Administration (VA) treadmill score. These models may assist in determining the proper evaluation and follow-up of patients. The American College of Cardiology (ACC) and the American Heart Association (AHA) guidelines recommend the use of scores to enhance the predictive ability of exercise tests. Since many measured parameters (e.g., METs achieved, ST-segment depression, blood pressure response) are based on "all-cause" mortality data (includes death from any cause and not necessarily limited to cardiac causes), one must be cautious in applying such data to the specific patient under evaluation. These numerical statistical evaluations are useful when evaluating populations of patients but may not be appropriate in evaluating and managing an individual patient [17]. From this analysis simplified, user-friendly treadmill scores have been developed and validated which assist in risk-stratifying specific patients. Lastly, additional criteria have been developed which assist in risk-stratifying patients with chest pain.

Multivariate Analysis

Multivariate analysis is utilized in risk-stratifying patients with symptoms. Investigators have found that while ST-segment depression changes have diagnostic and prognostic relevance, one can improve the sensitivity, specificity and predictive value of the exercise stress test by combining additional parameters. Multivariate analysis evaluates and determines the relationship of variables such as historical, clinical, exercise stress testing end points and others. The analysis then validates the prognostic significance of the variables and is then utilized to develop a prognostic statement. The subsequent result then places the patient in either a low, moderate or high-probability category when risk-stratifying for coronary artery disease. This approach is more useful in the clinical setting when evaluating an individual patient. Instead of stating that the testing results are "negative" for coronary artery disease it is more appropriate to inform the patient that he is at a "low risk" for coronary artery disease in the near future. Most patients understand that the relative risk for future coronary artery disease depends on many factors including age, sex, history of smoking, hypertension, diabetes and current symptoms as well as the result of cardiac testing. This places the patient's risk on a continuum rather than an absolute "positive" or "negative". Further evaluation and management can then be recommended.

Ellestad's Multivariate Analysis

Greenberg et al. reviewed patients who underwent treadmill exercise stress tests and the gold standard for coronary artery disease was based on coronary angiograms [2]. In women 20 variables were evaluated while in men 21 variables were analyzed. From their analysis they found different variables were predictive of significant coronary artery disease based on gender. In women, five variables were significant: (1) age, (2) previous myocardial infarction by history, (3) previous myocardial infarction by ECG, (4) ST-segment depression with exercise stress testing and (5) angina during the exercise test. In men three variables were significant: (1) myocardial infarction by electrocardiogram, (2) duration of the exercise test and (3) ST-segment depression [1, 2, 18]. In women the sensitivity was 85%, the specificity was 94% and the predictive value was 90%. In men the sensitivity was 85%, specificity 86% and the predictive value of a positive test was 89%.

Cohn's Multivariate Analysis

Berman et al. also developed a multivariate approach to the interpretation of the exercise stress test by analyzing four variables: (1) anginal chest pain induced by exercise, (2) heart rate–blood pressure product (peak double product) at peak exercise, (3) persistence of ST-segment depression during recovery from exercise and (4) depth of ST-segment depression [9]. Treadmill exercise test results (Bruce protocol) were analyzed and coronary artery disease was defined as an obstructive coronary vessel with greater than 70% luminal diameter narrowing. The predictive value of a positive exercise stress test was 0.88 overall (0.78 if the ST-segment depression was less than 1.0–1.9 mm and 0.97 if it was equal to or greater than 2 mm). In addition, the parameters providing the best separation of the true positive tests from the false-positive tests were (1) exercise duration less than 6 min, (2) persistence of ST-segment change for >3 min into recovery and (3) a double product ≤23,000 [9]. For example, if the criterion of 1.0–1.9 mm of ST-segment depression was combined with a double product ≤23,000, exercise duration <6 min and ST-segment depression >3 min into recovery, the predictive value increased from 0.78 to 0.89. In contrast to other studies they found no augmentation in the predictive value for coronary disease if exercise-induced chest pain occurred during the test. Subsequently, prospective applications of this multivariate approach were reported.

Froelicher's Multivariate Analysis

Froelicher and his group developed a "simplified" score for evaluating both men and women [19–21]. This score combines personal risk factors with results of exercise testing (Tables 9.2 and 9.3). Each of these factors is "weighted" and a summation score is calculated. Based on this summation scoring system patients are placed into one of three groups of probability for coronary artery disease based on the angiographic finding of ≥50% stenosis in at least one coronary artery. The grouping of patients into low, intermediate and high probability for coronary artery disease is based on a simple mathematical calculation. Men with a score less than 40 have a low probability; men with a score between 40 and 60 have an intermediate probability; men with a score greater than 60 have a high probability of coronary artery disease. In a similar fashion a scoring system was developed for women. Women with a score less than 37 have a low probability; women with a score between 37 and 57 have an intermediate probability; women with a score greater than 57 have a high probability of coronary artery disease.

Treadmill Scores

Duke Treadmill Score

The Duke treadmill score developed by Mark et al. is utilized for estimating the likelihood of significant coronary artery disease in patients and the future risk of cardiac events [22, 23]. In the initial study inpatients underwent treadmill exercise

Table 9.2 Simple exercise test for men

Variable	Response	Score
Maximum heart rate	<100 bpm = 30 100–129 bpm = 24 130–159 bpm = 18 160–189 bpm = 12 190–190 bpm = 8	
		Subtotal
Exercise ST-segment depression	1–2 mm = 15 >2 mm = 25	
		Subtotal
Age	>55 years = 20 40–55 years = 12	
		Subtotal
Angina history	Definite/typical = 5 Probable/atypical = 3 Non-cardiac pain = 1	
		Subtotal
Hypercholesterolemia	Yes = 5	
		Subtotal
Diabetes	Yes = 5	
		Subtotal
Exercise test-induced angina	Occurred = 5 Reason for stopping test = 3	
		Subtotal
		Total

<40, Low probability; 40–60, intermediate probability; >60, high probability.
From Raxwal et al. [20], with permission from *Chest*.

testing utilizing a Bruce protocol within 6 weeks of cardiac catheterization. In this study Mark defined significant coronary artery disease as a 75% or greater stenosis of the lumen of a major coronary artery [22]. The development of the Duke treadmill score from this initial study of inpatients was later confirmed in an outpatient population [23].

The score is based on three components obtained during the exercise stress test: (1) exercise duration, (2) magnitude of ST-segment deviation and (3) anginal index. The Duke treadmill score allocates negative values for adverse prognostic factors (angina during exercise and ST-segment depression) and positive values for improved prognostic factors (longer exercise time or exercise capacity).

Mathematically, the Duke treadmill score is calculated as follows:

$$\text{Duke treadmill score} = \text{exercise duration} - (5 \times \text{ST-segment deviation})$$
$$- (4 \times \text{treadmill angina index})$$

where exercise duration is time in minutes; ST-segment deviation is in millimeters; and the angina index equals 0 for no angina with exercise, 1 for angina with exercise and 2 for angina causing cessation of the treadmill test (Table 9.4). The calculation

Table 9.3 Simple exercise test for women

Variable	Response	Score
Maximum heart rate	<100 bpm = 20 100–129 bpm = 16 130–159 bpm = 12 160–189 bpm = 8 190–190 = 4	
		Subtotal
Exercise ST-segment depression	1–2 mm = 6 >2 mm = 10	
		Subtotal
Age	>65 years = 25 50–65 years = 15	
		Subtotal
Angina history	Definite/typical = 10 Probable/atypical = 6 Non-cardiac pain = 2	
		Subtotal
Smoking	Yes = 10	
		Subtotal
Diabetes	Yes = 10	
		Subtotal
Exercise test-induced angina	Occurred = 9 Reason for stopping test = 15	
		Subtotal
Estrogen status	Positive = −5 Negative = 5	Total

<37, low probability; 37–57, intermediate probability; >57, high probability.
From Morise et al. [21], with permission from Elsevier.

Table 9.4 Duke treadmill score

Risk group	Treadmill exercise score	Average annual cardiac mortality (%)	5-year survival rate (%)
Low	≥ +5	0.25–0.50	97
Moderate	−10 to +4	1.25–2.0	91
High	≤ −11	5.0–7.0	72

From Mark [11], with permission from Elsevier.

is a numerical score which estimates the likelihood of significant coronary artery disease and future cardiac risk.

The Duke treadmill score provides practical information for the management of patients based on their likelihood of significant coronary artery disease. This score divides patients into three groups—low risk, intermediate or moderate risk and high risk of coronary artery disease—and then correlates this classification with future prognosis. In other words, the Duke treadmill score predicts the prognosis based on mortality at 1 and 5 years and *not* the presence or absence of coronary artery disease. A person in the low-risk group has an extremely low annual cardiac mortality rate and is treated with modification of risk factors and careful follow-up since the annual cardiac mortality rate in this low-risk group is 0.25–0.50%. In fact, any interventional treatment would potentially carry a statistically higher mortality rate due to possible complications from procedures. Those patients in the high-risk group need referral to the cardiologist for further management. Those patients in the intermediate group need further evaluation to assist with more definite risk stratification. This evaluation may include stress imaging testing, angiography or cardiology consultation.

For example, assume that a male patient exercises for 13 min on the treadmill (Bruce protocol), develops 1 mm of ST-segment depression and has no chest pain during the test. Even though this patient develops ST-segment depression, his Duke treadmill score of +9 places him in the low-risk group with an excellent prognosis (Table 9.4). Any risk factors are treated and modified, and he can be followed clinically unless new symptoms or clinical findings occur.

There are some limitations and exclusions to the Duke exercise score. First, the testing procedure initially utilized only a Bruce protocol and not all patients are able to exercise at this vigorous level. Later, Mark et al. developed and published a nomogram for calculating the prognosis based on the Duke treadmill score (see Fig. 5.11). This nomogram utilizes METs of oxygen consumption or work instead of minutes on the Bruce protocol. Thus, an alternative exercise protocol can be utilized in the calculation [23]. Second, patients with baseline electrocardiographic abnormalities (left bundle branch block or resting ST-segment abnormalities) were excluded. Third, patients with exercise-induced ST-segment elevation with pathologic Q waves were excluded if they had no other exercise-related ST-segment changes. Fourth, this system is not useful in those patients taking digoxin or unable to perform the required exercise, e.g., arthritis, musculoskeletal conditions, neurologic disorders. Lastly, this system may not apply to some older patients since the average age of the initial inpatient study group was 49 years with a range of 37–60 years whereas the average age in the outpatient group was 54 years with a range of 45–62 years [22, 23]. While this test is not suitable for every patient, it does provide a risk-stratifying system for eligible patients with suspected coronary artery disease. Furthermore, this test is valid in women. With this score primary care physicians can decide which patients are candidates for risk factor modification and which patients need referral for further evaluation and interventional therapy.

Veterans Administration Exercise Score

The VA exercise score developed by Morrow et al. at the Long Beach VA Hospital utilized different variables [24]. This score incorporated the history of congestive heart failure as well as a change in blood pressure while undergoing stress testing:

$$VA \text{ treadmill score} = 5 \times (CHF/digitalis) + \text{exercise-induced ST-segment depression}$$
$$+ \text{ change in systolic blood pressure score} - METs$$

where CHF/digitalis is yes $= 1$, no $= 0$; exercise-induced ST-segment depression is in millimeters; change in systolic blood pressure score is the following:0 $=$ greater than 40 mmHg increase in SBP,1 = greater than 30 mmHg increase in SBP,2 = greater than 20 mmHg increase in SBP,3 = greater than 10 mmHg increase in SBP,4 = between 0 and 10 mmHg increase in SBP,5 = decrease in SBP *below* resting standing SBP; and METs denote METs of work achieved during the exercise test [11, 23].

This score correlated with prognosis and identified three risk groups (Table 9.5). The sensitivity and specificity of this score was based on coronary angiography within 12 weeks of the exercise test. Significant angiographic coronary artery disease was defined as a 70% narrowing of the left anterior descending, left circumflex or right coronary arteries or their major branches or a 50% narrowing in the left main artery [6, 25]. Since all patients in the VA intermediate group underwent angiography, by definition this middle group was 100% correct with the further evaluation. This score was well validated and utilizes a history of congestive heart failure or use of digitalis together with three exercise stress test results—systolic blood pressure, ST-segment depression and exercise capacity—to risk-stratify patients for future cardiovascular death.

Table 9.5 VA treadmill score

Risk group	Treadmill exercise score	Average annual cardiac mortality over 3 years post-test (%)	Percent of studied population (%)
Low	< −2	< 2	77
Moderate	−2 to +2	7	18
High	> +2	15	6

Data from Morrow et al. [24].

However, the VA exercise score is limited by two factors. First, it is based on data derived from men in the VA hospital system. Second, although the score was correlated with coronary angiograms, the definition of a clinically significant coronary lesion varies from the definition of ≥75% narrowing of any major artery in the Duke treadmill score.

Other Stratification Criteria

Goldschlager Criteria

Goldschlager et al. described indicators of not only the presence but the *severity* of coronary artery disease based on the exercise stress test results [26]. In a population of patients aged 27–70 years (average age 48 years) referred for further diagnostic evaluation the type of ST-segment response, time of onset of ischemia and duration of ischemic changes with exercise stress testing were correlated with severity. Downsloping ST-segment depression, ischemic changes occurring in the first 3 min of exercise and ischemic changes persisting past 8 min in recovery were associated with a 91, 86 and 90% prevalence of two- to three-vessel or left main coronary disease, respectively. This referral patient population consisted of patients with both known pre-existing coronary artery disease and patients with chest pain without proven cardiac disease. In addition, normal volunteers served as a control population. All patients underwent exercise stress testing based on the Bruce protocol and all patients, save the normal volunteers in the control group, underwent coronary angiography. Four ST-segment responses—each correlating with a varying severity of disease in this study group of patients—were described (see Fig. 5.10). Horizontal ST-segment depression and downsloping ST-segment depression were associated with more severe coronary artery disease. Moreover, patients with early-onset ischemic ECG changes (during stage I of the Bruce protocol) and ischemic ST-segment changes lasting greater than 8 min into recovery had severe coronary disease.

Subsequently, Goldschlager summarized treadmill responses indicating severe, multi-vessel and/or left main coronary artery disease [27]. These responses include both ECG and non-ECG abnormalities seen with exercise stress testing (Table 9.6).

Table 9.6 Predictive treadmill test responses for diagnosis of severe, multi-vessel and/or left main coronary artery disease

ECG abnormalities
ST-segment response
Downsloping
Elevation
ST-segment depression exceeding 2.5 mm
Serious ventricular arrhythmias occurring at low (120–130/min) heart rates
Early onset (first 3 min) of ischemic ST-segment depression or elevation
Prolonged duration in the post-test recovery period ($\geq$8 min) of ischemic ST-segment depression
Non-ECG abnormalities
Low achieved heart rate (chronotropic incompetence) defined as $\leq$120/min
Hypotension* ($\geq$10 mmHg fall in systolic pressure)
Rise in diastolic pressure ($\geq$110–120 mmHg)
Low achieved rate–pressure product ($\leq$15,000)
Inability to exercise beyond 3 min

*In the absence of antihypertensive medications or hypovolemia of any cause.
Adapted from Goldschlager [27].

McNeer Criteria

McNeer et al. at Duke evaluated a cohort of 1,472 patients who underwent exercise stress testing and coronary angiography within 6 weeks. Significant coronary artery disease was defined as greater than 50% occlusion. He found that those patients who exercise either more than 12 min or achieve a heart rate of 160/min or greater or both had only a 15% prevalence of severe three-vessel disease irrespective of the ST-segment response with the exercise stress test [28]. In addition, these patients had an excellent prognosis of 1% mortality per year and 7% mortality at 4 years. McNeer defined the significance of exercise intolerance and was the first to identify a patient group with severe disease identified as an abnormal test at a low level of exertion.

Coronary Artery Surgery Study Criteria

In the CASS good left ventricular function correlated with prognosis. This study evaluated medically treated patients with symptomatic coronary artery disease. In a subset 16% of the enrolled 4,083 patients were analyzed and their subsequent prognosis was based on clinical parameters and exercise stress testing. During a 4-year follow-up 5% died representing a low annual mortality rate. Those patients with three-vessel coronary artery disease and preserved left ventricular function (able to achieve 10 METs of work) had a 100% 4-year survival rate while those achieving only stage 1 (4.2 METS) or stage 2 (5.8 METs) had a 53% 4-year survival rate. Left ventricular function was important in determining prognosis, and the single most potent clinical predictor of survival at 4 years was the presence or absence of congestive heart failure [29, 30].

Recovery-Only ST-Segment Depression Criteria

"Recovery-only ST-segment depression" changes associated with severe disease were confirmed by Lachterman et al. in 1990 [31] These patients often have risk factors and complain of exercise-associated symptoms. Many times they perform well with formal exercise stress testing and achieve a high workload. ST-segment changes occurring only with exercise are usually associated with less severe angiographic coronary artery disease. In fact, the rank order of the positive predictive value for three-vessel or left main disease was greatest with ST-segment changes during both exercise and recovery, followed by ST-segment changes during recovery only and finally by changes during exercise only.

Savage et al. also studied recovery-only ST-segment depression and found that most patients were men with an average age of 58 years [32]. This study concluded that ST-segment depression was not a false-positive response and was usually associated with coronary artery disease, often indicated multi-vessel disease and men were more likely to have positive thallium scans.

Morise Clinical Score Criteria

In 1997 Morise et al. published a clinical score based on a population of 915 men and women seen at the West Virginia University School of Medicine [8]. Patients in the study had no prior history of coronary artery disease, a normal resting electrocardiogram but were evaluated for suspected coronary artery disease. Patients who underwent exercise testing and subsequent coronary angiography within 3 months were included in the study. Patients with a history of previous myocardial infarction (based on clinical history or electrocardiogram) or prior cardiomyopathy, valvular heart disease, coronary angiography or diagnosed coronary artery disease were excluded. The Morise scoring method is based on clinical findings and places patients into three categories of risk for coronary artery disease—low, intermediate and high probability (Table 9.7). Based on this clinical score 4,300 patients were subsequently evaluated. About one-half of

Table 9.7 Morise scoring system

	9 points	6 points	3 points
Men	>55 years	40–55 years	<40 years
Women	>65 years	50–65 years	<50 years
Symptoms	Typical angina	Atypical angina	Nonanginal
	5 points	3 points	1 point
Estrogen status	Positive	Negative	Male/unknown
	−3 points	+3 points	0 points
Diabetes	2 points		
Hypertension	1 point		
Smoking	1 point		
Hyperlipidemia	1 point		
Family history	1 point		
Obesity	1 point		

Low probability: 0–8 points; intermediate probability: 9–15 points; high probability: 16–24 points.
From Morise et al. [8], with permission from Elsevier.

these patients (49%) were categorized as low probability including 55% of the women. These patients at low probability for coronary artery disease were evaluated with exercise electrocardiography. In the validation group the prevalence of significant coronary disease was 69% in the high-probability group, 44% in the intermediate-probability group and 16% in the low-probability group. Based on the clinical probability classifications one can determine further appropriate diagnostic testing including exercise stress testing, stress testing with imaging or coronary angiography.

Historical Dyspnea Criteria

In 2005 Abidov et al. reported a study group of almost 18,000 patients who were evaluated with exercise and pharmacologic stress testing together with myocardial perfusion imaging [33]. This clinical outcomes study evaluated the historical incidence of dyspnea in patients and correlated this symptom with death from cardiac causes ($p < 0.001$) and all-cause mortality ($p < 0.001$) over the follow-up period of 2.7 ± 1.7 years. Among patients with no known history of coronary artery disease there was a four times increased risk of death from cardiac causes in those with dyspnea. Among patients with typical angina there was more than twice the increased risk of death from cardiac causes in those with dyspnea. The authors noted that while dyspnea is commonly associated with both pulmonary diseases and left ventricular systolic dysfunction, this simple symptom was useful in determining the prognosis of the patients undergoing study.

From the previous exercise scores and other criteria one can stratify patients into low-risk and high-risk groups (Tables 9.8 and 9.9). One can outline and develop management plans based on the stress test characteristics of these identified groups.

Table 9.8 Identification of low-risk groups of patients with exercise testing

Low-risk criteria	Prevalence (%)	Average annual mortality rate (%)
Duke TM score ≥ +5	34 (inpatients)	0.6
	62 (outpatients)	0.3
VA exercise score	< −2	< 1
CASS registry		
Stage ≥ 3, ST < 1 mm	32 (inpatients)	1.0
Yale registry		
Normal quantitative planar TI^{201}	28	0*
University of Virginia registry		
Normal quantitative planar TI^{201}	35	0.5
Duke exercise RNA		
Exercise EF ≥ 50%	62	0.6

VA = Veterans Administration; CASS = coronary artery surgery study; EF = ejection fraction;
RNA = radionuclide angiography; TM = treadmill
*2-year follow-up.
From Mark [11], with permission from Elsevier.

Table 9.9 Identification of high-risk groups of patients with exercise testing

Exercise score/study	High-risk criteria
Duke treadmill score	≤ −11
VA treadmill score	> +2
Goldschlager criteria	1. Downsloping ST-segment depression during exercise or recovery
	2. Ischemic changes during initial 3 min of exercise
	3. Ischemic changes lasting longer than 8 min into recovery
CASS Registry	<Stage II of Bruce protocol
Lachtermann criteria	Recovery-only ST-segment depression

Approach to the Patient with Chest Pain

When a patient presents with chest pain, the primary care physician must evaluate four general subjects—diagnosis, prognosis, functional evaluation and treatment. Patients may present to either the outpatient office or to the emergency department for evaluation of symptoms.

Diagnosis

Does the presenting patient have coronary artery disease or what is the likelihood of coronary artery disease? Patients are stratified into four groups: (1) non-cardiac pain, (2) stable angina, (3) possible acute coronary syndrome (ACS) and (4) definite ACS.

Prognosis

The determination relates to the diagnosis and focuses on the relative mortality risk in the future. Is the presenting patient at risk for death from a cardiac event in the next few days or the next 12 months or does the patient have a low mortality risk over the next 5 years? Does the presenting patient require immediate intervention or is medical treatment of coronary risk factors indicated?

Functional Evaluation

Is a functional evaluation indicated? This may be an exercise stress test with or without imaging studies to help not only define the diagnosis but also the prognosis as well as the prescribed level of activity in the future.

Treatment

Is procedural intervention required? Is the patient at such high risk that interventional therapy is indicated to decrease the immediate mortality rate? Or can risk factors for coronary artery disease be modified by lifestyle changes and medications? These are questions that may require consultation and evaluation by a consulting cardiologist.

Management of Patients with Chest Pain

Presenting patients with chest pain are categorized to one of four groups: (1) non-cardiac pain, (2) chronic stable angina, (3) possible ACS and (4) definite ACS. This chapter focuses on the patient with non-cardiac pain, chronic stable angina and possible ACS. Those patients with definite ACS are managed according to the American College of Cardiology guidelines with appropriate consultation.

There are published guidelines for the short-term risk of death or nonfatal myocardial infarction in patients with chest pain and unstable angina [25, 34–36] (Tables 9.10 and 9.11). The initial stratification of patients with chest pain or suspicion of coronary artery disease is based on history and physical examination along with resting ECG changes (ischemic changes involving ST segments or Q wave formation) and biomarkers (cardiac troponin I, cardiac troponin T, creatinine kinase-MB and myoglobin). Other possible parameters include chest x-ray findings (cardiomegaly or pulmonary congestion), B-type natriuretic peptide (BNP) elevation and C-reactive protein (CRP) elevation.

The patients with a non-cardiac diagnosis for presenting chest pain can be evaluated and treated appropriately on either an outpatient or inpatient basis. Common etiologies include esophageal discomfort, musculoskeletal discomfort, pulmonary embolus or cardiac pain but not caused by cardiac ischemia, e.g., pericarditis [37].

Table 9.10 Short-term risk of death or nonfatal myocardial infarction in patients with chest pain

Low risk	Intermediate risk	High risk
No high- or intermediate-risk feature but may have any of the following features:	No high-risk feature but must have either	At least one of the following features must be present:
1. Increased angina, frequency, severity or duration	1. Prolonged (>20 min) rest angina, now resolved, with moderate or high likelihood of CAD	1. Prolonged (>20 min) rest pain
2. Angina provoked at a lower moderate or high threshold	2. Rest angina (>20 min or relieved promptly with rest or NTG)	2. Pulmonary edema, most likely due to ischemia
3. New onset with onset 2 weeks to 2 months prior to presentation	3. Nocturnal angina	3. Angina at rest with ST changes (≥ 1 mm)
4. Normal ECG	4. New-onset CCSC III or IV angina in the past 2 weeks with moderate or high likelihood of CAD	4. Angina with S_3 or new/worsening rales
	5. Pathologic Q waves or resting ST-segment depression ≥ 1 mm in multiple lead groups (anterior, inferior, lateral)	5. Angina w/hypotension

CSCC = Canadian cardiovascular society class.
Data from Braunwald et al. [34].

Patients with chronic stable angina who develop no ECG or cardiac biomarker changes after serial monitoring are considered at a low risk and are evaluated prior to discharge or within 72 hours [37]. These patients can undergo functional cardiac stress testing (exercise or pharmaceutical) or noninvasive coronary imaging (coronary CT angiography). Some of these patients are managed conservatively [38]. If abnormalities are found on subsequent cardiac stress testing or noninvasive coronary imaging, further evaluation is done following cardiology consultation.

Acute coronary syndrome includes patients with ST-elevation myocardial infarction (STEMI), non-ST-elevation myocardial infarction (NSTEMI) or unstable angina (UA). Patients with symptoms of ACS include those patients with chest pain with or without radiation, heaviness, tightness, weakness, diaphoresis, nausea, indigestion, heartburn, lightheadedness or loss of consciousness. Non-ST-elevation myocardial infarction usually presents as prolonged, more intense rest angina or angina equivalent [37]. These patients require evaluation in a facility (emergency department or hospital outpatient department) where immediate evaluation and necessary biomarkers are obtained. Unfortunately, these patients sometimes present to the outpatient office of the primary care physician and should be transferred immediately via ambulance to an appropriate hospital facility. Following appropriate study and monitoring these patients usually fall into one of three groups: (1) acute myocardial infarction, (2) unstable angina or (3) rule out other cardiac diseases (Fig. 9.1) [37].

Table 9.11 Thrombolysis in myocardial infarction risk score for unstable angina/non-ST-segment elevation myocardial infarction

Historical	Points
Age ≥65	1
≥3 CAD risk factors (FHx, hypertension, increased cholesterol, diabetes mellitus, active smoker)	1
Known CAD (stenosis >50%)	1
ASA use in past 7 days	1
Presentation	
Recent (<24 hour) severe angina	1
Increased cardiac markers	1
ST deviation >0.5 mm	1
Risk score = total points (0–7)	
Risk of cardiac events (%) by 14 days in TIMI 11B*	

Risk score	Death or MI	Death, MI or urgent revascularization
Low risk		
0/1	3	5
2	3	8
Moderate to high risk		
3	5	13
4	7	20
5	12	26
6/7	19	41

*Entry criteria: UA or NSTEMII defined as ischemic pain at rest within past 24 hour, with evidence of CAD (ST-segment deviation or increased marker).
Adapted from Antman et al. [36], with permission. Copyright © 2000, American Medical Association. All rights reserved.

Acute Evaluation of ACS

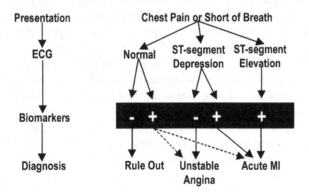

Fig. 9.1 Acute evaluation of acute coronary syndrome. (From Anderson et al. [37], with permission from Elsevier.)

These high-risk patients are admitted to the hospital for further evaluation and treatment. Coronary angiography and interventional therapy are frequently indicated for those with definite ACS (ST-elevation myocardial infarction) [37].

Unstable angina is defined as (1) rest angina, (2) new-onset (less than 2 months) severe angina and (3) increasing angina (in intensity, duration and/or frequency) [39]. Patients with possible or probable ACS (initial normal ECG and biomarkers) must be monitored in a dedicated chest pain unit or coronary care unit with continuous telemetry monitoring until the status is clarified with serial repeat ECGs and biomarkers.

Whether to then carry out this stratification process by an exercise or a pharmacological stress test depends on the patient. In addition, one may select an imaging component (nuclear or echocardiography) to complement the exercise or pharmacological stress test (see Chapters 7 and 8). Some patients may be receiving medications or have baseline ECG abnormalities that necessitate an imaging stress test (see Chapter 2). For example, baseline ECG changes from left ventricular hypertrophy with associated ST-segment changes cannot be interpreted accurately without simultaneous imaging since exercise-related changes could occur with either coronary artery disease or demand alterations. In those patients unable to exercise a pharmacologic stress test may be necessary. In the remaining patients an exercise stress test is the initial step. Combining the stress test with imaging can then be done if indicated.

Based on the Duke treadmill score results the physician can risk-stratify the patient. Patients are considered as low risk if the predicted annual mortality rate is less than 1%. Patients are considered as high risk if the predicted annual mortality rate exceeds 4% per year or if studies indicate three-vessel or left main coronary artery disease. Patients between these two groups are at intermediate risk [23, 25, 34].

Mark feels that the initial process should identify those in the low-risk group since these patients are treated medically by the primary physician with no further evaluation. While one cannot predict with complete accuracy that no severe cardiac event will occur in the low-risk group, cardiac angiography and intervention are not cost-effective when applied to the large numbers in this population. Mark et al. identified almost two-thirds of the patients in the outpatient study who were at low risk (annual mortality, 0.25% and average 4-year survival rate of 99%) [23]. Moreover, the risk of complications from interventional therapy in these low-risk patients is often greater than following them medically and modifying risk factors. Other methods of identifying patients in this low-risk group are listed in Table 9.8.

In the clinical outcomes utilizing revascularization and aggressive drug evaluation (COURAGE) trial 2,287 patients were randomized to either percutaneous coronary intervention (PCI) and optimal medical therapy or optimal medical therapy alone [40]. In this multi-center study, interventional therapy (PCI) with optimal medical therapy did not improve outcomes (risk of death, myocardial infarction or other major cardiovascular events) over treatment with optimal medical therapy alone.

Further evaluation of patients in the low-risk group would be indicated if the clinical situation changes or new symptoms occur. These patients are then stratified anew with a change in symptoms. The clinician can either perform further studies, i.e., exercise imaging studies, or seek consultation for those patients with an annual mortality rate of 2% or greater.

Patients in the intermediate-risk group can be further risk-stratified with a stress imaging study. With results from the stress imaging test (establishing a greater specificity for risk-stratifying patients for coronary artery disease) one can move many of these patients into the low-risk group or into the high-risk category discussed below. From this more specific information definitive treatment and management can be recommended.

High-risk patients with an average annual cardiac mortality of 4% or greater require consideration for cardiac consultation and catheterization [25]. Criteria for identifying patients in this high-risk group are listed in Table 9.9. These high-risk patients have a high annual mortality rate and a 5-year survival rate of 72%. Interventional therapy is often indicated in this group if technically possible.

Some patients postpone seeking medical evaluation until symptoms are severe and then present for evaluation in the emergency department with dire complaints. Emergency department patients at intermediate or high risk should be evaluated urgently. Those at low risk can be further stratified based on exercise stress testing.

Unfortunately, sudden death may present as the first sign or symptom of coronary artery disease in certain patients in our society [41, 42]. In 1998, a total of 719,456 cardiac disease deaths occurred among those persons ≥35 years of age and 63% were classified as sudden cardiac death [42]. Whether symptoms of cardiac disease were ignored by some patients is unknown. However, many of these patients with risk factors for coronary artery disease were never evaluated.

Case Presentations

Case 1

A 34-year-old Caucasian woman with a family history of premature heart disease (brother who had an acute myocardial infarction at age 52) presents for evaluation. The patient's only personal risk factor for heart disease is a 16 pack-year history of smoking. She denies any chest pain but requests an exercise stress test to rule out heart disease. Is an exercise stress test indicated in this patient?

Discussion

Her pre-test likelihood for coronary artery disease is 0.8 ± 0.3% [43]. Based on her extremely low pre-test probability of disease a positive exercise stress test result would be statistically a false-positive test. Exercise testing does not assist in risk-stratifying this patient. Thus, exercise stress testing is not indicated. One might undertake an exercise stress test for purposes of developing an exercise prescription since lifestyle changes (smoking cessation and regular exercise) would reduce her future risk for coronary artery disease.

Case 2

A 48-year-old Caucasian man with treated hypertension presents with chest pain associated with activity and relieved with rest. He has experienced this symptom for over 1 year with no change in the character of his pain. He continues to walk 5 out of 7 days with his wife and does not have to stop walking when he maintains a specific pace. He has a family history of premature heart disease (mother with an acute myocardial infarction at age 54 and his brother underwent stent placement at age 51) but no other personal cardiac risk factors. Should he undergo an exercise stress test?

Discussion

This patient presents with an excellent history for stable angina. Risk stratification of this patient is useful in recommending future management. For example, if he has 2 mm of ST-segment depression with exercise testing, must stop exercising due to severe angina and is only able to exercise for 7 min on the Bruce protocol, his Duke treadmill score is −11. This result places him in the high-risk group of patients with a poor prognosis and cardiology referral is indicated for further evaluation.

In contrast, if he has no ST-segment depression with exercise testing, experiences angina during the test but is able to exercise for 10 min on the Bruce protocol, his Duke treadmill score is +6. This places him in the low-risk group for a future event during the next year even though he has angina. His management would include careful treatment of his hypertension and continuation of his exercise program. He should be seen for re-evaluation and re-stratified if his symptoms change or new symptoms occur.

Case 3

A 54-year-old African-American man presents with chest pain occurring in his anterior chest associated with dyspnea and fatigue and relieved with rest. He notices this discomfort (heavy pressure sensation) most often when he climbs stairs. Over the past 2 weeks his symptoms have increased in severity and frequency and he now is unable to climb one flight of stairs due to discomfort. He is under treatment for hypertension, hyperlipidemia and has been told he has pre-diabetes. He has a positive family history for premature heart disease (father with an acute myocardial infarction at age 51 and brother with an acute myocardial infarction at age 48) and states that "everyone in my family has high blood pressure". Does he need an exercise stress test? His resting ECG demonstrates no ST-segment deviation, his chest film reveals "borderline cardiomegaly" and his myocardial source creatinine kinase (CK-MB) and troponin test results are normal.

Discussion

The initial treatment strategy, whether conservative or invasive, of patients with unstable angina is based on individual patient characteristics and thrombolysis in myocardial infarction (TIMI) or GRACE scores [36, 44] (Table 9.11). This patient, defined as a low-risk patient by his TIMI score, may be managed conservatively [37] (Table 9.12).

He can be managed in the outpatient setting and an exercise or pharmacological stress test based on his ability to exercise can be performed within 72 hours of presentation. Based on the stress test results (including non-electrographic parameters—exercise symptoms, blood pressure response, maximum double product during his test), his further management can be determined.

Case 4

A 66-year-old Caucasian woman presents to the emergency department with chest pain that has been increasing in frequency and severity over the past 10 days and is now intolerable. She has known coronary artery disease which has been stable over the past 2 years and previously has experienced chest pain only one to two times per year which has always been relieved with nitroglycerin. In addition, she has hypertension, type 2 diabetes mellitus and dyslipidemia. She is followed by her primary care physician every 3 months and by a cardiologist once yearly. How do you manage this patient?

Table 9.12 Treatment strategy of patients with unstable angina

Preferred strategy	Patient characteristics
Invasive	Recurrent angina or ischemia at rest or with low-level activities despite intensive medical therapy
	Elevated cardiac biomarkers (TnT or TnI)
	New or presumably new ST-segment depression
	Signs or symptoms of HF or new or worsening mitral regurgitation
	High-risk findings from noninvasive testing
	Hemodynamic instability
	Sustained ventricular tachycardia
	PCI within 6 months
	Prior CASG
	High-risk score (e.g., TIMI, GRACE)
	Reduced left ventricular function (LVEF less than 40%)
Conservative	Low-risk score (e.g., TIMI, GRACE)
	Patient or physician preference in the absence of high-risk features

From Anderson et al. [37], with permission from Elsevier.

Discussion

This patient has unstable angina characterized by recent increasing frequency and severity of symptoms with marked accentuation over the past 24 hours. In the emergency department she is evaluated for acute coronary syndrome, defined as ST-elevation myocardial infarction, unstable angina or non-ST-elevation myocardial infarction [45–50]. No abnormal markers of acute myocardial damage are found. The patient is felt to be at a moderate risk for short-term risk of death or nonfatal myocardial infarction based on history, physical examination and initial 12-lead resting ECG and cardiac markers and her TIMI score (Table 9.11).

This patient requires cardiology consultation since she is in the intermediate-risk group based on her TIMI score. Some of these patients are managed with conservative treatment and some require invasive therapy (Table 9.12). If conservative therapy is selected, she is treated with anticoagulant therapy, beta blockers and any additional indicated medications. If no subsequent symptoms or events (arrhythmias, hypotension, ECG changes) occur and her ejection fraction is greater than 40%, she can undergo a stress test.

This patient should undergo exercise or pharmacological stress testing within 72 hours either on an outpatient basis or during the hospitalization if an inpatient. In this intermediate-risk patient exercise stress testing can be performed when she is free of any active ischemic or congestive heart failure symptoms for a minimum of 8–12 hours [34, 48]. If the stress test is low risk with a good Duke treadmill score, she is managed medically. If the stress test does not place her in a low-risk group, diagnostic angiography is indicated [38].

Studies have confirmed that exercise testing is safe in low-risk patients and in carefully selected intermediate-risk patients who present to the hospital emergency department. High-risk patients usually require angiography and further evaluation [38, 48].

If the exercise stress test results based on the Duke treadmill score place the patient in an intermediate or high risk for mortality in the next year, angiography is indicated. Those stratified to the low risk can be managed medically subsequently. Patients presenting to the emergency department may be risk-stratified with imaging stress testing to increase the specificity of the test and reduce the incidence of false negatives.

Case 5

A 48 year-old Caucasian man presents to the office with severe indigestion currently treated with ranitidine. He requests a stronger medication since the symptoms are increasing in severity and now occurs both at rest and with activity. His family history includes an acute myocardial infarction in his mother at age 53. The patient's blood pressure is 120/68 and he has a 50 pack-year history of smoking. His blood glucose, lipid panel and resting ECG are normal. He exercises on a regular basis and is not overweight. Because of his history of exercise-associated indigestion, he is scheduled for an exercise stress test.

Discussion

This patient presents with complaints which suggest cardiac symptoms based on occasional relationship to activity. He is scheduled for an exercise stress test in the hospital outpatient department and on the day of the scheduled test volunteers that he ingested aluminum hydroxide/magnesium hydroxide/simethicone (*Maalox*) prior to leaving home. His resting ECG is normal and an exercise test is initiated with a Bruce protocol.

At 1:05 min into the exercise test he complains of epigastric pain. His ECG shows peaking of the T waves in V_3 and V_4 but no ST-segment changes. At 2:50 min into the test he suddenly develops ECG changes with ST-segment elevation in V_2 (3 mm), V_3 (6 mm), V_4 (3 mm) and V_5 (1 mm) with increasing epigastric symptoms. The test is terminated. His Duke treadmill score is −35 and this patient is in the high-risk category.

He is transferred to the hospital emergency department where an acute myocardial infarction is excluded and cardiology consultation is obtained. Subsequent angiography reveals a 95% lesion of the left anterior descending artery and a 90% lesion of the right coronary artery with normal left ventricular function. A double coronary artery bypass graft is performed and postoperatively he has no further symptoms of indigestion.

This patient has risk factors for coronary artery disease but presented with gastrointestinal complaints occasionally related to activity. Risk stratification with exercise stress testing of this patient defined his severe cardiac risk. Coronary artery disease must always be considered in patients presenting with exercise-associated symptoms.

Summary

Patients seen in the primary care setting with risk factors for coronary artery disease and possible cardiac symptoms can be further evaluated and risk-stratified for future events. The initial evaluation is based on the presenting history and physical examination along with a resting ECG and chest x-ray. Further evaluation tools and criteria, including exercise stress testing, have been developed to assist with this process. The resultant risk stratification determines subsequent medical management or cardiology consultation. The primary care physician must be adept at delineating those patients with an excellent prognosis and a low likelihood of significant coronary artery disease. This identified group of patients may be managed by the primary care physician.

The initial evaluation of patients who present with acute coronary artery syndrome in the office or emergency department is based on history, clinical examination, resting electrocardiogram, biochemical cardiac markers and other appropriate laboratory tests. These patients are then categorized into ST-segment elevation myocardial infarction, non-ST-segment myocardial infarction or unstable angina. Patients with myocardial infarction are then managed according to published treatment guidelines.

Those remaining patients with unstable angina are then classified into low, intermediate or high risk for subsequent myocardial disease. Exercise testing with or without imaging is an integral part of this process and from these studies one can determine subsequent treatment and management. The 2007 guidelines for the management of patients with unstable angina and non-ST-elevation myocardial infarction from the American College of Cardiology and the American Heart Association is an excellent resource for the management of these patients [37].

References

1. Greenberg PS, Cangiano B, Leamy L, et al. Use of the multivariate approach to enhance the diagnostic accuracy of the treadmill stress test. J Electrocardiology 1980;13:227–36.
2. Greenberg PS, Ellestad MH, Clover RC. Comparison of the multivariate approach to enhance the diagnostic accuracy of the treadmill stress test. Am J Cardiol 1984;53:493–496.
3. Diamond, GA, Staniloff HM, Forrester JS, et al. Computer assisted diagnosis in the non-invasive evaluation of patients with suspected coronary artery disease. J Am Coll Cardiol 1983;1:444–55.
4. Detrano R, Janosi A, Lyons KP, et al. Factors affecting sensitivity and specificity of a diagnostic test: the exercise thallium scintigram. Am J Med 1988;84:699–710.
5. Shaw LJ, Peterson ED, Shaw LK, et al. Use of prognostic treadmill score in identifying diagnostic coronary disease subgroups. Circulation 1998;98(16):1622–30.
6. Do D, West JA, Morise A, Atwood JE, Froelicher VF. A consensus approach to diagnosing coronary artery disease based on clinical and exercise data. Chest 1997;111:1742–9.
7. Lipinski M, Froelicher V, Atwood E, et al. Comparison of treadmill scores with physician estimates of diagnosis and prognosis in patients with coronary artery disease. Am Heart J 2002;143:650–8.
8. Morise AP, Haddad WJ, Beckner D. Development and validation of a clinical score to estimate the probability of coronary artery disease in men and women presenting with suspected coronary disease. Am J Med 1997;102:350–6.
9. Berman JL, Wynne J, Cohn PF. A multivariate approach for interpreting treadmill exercise tests in coronary artery disease. Circulation 1978;58:505–12.
10. Mark DB. Ischemic heart disease. In Conn RB (ed) Current Diagnosis 8. WB Saunders, 1991, Philadelphia, PA, pp 416–27.
11. Mark DB. Risk stratification in patients with chest pain. Primary Care 2001;28:99–118.
12. Kligfield P and Lauer MS. Exercise electrocardiogram testing: Beyond the ST segment. Circulation 2006;114:2070–82.
13. Ellestad, M: Stress Testing: Principles and Practices. 5th ed. Oxford University Press; 2003; New York, NY 43–75.
14. Sambuceti, G, Marzilli M, Fedele, et al. Paradoxical increase in microvascular resistance during tachycardia downstream from a severe stenosis in patients with coronary artery disease: reversal by angioplasty. Circulation 2001;103;2352–60.
15. Wei K, Ragosta M, Thorpe J, et al. Noninvasive quantification of coronary blood flow reserve in humans using myocardial contrast echocardiography. Circulation 2001;103:2560–5.
16. White CW, Wright CB, Doty DB, et al. Does visual interpretation of the coronary arteriogram predict the physiologic importance of a coronary stenosis? N Engl J Med 1984;310:819–24.

17. Ellestad, M: Stress Testing: Principles and Practices. 5th ed. Oxford University Press; 2003; New York, NY 271–303.
18. Greenberg PS, Bible M, Ellestad MH. Prospective application of the multivariate approach to enhance the accuracy of the treadmill stress test. J Electrocardiology 1982;15:143–8.
19. Raxwal V, Shetler, Do D, et al. A simple treadmill score. Chest 2000;113:1933–40.
20. Raxwal V, Shetler K, Morise A, et al. Simple treadmill score to diagnose coronary disease. Chest 2001;119:1933–40.
21. Morise AP, Lauer MS, Froelicher VP. Development and validation of a simple exercise test for use in women with symptoms of suspected coronary artery disease. Am Heart J 2002;144;818–25.
22. Mark DB, Hlatky MA, Harrell FE Jr, et al. Exercise treadmill score for predicting prognosis in coronary artery disease. Ann Intern Med 1987;106:793–800.
23. Mark DB, Shaw L, Harrell FE, et al. Prognostic value of a treadmill exercise score in patients with suspected coronary artery disease. N Engl J Med 1991;325:849–53.
24. Morrow K, Morris CK, Froelicher VF, et al. Prediction of cardiovascular death in men undergoing noninvasive evaluation for coronary artery disease. Ann Intern Med 1993;118:689–95.
25. Braunwald E, Jones RH, Mark DB, et al. Diagnosing and managing unstable angina. Agency for Health Care Policy and Research. Circulation 1994;90:613–22.
26. Goldschlager N, Selzer A, Cohn K. Treadmill stress tests as indicators of presence and severity of coronary artery disease. Ann Intern Med 1976;85:277–86.
27. Goldschlager N. Use of the treadmill test in the diagnosis of coronary artery disease in patients with chest pain. Ann Intern Med 1982;97:383–8.
28. McNeer JF, Margolis JR, Lee KL, et al. The role of the exercise test in the evaluation of patients for ischemic heart disease. Circulation 1978;57:64–70.
29. Froelicher VF, Myers J: Exercise and the heart. 5th ed. Sanders-Elsevier, 2006; Philadelphia, PA, p 253–4.
30. Weiner DA, Ryan T, McCabe CH. Prognostic importance of a clinical profile and exercise test in medically treated patients with coronary artery disease. J Am Coll Cardiol 1984;3:772–9.
31. Lachterman B, Lehmann KG, Abrahamson D, Froelicher VF. "Recovery only" ST-segment depression and the predictive accuracy of the exercise test. Ann Intern Med 1990;112:11–6.
32. Savage MP, Squires LS, Hopkins JT, et al. Usefulness of ST-segment depression as a sign of coronary artery disease when confined to the postexercise recovery period. Am J Cardiol 1987;60:1405–6.
33. Abidov A, Rozanski A, Hachamovitch R, et al. Prognostic significance of dyspnea in patients referred for cardiac stress testing. N Engl J Med 2005;353:1889–98.
34. Braunwald E, Mark DB, Jones RH, et al. Unstable Angina: Diagnosis and management: Clinical practice Guideline No. 10 AHCPR Publication NO. 94-0602, Rockville, MD: Agency for Health Care Policy and Research, March 1994.
35. Gibbons RJ, Balady GJ, Bricker JT, et al. ACC/AHA 2002 guideline update for exercise testing: summary article: A report of the American College of Cardiology/ American Heart Association task force on practice guidelines (committee to update the 1997 exercise testing guidelines). J Am Coll Cardiol 2002;40:1531–40.
36. Antman EM, Cohen M, Bernik PJLM et al. The TIMI risk score for unstable angina/non-ST elevation MI: A method for prognostication and therapeutic decision making. JAMA 2000;284:835–42.
37. Anderson JL, Adams CD, Antman EM, et al. ACC/AHA 2007 Guidelines for the management of patients with unstable angina/Non ST-elevation myocardial infarction executive summary: a task force on practice guidelines. J Am Coll Cardiol 2007;50:652–726.
38. Fraker TD, Fihn SD. 2007 Chronic angina focused update of the ACC/AHA 2002 guidelines for the management of patients with chronic stable angina. Circulation 2007;116:2762–72.
39. Braunwald E. Unstable angina: A classification. Circulation 1989;80:410–4.
40. Boden WE, O'Rourke RA, Teo KK, et al. for the COURAGE Trial Research Group. Optimal Medical Therapy with or without PCI for stable coronary disease. N Engl J Med 2007;356:1503–16.

41. Zipes DP, Wellens HJJ. Sudden cardiac death. Circulation 1998;98:2334–51.
42. Zheng ZJ, Croft JB, Giles WH, et al. Sudden cardiac death in the United States, 1989 to 1998. Circulation 2001;104:2158–63.
43. Diamond GD, Forrester JS. Analysis of probability as an aid in the clinical diagnosis of coronary-artery disease. N Engl J Med 1979:300:1350–8.
44. Goncalves PA, Ferreira J, Aguiar C, et al. TIMI, PURSUIT, and GRACE risk scores: sustained prognostic value and interaction with revascularization in NSTE-ACS. Eur Heart J 2005;26:865–72.
45. Achar SA, Kundu S, Norcross WA. Diagnosis of acute coronary syndrome. Am Fam Physician 2005;72:119–26.
46. Swap CJ, Nagurney JT. Value and limitations of chest pain history in the evaluation of patients with suspected acute coronary syndromes. JAMA 2005;294;2623–9.
47. Stein RA, Chaitman BR, Balady GJ, et al. Safety and utility of exercise testing in emergency room chest pain centers: an advisory from the Committee on Exercise, Rehabilitation, and Prevention. Council on Clinical Cardiology, American Heart Association. Circulation2000;102:1463–7.
48. Braunwald E, Antman EM, Beasley JW, et al. ACC/AHA 2002 guideline update for the management of patients with unstable angina and non-ST-segment elevation myocardial infarction: a report of the American College of Cardiology/ American Heart Association Task Force on Practice Guidelines (Committee on the Management of Patients with Unstable Angina). J Am Coll Cardiol 2002;40:1366–74.
49. American Heart Association. 2005 International Consensus Conference on Cardiopulmonary Resuscitation and Emergency Cardiovascular Care Science with Treatment Recommendations. Part 5. Acute Coronary Syndromes. Circulation 2005;112 (Supplement):III-55–72.
50. Farkouh ME, Smars PA, Reeder GS, et al., for the Chest Pain Evaluation in the Emergency Room (CHEER) Investigators. A clinical trial of a chest-pain observation unit for patients with unstable angina. N Engl J Med 1998;339:1882–8.

Chapter 10
Exercise Testing as Applied to the Preoperative Patient

H. Jack Pyhel

In the course of a month you are asked to see three patients preoperatively for surgical clearance. The following three cases are probably representative of patients you see on a daily basis in the office.

Case Studies

Case 1

A 59-year-old man is found to have a 6 cm abdominal aortic aneurysm on a routine x-ray he had obtained for low back pain. This was confirmed with an abdominal ultrasound. He is one of your regular patients and now sent to you by the surgeon for preoperative clearance. On review of your records you note that he has been hypertensive with fairly good control for approximately 7 years and on oral agents for type 2 diabetes for 5 years. Not surprisingly he also has a metabolic dyslipidemia treated with a statin drug. Unfortunately he continues to smoke and has a 30 pack-year tobacco history presently smoking one pack per day. There is no outward evidence of chronic pulmonary disease and he has never experienced chest pain to suggest ischemic heart disease. Physical examination reveals normal vital signs, no auscultatory evidence of pulmonary or cardiac valve disorder, some abdominal adiposity with an enlarged abdominal aorta and absent pedal pulses with no prior history of claudication. What would you recommend?

Case 2

A 74-year-old man presents with an abnormal electrocardiogram suggesting an old inferior myocardial infarction which by history would appear to be "silent".

H.J. Pyhel (✉)
University of South Florida Medical School, Bayfront Medical Center, 701 Sixth St. South, St. Petersburg, FL 33701, USA
e-mail: Hjp@tampabay.rr.com

C.H. Evans, R.D. White (eds.), *Exercise Testing for Primary Care and Sports Medicine Physicians,* DOI 10.1007/978-0-387-76597-6_10
© Springer Science+Business Media, LLC 2009

Review of recent laboratory studies reveals mild renal insufficiency with a serum creatinine of 1.6 mg/dL. Serum glucose, electrolytes, and hepatic enzymes are normal. He is hypertensive controlled on medication. There is no history of angina pectoris and he is not diabetic. Presently he is in the hospital after suffering a small transient ischemic attack (TIA) and found to have left carotid stenosis. You are asked to clear him for carotid endarterectomy. What would you recommend?

Case 3

An 82-year-old woman presents with a left hip fracture sustained in a nonsyncopal fall. She appears older than her stated age and has very poor functional capacity. On physical examination you find her to be mildly hypertensive with a blood pressure of 152/68 and a mild resting tachycardia at 86 beats per minute. The remainder of the physical exam is normal. She has no history of any previous cardiac event and is a nonsmoker. What would you recommend?

Introduction

Preoperative cardiovascular evaluation is frequently requested prior to noncardiac surgery. Your job is not simply to *clear* the patient, but to make some estimation of the risk for major cardiovascular complications. If you can identify the patient who is at high risk, then therapeutic measures can be undertaken to minimize this risk. This review will address clinical risk assessment and identify the most appropriate testing and treatment to optimize care of the patient.

In 1996 [1], 2002 [2], and most recently in 2007 [3], the American College of Cardiology and American Heart Association developed clinical guidelines for preoperative evaluation for noncardiac surgery. Using these guidelines for preoperative identification of high-risk patients and exclusion of low-risk patients may prevent the use of unnecessary tests and reduce costs. The goal of this text is to identify the high-risk patient and determine what preoperative tests or therapy is best for that patient.

Preoperative Cardiac Risk Stratification

When evaluating a preoperative patient, the purpose may be to clear for elective or emergent surgery. It is much more important to evaluate and implement measures to prepare higher risk patients for surgery and identify the high-risk patient. It has been shown that outpatient medical evaluation can reduce length of hospital stay and minimize postponed or canceled surgery [4]. Patients undergoing major noncardiovascular surgery have an almost 6% risk of postoperative cardiac death or major cardiac complications [5].

Ideally the patient should be evaluated several weeks prior to surgery. A careful history will almost always identify patients who fall into a high surgical risk category. Modifiable risk factors for coronary artery disease should be noted with evidence of associated disease such as peripheral artery disease, cerebrovascular disease, diabetes, renal impairment, and chronic pulmonary disease. If the patient has a known cardiac history, recent change in symptoms as well as current medications and doses should be ascertained. Most importantly an assessment of functional capacity should be made as part of the history also. Performance of daily tasks will correlate closely with maximal oxygen uptake by treadmill testing. By estimating the energy equivalent in "metabolic equivalents" or METS it is easy to separate moderate from poor functional status. A patient who can walk a block on level ground at 2–3 mph or climb a flight of stairs has an approximate functional capacity of 4 METS which separates poor from moderate functional status. Perioperative risk is increased in those unable to meet a 4 MET demand during most normal daily activity.

The general appearance provides evidence of the patient's overall health status. A careful cardiovascular examination should be completed with assessment of vital signs, carotid pulse contour and bruits, jugular venous pressure, and pulsations. Cardiac auscultation and palpation are essential to exclude significant aortic stenosis placing the patient at high risk for noncardiac surgery. Auscultation of the lungs and palpation of the abdomen for abdominal aortic aneurysm, and evaluation of extremities for edema and vascular integrity should complete the physical examination. The presence of associated vascular disease should heighten suspicion of occult coronary artery disease.

Obtaining or reviewing, if complete, a few simple tests will allow for thorough risk stratification. The electrocardiogram, chest x-ray, complete blood count (CBC), and metabolic profile will allow identification of potentially serious cardiac disorders to include coronary artery disease, congestive heart failure, potentially serious arrhythmia, anemia, diabetes, and renal insufficiency. Physical findings or review of the blood chemistry may indicate the necessity for other preoperative tests. These may include an echocardiogram to evaluate aortic stenosis, other cardiac murmur, or left ventricular function if clinically suspect. A hemoglobin AlC indicates level of diabetic control.

Once the history, physical examination, and review of appropriate ancillary studies are done, perioperative risk stratification can be completed. Tables 10.1 and 10.2 taken from the ACC/AHA guidelines update for perioperative cardiovascular evaluation for noncardiac surgery [2] will allow you to predict your patient's risks. Note that in addition to clinical predictors there are surgery-specific risks. Table 10.2 emphasizes two important factors: the type of surgery itself and the degree of hemodynamic stress associated with the procedure.

From a review of Table 10.1, major clinical predictors would preclude surgery until further cardiovascular consultation and evaluation could be obtained. Certain emergent surgeries, for example, ruptured abdominal aortic aneurysm or acute ischemic leg, will not allow for adequate preoperative screening since the risk of delaying surgery is worse than proceeding directly to the operating room. In these people postoperative risk stratification may be appropriate. From the two tables the patients who would most benefit from further noninvasive testing fall into the "high"

Table 10.1 Major, intermediate, and minor predictors for perioperative cardiovascular evaluation

Major predictors that require intensive management and may lead to delay in or cancellation of the operative procedure unless emergent

- Acute myocardial infarction (within 7 days) in patients with evidence of important ischemic risk as determined by symptoms or noninvasive testing
- Recent myocardial infarction (within 8–30 days) in patients with evidence of important ischemic risk as determined by symptoms or noninvasive testing
- Unstable angina
- Severe angina (Canadian Cardiovascular Society class III or IV); may include patients with stable angina who are usually sedentary
- Decompensated heart failure
- High-grade atrioventricular block
- Symptomatic ventricular arrhythmias in patients who have underlying heart disease
- Supraventricular arrhythmias with a poorly controlled ventricular rate
- Severe heart valve disease

Intermediate predictors that warrant careful assessment of current status

- Mild angina (Canadian Cardiovascular Society class I or II)
- Previous myocardial infarction as determined from the history or the presence of pathologic Q waves
- Compensated heart failure or a prior history of heart failure
- Diabetes mellitus, particularly in patients who are insulin dependent
- Reduced renal function, which is defined as a serum creatinine $>2.0\,\mathrm{mg/dL}$ (177 μmol/L) or a $\geq 50\%$ increase above an abnormal baseline concentration

Minor predictors that have not been proven to independently increase perioperative risk

- Advanced age
- Abnormal ECG (left ventricular hypertrophy, left bundle branch block, ST-T abnormalities)
- Rhythm other than sinus rhythm (e.g., atrial fibrillation)
- Low functional capacity (e.g., inability to climb one flight of stairs with a bag of groceries)
- History of stroke
- Uncontrolled hypertension

From Eagle et al. [2], with permission from Elsevier.

cardiac risk surgical procedures and have "intermediate" clinical predictors of perioperative cardiovascular risk. If the patient has previously undergone coronary bypass surgery within the last 5 years and is stable with no recurrent symptoms further testing is not necessary [6]. Likewise, if a cardiac stress test was normal in the past 2 years, no further assessment is necessary [1] unless new symptoms are present. Patients with good functional capacity and intermediate clinical risk present very low surgical risk and probably would not benefit from further noninvasive testing. Conversely, patients with poor functional capacity and any intermediate risk may benefit from noninvasive testing for high or intermediate surgical procedures.

Table 10.2 ACC/AHA guidelines: cardiac risk stratification for noncardiac surgical procedures[a]

High risk (reported cardiac risk often greater than 5%)
Emergent major operations, particularly in the elderly
Aortic and other major vascular surgery
Peripheral vascular surgery
Anticipated prolonged surgical procedures associated with large fluid shifts and/or blood loss
Intermediate risk (reported cardiac risk generally less than 5%)
Carotid endarterectomy
Head and neck surgery
Intraperitoneal and intrathoracic surgery
Orthopedic surgery
Prostate surgery
Low risk (reported cardiac risk generally less than 1%)[b]
Endoscopic procedures
Superficial procedure
Cataract surgery
Breast surgery

[a]Combined incidence of cardiac death and nonfatal myocardial infarction.
[b]Do not generally require further preoperative cardiac testing.
From Eagle et al. [2], with permission from Elsevier.

Patients who have had PTCA or coronary stenting within the last 6 months probably require cardiac re-evaluation or consultation. Diabetes, representing a coronary risk marker, should indicate need for further testing in high and intermediate surgical risk procedures as should the presence of peripheral artery disease [7–12].

To summarize, preoperative cardiac testing and further cardiac evaluation are determined by the clinical risk predictors along with the history, physical examination, electrocardiogram, and functional status as well as the risks and urgency of the surgical procedure. Remember, do not let the risk of coronary intervention or even corrective cardiac surgery exceed the risk of the noncardiac surgery.

Noninvasive Cardiac Testing: What to Do with the Results

Results of noninvasive cardiac testing can be used to determine the need for additional preoperative testing and treatment. The routine treadmill stress test has a high negative predictive value but a low positive predictive value, 6–67% [13]. In one study, dipyridamole-thallium myocardial perfusion imaging prior to vascular surgery resulted in a negative predictive value of 98% but a positive value of only 18% [14]. The predictive value of a positive test will be much lower if therapy that prevents adverse cardiac outcomes such as coronary bypass surgery, appropriate preoperative medical treatment, and close monitoring during the perioperative period is undertaken.

Since functional capacity is a very important determinate of preoperative risk, if at all possible, exercise is the preferred stress. Exercise tolerance is a more important predictor of outcome than the electrocardiographic response. Pharmacologic stress testing, currently adenosine myocardial perfusion imaging, or dobutamine myocardial scintigraphy or echocardiography can be done in patients who cannot exercise. The choice of test should be determined by local experience and availability.

Exercise electrocardiographic testing is most valuable with associated perfusion imaging or echocardiography since imaging will identify high-risk patients who would need referral for angiography. This would be essential if there were resting electrocardiographic abnormalities, not limited to but including, a paced rhythm, left bundle branch block, left ventricular hypertrophy, or use of digitalis. Abdominal aortic aneurysm measuring greater than 6 cm may be an exception to exercise stress because of the increase in systolic blood pressure and heart rate and perhaps an adenosine pharmacologic stress test may be preferred [15].

Since vascular surgery seems to impose the greatest perioperative risk, stress testing would be the most beneficial in these patients. Moreover, myocardial perfusion imaging would give the most information. In one study the extent of ischemia rather than only its presence is related to the risk of myocardial infarction or cardiac death [16]. In another study of 355 patients postoperative events varied from 1.3% in 225 patients with normal dipyridamole-thallium imaging to as high as 52% in the 29 patients with reversible defects in all three segments or at least one severe reversible defect or transient left ventricular dilatation [17].

The resting electrocardiogram which is usually included in the preoperative examination also has been demonstrated to offer some prognostic information in patients undergoing noncardiac surgery [18]. Likewise, resting echocardiography may be indicated to quantify valve dysfunction in patients with a murmur or to evaluate left ventricular function in heart failure or assess the degree of pulmonary hypertension. Routine echocardiography is not recommended [19].

If after noninvasive testing it appears there is an indication for cardiac revascularization or percutaneous coronary intervention, the potential benefit must be balanced against the delay of surgery in the former and a requirement for aggressive antiplatelet therapy possibly prohibiting surgery in the latter. There are little data regarding appropriate timing of noncardiac surgery after percutaneous coronary intervention and there appears to be a high incidence of complications of noncardiac surgery when surgery is performed within 6 months of stenting [20, 21]. High rates of perioperative morbidity and mortality occurred with either PTCA alone or with stenting if performed within 2 weeks of noncardiac surgery and both procedures resulted in a similar percentage of events [22]. There is little evidence to support prophylactic coronary intervention before noncardiac surgery. Even coronary bypass grafting, the gold standard, may not reduce the risk of noncardiac surgery as believed by many [23]. Even today there is uncertainty regarding the time interval of revascularization and noncardiac surgery. Using bare metal stents a delay of at least 2 weeks and ideally 4–6 weeks would appear appropriate [21]. Similar data for drug-eluting stents are not available but considering the necessity of prolonged antiplatelet therapy even a minimum delay of 6 months may not be adequate. If the risk of revascularization is greater than the risk of noncardiac surgery without it, preoperative medical therapy is a better option. Although controversial, numerous studies have shown significant reductions of perioperative morbidity with the use of beta-blockers [24–28].

Summary

Cardiac complications are one of the most significant risks to patients undergoing noncardiac surgery. Depending on the cardiac risk of the surgery and the perioperative risks of the patients, postoperative cardiac complications may range from less than 1% to as high as 6%. A carefully obtained history and brief assessment of functional capacity along with the risk associated with the operation itself will allow the clinician a reasonable approach to preoperative testing. Use of invasive and noninvasive testing should be limited to situations where the results will affect patient management. The treadmill or other noninvasive tests should refine the clinical risk assessment and lead to efforts to reduce events in high-risk patients.

Remember that even in high-risk surgery the postoperative event rate is usually less than 6% so a positive preoperative noninvasive test will give a low positive predictive value for events. On the other hand a negative stress test is very reassuring with up to a 98% negative predictive value [13]. Remember also that cardiac interventions may not reduce risks as much as might be anticipated [20–23]. Only patients who would benefit regardless of noncardiac surgery should undergo cardiac interventions [7].

Recommendations of Three Presenting Cases

Case 1

This 59-year-old gentleman with a large aortic aneurysm, peripheral artery disease, diabetes mellitus, hypertension, dyslipidemia, and heavy tobacco use almost certainly has extensive coronary disease that imposes a high risk. You recommended routine treadmill exam which demonstrates very significant, asymptomatic, ST-segment depression early in the Bruce protocol which was terminated after only 2 min and 20 s. The patient went on to have cardiac catheterization revealing three-vessel disease and a 95% proximal LAD obstruction. Coronary revascularization with four bypasses was done and 6 weeks later successful abdominal aortic aneurysmectomy.

Case 2

This 74-year-old gentleman with carotid stenosis, post-transient ischemic attack, and several risks as well as an abnormal electrocardiogram suggesting an old inferior myocardial infarction is an intermediate perioperative risk as well as intermediate noncardiac surgical procedure risk. He underwent a screening treadmill and had excellent exercise capacity, 8 METS, and only minimal (less than 1 mm) ST-segment depression at peak exercise (asymptomatic). He was started on perioperative beta-blocker therapy, bisoprolol 5 mg daily, and continued 30 days postoperatively. He encountered no problem with his surgery.

Case 3

Despite this elderly woman's poor functional capacity there is little evidence to pursue noninvasive testing especially since there would appear to be no indications for cardiac intervention if noncardiac surgery were not planned. Adding a preoperative beta-blocker as in case 2 may be helpful considering her tachycardia and elevated blood pressure. She did well with her surgery and suffered no perioperative complications.

References

1. Eagle KA, Brundage BH, Chaitman BR, et al. Guidelines for perioperative cardiovascular evaluation for noncardiac surgery. Report of the American College of Cardiology/American Heart Association Task Force on Practice Guidelines. Committee on Perioperative Cardiovascular Evaluation for Noncardiac Surgery. Circulation 1996;93:1278–1317.
2. Eagle KA, Berger P, Calkins H, et al. ACC/AHA guidelines update for perioperative cardiovascular evaluation for noncardiac surgery – executive summary. J Am Coll Cardiol 2002;39: 542–53.
3. Fleisher LA, Beckman JA, Brown KA, et al. ACC/AHA 2007 Guidelines on perioperative cardiovascular evaluation and care for noncardiac surgery: executive summary. J Am Coll Cardiol 2007; 50: 1707–25.
4. Macpherson DS, Lefgren RP. Outpatient internal medicine preoperative evaluation: a randomized clinical trial. Med Care 1994;32:498–507.
5. Goldman L, Caldera D, Nussbaum S, et al. Multifactorial index of cardiac risk in noncardiac surgical procedures. N Engl J Med 1977;297:845–50.
6. Mahar LJ, Steen PA, Tinker JA, et al. Perioperative myocardial infarction in patients with coronary artery disease with and without aorta-coronary bypass grafts. J Thorac Cardiovasc Surg 1978;76:533–7.
7. DiCarli, MF, Hochamovitch R. Should we screen for occult coronary disease among asymptomatic patients with diabetes? J Am Coll Cardiol 2005;45:50–53.
8. Anand DV, Lim A, Lahiri A, et al. The role of non-invasive imaging in the risk stratification of asymptomatic diabetic patients. Eur Heart J 2006;27(8):905–12.
9. Scognamiglio R, Negut C, Ramondo A, et al. Detection of coronary artery disease in asymptomatic patients with Type 2 Diabetes Mellitus. J Am Coll Cardiol 2006;47(1):65–71.
10. Giri S, Shaw LJ, Murthy DR, et al. Impact of diabetes on the risk stratification using stress single-photon emission computed tomography myocardial perfusion imaging in patients suggestive of coronary artery disease. Circulation 2002;105:32.
11. Bax Ro, Bonow D, Tschope SE, et al. The potential of myocardial perfusion scintigraphy for risk stratification of asymptomatic patients with Type 2 Diabetes. J Am Coll Cardiol 2006;48(4):754–60.
12. Kumar R, McKinney WP, Raj G, et al. Adverse cardiac events after surgery: assessing risk in a veteran population. J Gen Intern Med 2001;16:507.

13. Auerbach A, Goldman L. Assessing and reducing the cardiac risk of noncardiac surgery. Circulation 2006;113:1361.
14. Mangano DT, Goldman L. Preoperative assessment of patients with known or suspected coronary disease. N Engl J Med 1995;333:1750.
15. Best PJ, Tajik AJ, Gibbons RJ, et al. The safety of treadmill exercise stress testing in patients with abdominal aortic aneurysms. Am Intern Med 1998;129:628.
16. Etchells E, Meade M, Tomilinson G, et al. Semiquantitative dipyridamole myocardial stress perfusion imaging for cardiac risk assessment before noncardiac vascular surgery: a meta-analysis. J Vasc Surg 2002;36:534.
17. Lette J, Waters D, Cerino M, et al. Preoperative coronary artery disease risk stratification based on dipyridamole imaging and a simple three-step, three-segment model for patients undergoing noncardiac vascular surgery or major general surgery. Am J Cardiol 1992;69:1553.
18. Jeger R, Probst C, Arsiner R. Long-term prognostic value of preoperative 12-lead electrocardiogram before major noncardiac surgery in coronary artery disease. Am J Cardiol 2006;151(2):1508–13.
19. Devereaux PJ, Goldman L, Yusef S, et al. Surveillance and prevention of major perioperative ischemic cardiac events in patients undergoing noncardiac surgery: a review. CAMJ 2005;173:779.
20. Kaluza GL, Joseph J, Lee JR, et al. Catastrophic outcomes of noncardiac surgery soon after coronary stenting. J Am Coll Cardiol 2002;35:1288–94.
21. Wilson SH, Fasseas P, Orford JL, et al. Clinical outcome of patients undergoing noncardiac surgery in the two months following coronary stenting. J Am Coll Cardiol 2003;42:234–40.
22. Leibowitz D, Cohen M, Planer D, et al. Comparison of cardiovascular risk of noncardiac surgery following coronary angioplasty with versus without stenting. Am J Cardiol 2006;97:1188–91.
23. McFall EO, Ward HB, Moritz TF, et al. Coronary artery revascularization before elective major vascular surgery. N Engl J Med 2004;351:2795–2804.
24. Fleisher LA, Beckman JA, Brown KA, et al. ACC/AHA Guidelines update on perioperative cardiovascular evaluation for noncardiac surgery: focused update on perioperative beta-blocker therapy. J Am Coll Cardiol 2006;47:2343–55.
25. Lindenauer PK, Pekow P, Wang K, et al. Perioperative beta-blocker therapy and mortality after major noncardiac surgery. N Engl J Med;353:349–61.
26. Poldermans D, Boersma F, Bax JJ, et al. The effect of bisoprolol on perioperative mortality or myocardial infarction in high-risk patients undergoing vascular surgery. N Engl J Med 1999;341:1789–94.
27. Devereaux PJ, Beattie WS, Choi PT, et al. How strong is the evidence for use of perioperative beta-blockers in non-cardiac surgery? Systematic review and meta-analysis of randomized controlled trials. BMJ 2005;313–21.
28. Pasternack PF, Grossi EA, Baumann FG, et al. Beta-blocker to decrease silent myocardial ischemia during peripheral vascular surgery. Am J Surg 1989;158:113–6.

Chapter 11
Exercise Testing and Other Tools for Risk Stratification in Asymptomatic Patients

Corey H. Evans and Victor F. Froelicher

Reasons for Using Tools to Identify Asymptomatic Patients at Risk for Cardiac Events

There are several reasons to desire tools to help identify asymptomatic patients who are at increased risk for future cardiac events or premature mortality. If one could identify asymptomatic patients who are developing premature coronary disease then medical treatment could begin earlier. One would also wish to identify asymptomatic patients who are at such increased risk that surgical/intra-coronary artery interventions would increase survival and prevent cardiovascular (CV) events. Lastly, there are certain patients in high-risk occupations where a coronary event would threaten the lives of others. These patients should be identified.

Is There a Need to Detect CAD Earlier?

Despite declining mortality for coronary artery disease (CAD) in the United States, it is still the leading cause of death. The lifetime risk for CAD is still very high, approximately 50% for men and 32% for women [1]. In the United States there is a large burden of individuals with risk factors that increase their risk for CAD. For example, when the Framingham risk stratification is applied to a general US male population, one finds that about 62% of men aged 50–59 and 90% of men aged 60–69 are at intermediate or high risk for CAD. This is very well demonstrated in Fig. 11.1.

One would expect that the early identification of those at risk would enable earlier treatment of disease and prevention of premature mortality. This approach is suggested by the large amount of evidence showing the difference in mortality when comparing an asymptomatic population without risk factors to those with multiple

C.H. Evans (✉)
St. Anthony's Hospital, St. Petersburg, FL; Florida Institute of Family Medicine, St. Petersburg, FL, USA
e-mail: email@coreyevansmd.com

C.H. Evans, R.D. White (eds.), *Exercise Testing for Primary Care and Sports Medicine Physicians*, DOI 10.1007/978-0-387-76597-6_11

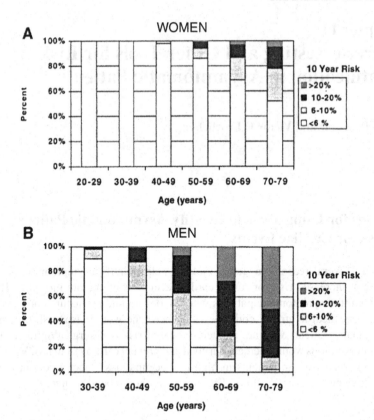

Fig. 11.1 (**A** and **B**) Data from the Framingham Heart Study seen in Bethesda conference. The 10-year risk of myocardial infarction or CHD death based upon age and sex. A majority of men aged 50–80 have an intermediate risk from 6 to 20% (From Pasternak RC, Abrams J, Greenland P, et al., 34th Bethesda Conference: Task force #1 – Identification of coronary heart disease risk: is there a detection gap? *J Am Coll Cardiol* 2003 Jun 4; 41(11):1863–74, with permission from Elsevier.)

risk factors. In general, men with multiple risk factors have a 5–8 times increase in CAD mortality compared to men without risk factors. There is ample evidence that statin therapy alone in high-risk patients can cut the CAD mortality by about 50%. The increasing effectiveness of early intervention encourages the use of tools for the early identification of those at high risk.

Discussion of Cost Effectiveness

Whenever one considers using tests to stratify asymptomatic patients, one needs always to consider the benefit of the test compared to the risk to the patient and the cost effectiveness of the testing. For tests to be useful in this respect, the test should be inexpensive enough to allow widespread use, safe, sensitive to identify high-risk individuals, and acceptable to patients. When analyzed, the screening costs per year of life saved should meet established standards. There are several excellent discussions of screening for the early detection of coronary disease. One such is the 34th Bethesda Conference: "Can Atherosclerosis Imaging Techniques Improve the Detection of Patients at Risk for Ischemic Heart Disease?" [2]

Overview of Tools

This chapter reviews the available tools to stratify asymptomatic patients for their risk of coronary events and premature mortality. First, the global risk appraisal systems will be reviewed. Next, tests to image the coronary arteries, CT coronary calcium scores, and rapid sequence CT angiography will be reviewed. Intimal medial thickness scoring is an indirect way to determine arterial health and, by inference, coronary artery health. Finally exercise testing will be reviewed as a tool to stratify asymptomatic patients.

Using Global Risk Assessment for Risk Stratification

Numerous risk scoring tools have been developed using risk factors to predict future CV events and to stratify individuals into low-, intermediate-, or high-risk groups. Collectively these computer-generated scoring systems are known as global risk scores. Some of the better known ones are the NCEP ATP III global risk score, the Framingham risk score, and the British Regional Heart Study risk score. Some are available for free and some are commercially available such as STAT cholesterol by STAT Coder. These scores use such factors as age, sex, blood pressure, total cholesterol, LDL, HDL, smoking, diabetes, family history of CAD, and even abdominal girth size to calculate the risk for patients. Typically the risk is expressed as the risk of myocardial infarction or death from cardiovascular disease within the next 10 years, expressed as a 10-year risk percent. Most agree that those with a greater than 20% 10-year risk are at high risk (the same risk as those with known CAD) and those with less than a 6% risk are at low risk.

Certainly those at high risk by these scores need aggressive therapy and those at low risk are not candidates for aggressive therapy. The problem is that many patients are at intermediate risk (as shown in Fig. 11.1), and it is not clear how they should be handled. The advantage of global risk assessment is the low cost of applying this tool using widely available data. Thus, most organizations strongly advise the use of global risk assessment tools in the initial evaluation of patients' CAD risk and for consideration of aggressive medical therapy. Global risk assessment has been endorsed by the American Heart Association, the American College of Cardiology, and ATP III [3, 4].

Several important questions remain to be answered about global risk assessment. First, are there high-risk individuals who should be further tested and stratified to identify those who would benefit from intervention beyond aggressive risk factor modification such as coronary artery revascularization? Second, for the large number of intermediate-risk patients, should this group be further stratified with additional testing, and if so how? Given the large number of patients that fall into the intermediate-risk category, further testing that would allow an intermediate-risk patient to be moved into a low- or high-risk group would be very valuable. The following discussion will look at tools that can be used to further stratify those with intermediate-risk scores.

Coronary Calcium Scores to Identify Coronary Artery Disease

Calcification of the coronary arteries has been noted for years. This calcification of the coronary arteries can be seen on chest radiographs, at coronary angiography, fluoroscopy, and other imaging techniques. This calcification of coronary arteries occurs in atherosclerotic plaques. The amount of calcification is strongly correlated with the presence and amount of significant coronary artery disease. There is also an excellent correlation between the amount of coronary calcification and overall plaque burden [5].

To image the calcium in the coronary arteries, scanning equipment must rapidly acquire numerous scans in one or two breath holds to eliminate motion artifact. These scans are also gated to the ECG during diastole to eliminate cardiac motion. Currently these scans can be obtained using ultrafast computed tomography with an electron gun (called electron-beam CT or EBCT) or using a rapid helical CT scanner. The calcifications of the coronary arteries can be well visualized and the scanner software calculates the total calcium area and density giving a coronary calcium score. One limitation of CT coronary scans is that they do not demonstrate the location of areas of luminal narrowing in the vessels, for example, a circumflex artery with a high amount of coronary calcification may or may not have luminal narrowing on angiography.

Numerous studies have demonstrated that the presence of coronary artery calcifications is a marker for increased future cardiovascular events and decreased survival. Arad [6] followed 1,173 individuals after EBCT scanning for 19 months and found increasing coronary calcium scores an independent marker for future CV events above traditional risk factors. Others have looked at the 5-year survival of asymptomatic individuals and found that increasing coronary calcium scores predict decreased survival, with scores of 0–10, 100–400, and >1000 having 4.5 year survivals of 99, 94, and 85%, respectively, in men. In women, the respective survival rates are 99, 91, and 80% for the same coronary score groups [7].

Do coronary calcium scores add prognostic information to that already obtained with global assessment tools? It seems the answer is yes. Greenland [8] followed 1,461 asymptomatic adults with Framingham risk scores (FRS) and coronary calcium scores by EBCT. Calcium scores were predictive of risk in patients with a FRS of >10%, but not less than 10%. This suggests that coronary calcium scores help further stratify those at intermediate and high risk by global risk assessment. This is especially important for those at intermediate risk where decision-making regarding aggressive therapy is unclear. This approach, using coronary calcium scores to further stratify intermediate-risk patients, is supported by the recent Clinical Expert Consensus Document on coronary artery calcium scoring [9]. This document also did not recommend coronary calcium scores to investigate low-risk or high-risk individuals per global risk assessment.

Rapid Sequence CT Coronary Angiography

With the development of rapid 64- and 128-slice CT scanners it is now possible to obtain CT angiography without cardiac catheterization. These scanners allow visualization of the coronary arteries to demonstrate luminal narrowing and coronary artery disease. This technology is now becoming available in community hospitals. As this technique becomes validated and available, there will be comparisons with cardiac catheterization. The scans have about one-quarter the resolution of the coronary artery lumen when compared to standard catheterization, especially using 64-slice CT scanners. Several problems exist with this procedure including exposure to ionizing radiation and exposure to iodinated contrast material which can lead to contrast-induced nephropathy especially in diabetics and those with pre-existing renal disease. Also many patients need B-blockade to achieve a heart rate of less than 60 for the test. Another problem with rapid sequence CT coronary angiography is that if there is calcium in the coronary artery, then the calcium limits the ability of the test to see coronary narrowing in that area. The test is more helpful in those without coronary calcification. More information on this emerging technology should be available in the next few years [10], especially its value to help stratify patients for future risk of CV events.

Screening for Peripheral Vascular Disease

Measuring the ankle-brachial blood pressure index (ABI) has long been a technique for evaluating the lower extremities for the presence of obstructive arterial disease. It is also recognized that the presence of peripheral lower extremity disease (PAD) increases the chance of having myocardial events and increased cardiovascular mortality. The ABI is a simple office test and has a good sensitivity (about 90%) and specificity (about 98%) for arterial occlusion of at least 50% narrowing [11], especially in older patients.

The test can be performed in the office with a blood pressure cuff and a handheld Doppler. The blood pressure cuff is used to measure the systolic BP in both arms by Doppler of the brachial artery. Then the BP cuff is placed around the ankle and the Doppler is used to measure systolic BP using the dorsalis pedis and posterior tibial arteries in both legs. The ABI for each leg is the higher of the two pedal pressures in that leg divided by the average of the arm blood pressures. An ABI of <90% in either leg is considered evidence for significant PAD.

Criqui et al. [12] found that ABI-detected PAD in men and women when followed for 10 years had a markedly increased risk of CVD and CHD mortality (RR 6.3 and 4.8, respectively). Thus, the presence of a positive ABI screen would increase one's risk of CV events and help risk stratification. Unfortunately, the ABI test is rarely positive in patients younger than 50, so it should be used in patients above the age of 50.

Carotid Intimal Medial Thickness Testing

Recently high-resolution B-mode ultrasonography is being used to assess atherosclerosis by measuring thickness of the intima and the media of the carotid arteries, called carotid intima-media thickness (IMT). The equipment is widely available, there is no radiation, and the scans can be performed in approximately 15 minutes. The small size of the IMT, usually less than 1 mm, necessitates computer-assisted measurements of the intima and media, using electronic calipers, and computer-assisted edge detection algorithms are used. This requires a special software package, and whereas ultrasound is widely available, the software for IMT is not as widely available. Figure 11.2 is an example of a typical report from an IMT test.

Cross-sectional studies have shown that the presence of an abnormal IMT is a surrogate marker for the presence of coronary artery disease. Thus, atherosclerotic thickening of the carotid intima and media reflects generalized atherosclerosis. Similarly, the presence of an abnormal IMT is an independent predictor for future CV events and stroke. One of the best studies, the atherosclerosis risk in communities (ARIC) study, followed 12,800 men and women after IMT over 4–7 years [13]. When those with IMT > 1 mm were compared to those with IMT < 1, the hazard ratio was 5.07 for women and 1.85 for men. In the ARIC study and the cardiovascular health study [14] there was a graded association between increasing IMT measurements and risk. In the cardiovascular health study, the association between CV events and IMT measurements remained after adjustment for traditional risk factors. Thus, it seems IMT measurements can provide additional helpful information to that from stratification by global risk assessment.

In addition, IMT testing is sensitive enough to be used as a monitor for the progression or regression of atherosclerotic arteries in clinical intervention trials. Although standardization of technique can be controlled in research trials allowing the use of this test for monitoring patients, it has yet to be shown that this same degree of reliability is achievable in community IMT testing.

One other advantage of B-mode imaging of the carotid arteries is that in addition to the amount of plaque, one also gets data on the nature of the plaque. Fibrous connective tissues such as collagen and minerals plus cholesterol monohydrate crystals are highly echogenic. On the other hand, hypoechogenic areas of plaque include necrotic areas, recent hemorrhage into plaques, and lipid-filled cores. Plaques with large amounts of hypoechogenic areas plus a thin fibromuscular cap, especially

A

CardioRisk™ Scan Patient Results©

PATIENT NAME:	REPORT, SAMPLE
GENDER:	M
DATE OF EXAM:	12/31/2005
DATE OF BIRTH:	2/28/1948
Physician:	Dr. Sample

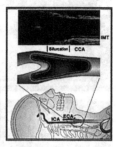

Patient Age	57	Patient IMT	0.86 mm
Arterial Age	74	Normal IMT	< .50mm

Test Criteria:	CV Event Risk			All measurements in mm	
	Normal	Moderate	High	Last Visit [+]	Alert Value [*]
Early Event Risk [++]			4.9		2.00
Average CCA Mean IMT		0.86			0.73
Average CCA Max Region			1.10		0.75
Plaque Burden [**]			11.0		

COMMENTS: The following values are the largest intima-media thickness (IMT) measurements found in each carotid artery segment. Any measurement equal to or exceeding 1.3mm is defined as 'plaque' and is characterized as plaque:
S = Soft; H = Heterogeneous; or E = Echogenic (includes mineral deposits like Calcium). (All measurements are in millimeters.)

Left: Common Carotid: 0.88; Bifurcation: 2.68 S; Internal Carotid: 1.49 H
Right: Common Carotid: 0.89; Bifurcation: 4.92 S; Internal Carotid: 1.95 E

++ Early Event Risk refers to a patient's increased risk of having an event in the next 5.1 years ± 2.3 years. It does not suggest the patient will have an event in that time frame, only that the hazard ratio significantly increases (from 1 to between 4.1 and 6.7 depending on the patient's Framingham risk score) (D Baldassare et al / Atherosclerosis xxx 2006 xxx-xxxx)

+ A progression rate of .034 mm or greater in the thickness of the mean IMT per year, increases the risk of future events significantly.
(Hodis HN, et al / Ann Intern Med 1998;128:262-9)

* The Alert Value is the threshold measurement at which this patient's risk is inflated beyond a 'Normal' reading.

** Plaque Burden is the sum of the plaques found and measured. It does not have an Alert Value because plaques of any size are atherosclerotic and increase patient risk. The Plaque Burden score is intended to help physicians track progression of disease over time.

Patients with values in Yellow or Red on ANY risk test criteria have inflated risk.

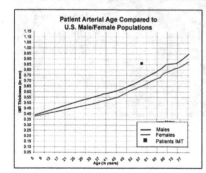

Your Doctor should interpret the results from this report in conjunction with your other risk factors. Medical decision making takes a multitude of factors into account, and risk factor modification should be made in consultation with your Doctor. ♦ Arterial Age™: The mean distal 1 cm common carotid artery (CCA) IMT measured looks like the average same gender person in a general population which had no coronary heart history expressed as Arterial Age above. The risk assessment data provided above should be used with caution. Data from five different studies which used different criteria for participation, different training methods, and different scanning and reading protocols [A: Tonstad, S (1996) Arterioscler Thromb; B: Urbina, E (2002) Am J Cardiol; C: Oren, A. (2003) Arch Intern Med.; D: Tonstad, S. (1998) Eur J Clin Invest; E: Aminbakhsh, A (1999) Clin Invest Med] were used to create an approximate arterial age compared to normal populations found in these studies. Regression analyses was used to estimate population age over time based on the cited studies above. In a careful literature review, the data cited above is an approximation of the relationship between CIMT and age in epidemiologic studies. The above data relating age to CIMT is useful in comparing a single patient's result with a population mean, and takes on additional meaning when comparing a current CardioRisk CIMT score with a previous CardioRisk CIMT score on the same patient. It is important to note that these studies do not account for the highest risk patients, those who died from the disease.

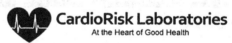 **CardioRisk Laboratories**
At the Heart of Good Health

9690 South 300 West   Sandy, UT. 84070 ♥ Office: 801.957.5445 ♥ Fax: 801.858.4512 ♥ www.cardiorisk.us   MKT-PR-v5J-10302007

Fig. 11.2 Typical report example of an IMT scan (Courtesy of CardioRisk Laboratories, Salt Lake City, UT.)

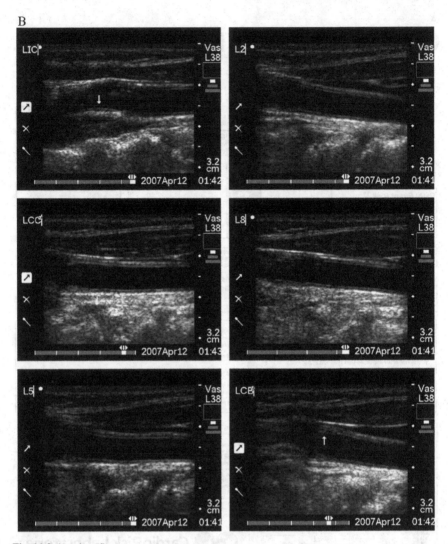

Fig. 11.2 (continued)

when combined with abnormal IMT measurements, are useful to identify unstable plaques prone to rupture. Honda [15] examined 286 consecutive patients with CAD, 71 with acute coronary syndromes (ACS), and 215 with stable CAD, with IMT and coronary artery catheterization. The plaque was analyzed using integrated backscatter (IBS) analysis as a quantitative way to measure the nature of the plaque, with lower IBS values indicating hypoechogenic or echolucent plaque. These patients were also followed for new cardiac events over 30 months. Echolucent plaque by IBS was strongly correlated with angiographic complex coronary plaques and with more cardiac events. There were 29 total coronary events in those with echolucent plaque versus 4 in those without (p < 0.001). This finding is especially interesting since the IMT values of each group were the same (2.2 mm).

The composition of plaque is also being investigated by magnetic resonance imaging (MRI). MRI imaging of the carotid arteries before carotid endarterectomy showed a good correlation between the MRI images and the pathology [16]. The aorta is also being evaluated by MRI to analyze the type of plaque. Here again the goal would be to identify patients with plaque characteristics correlating with instability and tendency to rupture. Many questions remain about this area: specifically, how strong will be the predictive value of different plaque types, and which imaging modality will prove to be superior for plaque imaging.

Exercise Testing as a Tool for Risk Stratification

There is a wealth of data using the exercise test (ET) to evaluate and stratify asymptomatic patients. A positive exercise test is an independent risk factor for increased CV mortality and events in asymptomatic patients, with a relative risk ratio usually in the 3–6 range compared to those with a negative test [17]. The multiple risk factor intervention trial (MRFIT) [18] with 12,866 participants only looked at the hard endpoint of cardiac death. Those with a positive ET had a three times greater risk of death than those with a negative ET. It is also clear that when one takes into account the presence of traditional risk factors with an abnormal exercise test the predictive power is much greater. Gibbons et al. from the Cooper Clinic [19] reported on a prospective study of 25,927 healthy men who underwent ET and were followed for 8.4 years. The age-adjusted relative risk in those with an abnormal ET was 21 times greater in those without risk factors, 27 times if one risk factor, 54 times if two risk factors, and 80 times if three or more risk factors were present. Finally, in the Framingham heart study offspring cohort, among 3,043 members free of CHD and followed for 18 years, those with ST-segment depression or failure to achieve target heart rate had a double risk of CHD. In this same study, a greater exercise capacity predicted lower CHD risk [20].

The exercise test provides multiple variables that are prognostically important. Four important exercise variables include (1) exercise duration less than 6 METS, (2) ST-segment depression, (3) heart rate impairment, and (4) chest pain at maximal exertion. Dyspnea should also be added as an important prognostic variable. Bodegard [21] reported on 2,014 asymptomatic men followed for 26 years. Those who terminated the exercise test for dyspnea as opposed to fatigue had a 2-fold increased risk of dying from CAD and a 3.5-fold increased risk of dying from pulmonary disease. As the number of these abnormal exercise variables increases in any given asymptomatic patient, the relative risk and predictive value increase. This is also true when both traditional risk factors and abnormal exercise variables are combined.

Thus, the exercise test provides important information that can further stratify asymptomatic patients who are at intermediate risk by global risk assessment (GRA). Intermediate-risk patients by GRA who have an abnormal ET will certainly move into the high-risk category where aggressive medical treatment is indicated.

(GRA). Intermediate-risk patients by GRA who have an abnormal ET will certainly move into the high-risk category where aggressive medical treatment is indicated.

Will exercise testing in intermediate-risk asymptomatic patients identify some patients who are at such high risk that they should be referred for interventional procedures to improve life expectancy? The answer is yes but rarely. Most asymptomatic patients with abnormal ETs will have mild coronary disease. At the USAFMC, Froelicher [22] reported on the catheterization results of 111 asymptomatic men with abnormal ETs. Only one-third of those catheterized had one or more lesions greater than 50% stenosed. Approximately 1–2 % of asymptomatic patients with abnormal ET will have severe three-vessel disease. These patients will be recognized by the indicators of severe ischemia as discussed in Chapter 5; myocardial ischemia at a low MET level, more than 2.5 mm ST-segment depression, downsloping ST-segment depression, ST-segment depression lasting more than 8 minutes into recovery, exercise-induced hypotension, or a high-risk exercise treadmill score. These severe ischemic responses will rarely be seen in asymptomatic patients but would merit further evaluation with nuclear imaging or catheterization with consideration for revascularization.

In summary, the exercise test is an excellent tool to help stratify asymptomatic patients. As the above studies demonstrate, there are more prognostic data on exercise testing over a longer period of time than with the other tools discussed for risk stratification. In addition, the exercise test is the only tool to provide the patients' aerobic capacity, which also has strong prognostic implications. Discovering a low aerobic capacity can motivate individuals to improve, as each MET increase in exercise capacity equates to a 10–15% increase in survival [23]. Considering all this new information, Froelicher [24] has recently recommended that all asymptomatic individuals (men over 40 years and women over 50 years) should undergo exercise testing on a regular basis in addition to traditional risk factor assessment [25].

Biochemical Markers for Risk Stratification

Recently there has been considerable discussion about the use of biochemical markers to help identify patients at increased risk for cardiac events and death. Since atherosclerosis can be considered an inflammatory response to vessel injury, many of these markers are inflammatory markers. Markers have included soluble adhesion molecules, cytokines, and acute-phase reactants. Since soluble adhesion molecules and cytokines are unstable making assays difficult, more research involves the acute-phase reactants such as high-sensitivity C-reactive protein (hs-CRP), fibrinogen, serum amyloid A (SSA), and the white blood count (WBC). Many questions arise about the use of biochemical markers:

1. Which are the best markers to be measured, if any?
2. Do the markers add independent prognostic information to the available traditional risk factors?

3. If they do, what is the best use of the markers?
4. Can the markers be used to monitor therapy?

These questions were addressed in the AHA/CDC scientific statement on markers of inflammation and cardiovascular disease [26]. The consensus statement recommended that hs-CRP had the best data and availability and recommended its use over other markers. Hs-CRP was an independent risk factor, even when other risk factors were controlled. There seems to be a dose–response relationship between the level of hs-CRP and the risk of coronary events. There is a 2-fold increase in major coronary events when patients with the lowest tertile of hs-CRP are compared to the upper tertile. These tertiles correspond to values of low risk (<1.0), average risk (1.0–3.0), and high risk (>3.0). The AHA/CDC Writing Group recommended measuring hs-CRP only after standard global risk appraisal, and only in selected individuals. Hs-CRP might be helpful to further stratify those at intermediate risk, to decide if aggressive therapy is needed. They recommended against using hs-CRP in all individuals, or in those already stratified as high risk, and felt hs-CRP is not indicated for monitoring of therapy.

More recently a study by Wang [27] and associates supported these recommendations. In this study 3,209 participants of the Framingham offspring group had 10 biomarkers measured and were followed for 7.4 years. They evaluated the predictive ability of individual markers plus a calculated multimarker score. Individually, the B-natriuretic peptide and hs-CRP were the best predictors of future events. However, the use of individual markers or a multimarker score added little to the classification of risk by conventional risk factors as measured by the C statistic. James Ware [28], in an editorial discussing these findings states, "this group of biomarkers makes a substantial contribution to the proportional-hazards model for predicting death from any cause, but it is of limited value for the risk stratification of individual patients." These articles emphasize the importance of using conventional risk factors for risk stratification in asymptomatic patients.

A Better Approach

Froelicher has proposed that exercise testing should be used for screening healthy, asymptomatic individuals along with risk factor assessment for the following reasons:

- A number of contemporary studies (previously discussed) have demonstrated remarkable risk ratios for the combination of the standard exercise test responses and traditional risk factors.
- Other modalities without the favorable test characteristics of the exercise test (i.e., EBCT) are being promoted for screening.
- Physical inactivity has reached epidemic proportions, and the exercise test provides an ideal way to make patients conscious of their deconditioning and to make physical activity recommendations.

- Adjusting for age and other risk factors, each MET increase in exercise capacity equates to a 10–25% improvement in survival.

Summary and Recommendations

All asymptomatic patients should be initially risk-stratified using one of the global risk assessment tools. These tools are readily available and inexpensive to apply. Using these tools patients who are at low risk for CV events and decreased mortality should continue to have therapeutic lifestyle changes including appropriate diet, weight loss, and exercise advice and are not candidates for aggressive drug treatment.

High-risk asymptomatic patients based on global risk assessment should have aggressive medical treatment to recommended goals. Further testing is usually not indicated as the goals of treatment are evident. Testing in these patients could be useful to look for signs of severe ischemia where surgical intervention would be life-prolonging, for instance, patients who show signs of severe ischemia on an exercise test or have a high-risk exercise treadmill score. Exercise testing in these high-risk asymptomatic patients might also be indicated to clear patients for a moderate intensity exercise program, say especially in high-risk diabetic patients [29] (see Chapter 4, Testing Special Populations). Finally, further testing could be used to follow the effectiveness of the therapeutic regimen, for example, using serial IMT measurements.

Many patients will have intermediate scores based on global risk scoring. These patients are ideally further stratified by testing to decide which ones need aggressive therapy. All of the tools discussed above can be helpful in varying degrees to further

Table 11.1 Probability of a coronary event within 10 years calculated on the basis of the results of electron-beam CT or of exercise electrocardiography

Pretest probability of a coronary event within 10 years	Probability within 10 years according to results of electron-beam CT		Probability within 10 years according to results of exercise electrocardiography	
	Calcium score ≥80 (%)	Calcium score <80 (%)	Abnormal (%)	Normal (%)
1.0	3.0	0.2	4.0	0.4
2.0	6.5	0.4	8.0	0.9
3.0	9.5	0.6	12.0	1.3
4.0	12.5	0.9	15.0	1.9
5.0	15.0	1.0	19.0	2.3
6.0	18.0	1.2	22.0	2.8
7.0	20.0	1.4	25.0	3.3
10.0	27.0	2.2	33.0	4.8
15.0	38.0	3.4	44.0	7.4
20.0	46.0	4.8	52.0	10.0

From Greenland P, Graziano JM [30], by permission of *N Engl J Med*.

stratify these patients. The evidence is greatest for exercise testing, and then CT coronary scores, followed by the other tools.

Greenland and Gaziano [30] discussed using the exercise test or coronary calcium scores to further stratify patients after global risk assessment. They presented a table showing how the risk percent changed when the results of each test were applied. This approach is especially useful for the patients with an intermediate-risk level and is recommended (Table 11.1).

Arguments can be made for each of the above tests as the best test to further stratify patients. There are no prospective studies that compare these tests against each other for the purpose of determining the best, most cost-efficient approach to stratifying the asymptomatic patient. Due to the wealth of information available from the maximal exercise test on amount of ischemia, presence of severe ischemia, hemodynamic responses, and aerobic capacity, one would be hard-pressed not to recommend the ET as the best test for further risk stratification in the patient who is at intermediate risk by global risk assessment.

Finally, as discussed previously, and further in Chapters 15 and 16, the exercise test is a very effective means of evaluating the fitness level and then prescribing an appropriate exercise prescription to help our patients achieve a higher level of fitness and the resulting health benefits.

References

1. O'Rourke RA, Brundage BH, Froelicher VF, et al. American College of Cardiology/American Heart Association Expert Consensus document on electron-beam computed tomography for the diagnosis and prognosis of coronary artery disease. Circulation 2000; 102:126–40.
2. Taylor AJ, Bairey Merz CN, Udelson JE, et al. Can Atherosclerosis Imaging Techniques Improve the Detection of Patients at Risk for Ischemic Heart Disease? Presented at the 34th Bethesda Conference, Bethesda, Maryland, October 7, 2002, J Am Coll Cardiol 2003; 41:1855–917.
3. Grundy SM, Pasternak R, Greenland P, et al. Assessment of cardiovascular risk by use of multiple-risk-factor assessment equations: a statement for healthcare professionals from the American Heart Association and the American College of Cardiology. Circulation 1999; 100:1481–92.
4. Executive Summary of the Third Report of the National Cholesterol Education Program (NCEP). Expert Panel on Detection, Evaluation and Treatment of High Blood Cholesterol in Adults (Adult Treatment Panel III). JAMA 2001; 285:2486–97.
5. Burde and Virmani et al. Pathologic Basis for New Atherosclerosis Imaging Techniques, in 34th Bethesda Conference, ibid. p 1881.
6. Arad Y, Spadaro LA, Goodman K, et al. Predictive value of electron beam CT of the coronary arteries: 19 month follow-up of 1173 asymptomatic subjects. Circulation 1996; 93:1951–1953.
7. Redberg, RF and Vogel RA, What is the Spectrum of Current and Emerging Techniques for the Noninvasive Measurement of Atherosclerosis? 34th Bethesda Conference, ibid, page 1889.
8. Greenland P, LaBree L, Azen SP, et al. Coronary artery calcium score combined with Framingham score for risk prediction in asymptomatic individuals. JAMA 2004; 291:210–215.
9. Greenland P, Bonow RO, Brundage BH, et al. ACCF/AHA 2007 clinical expert consensus document on coronary artery calcium scoring by computed tomography in global cardiovascular risk assessment and in evaluation of patients with chest pain: a report of the American College of Cardiology Foundation Clinical Expert Consensus Task Force. J Am Coll Cardiol 2007; 49: 378–402.

10. ACC/AHA Clinical Competence Statement of Cardiac Imaging with Computed Tomography and Magnetic Resonance. JACC 2005;46:383–402.

11. Greenland P, et al. Prevention Conference V: Beyond Secondary Prevention; Identifying the High-Risk Patient for Primary Prevention, Noninvasive Test of Atherosclerotic Burden. Circulation 2000; 101: e16–e22.

12. Criqui MH, Langer RD, Fronek A, et al. Mortality over a period of 10 years in patients with peripheral arterial disease. N Engl J Med 1992; 326:381–6.

13. Chambless LE, Heiss G, Folsom AR et al. Carotid arterial wall thickness and major risk factors: the Atherosclerosis Risk in Communities (ARIC) Study 1987–1993. Am J Epidemiol 1997; 146:483–494.

14. O'Leary DH, Polak JF, Kronmal RA, et al. Carotid-artery intima and media thickness as a risk factor for myocardial infarction and stroke in older adults: Cardiovascular Health Study. N Engl J Med 1999; 340:14–22.

15. Honda O, Sugiyama S, Kugiyama K, et al. Echolucent carotid plaques predict future coronary events in patients with coronary artery disease. J Amer Coll Cardiol 2004; 43: 1177–84.

16. Toussaint JF, LaMuraglia GM, Southern JF et al. Magnetic resonance images lipid, fibrous, calcified, hemorrhagic and thrombotic components of human atherosclerosis in vivo. Circulation 1996; 94: 932–8.

17. Froelicher VF and Myers J. Exercise and the Heart, 5th Ed. Saunders Elsevier, Philadelphia, 2006, 361–6.

18. Multiple Risk Factor Intervention Research Group: Exercise electrocardiogram and coronary heart disease mortality in the multiple risk factor intervention trial. Am J Cardiol 1985;55: 16–24.

19. Gibbons LW, Mitchell TL, Wei M, et al. Maximal exercise test as a predictor of risk for mortality from coronary heart disease in asymptomatic men. Am J Cardiol 2000; 86: 53–58.

20. Balady GJ, Larson MG, Vasan RS, et al. Usefulness of exercise testing in the prediction of coronary disease risk among asymptomatic persons as a function of the Framingham risk score. Circulation 2004; 10:1920–25.

21. Bodegard J, Erikssen G, Bjornhold JV, et al. Reasons for terminating an exercise test provide independent prognostic information. 2014 apparently healthy men followed for 26 years. Eur Hear J doi: 10.1093/eurheartj/ehi278.

22. Froelicher VF and Myers J. Exercise and the Heart, 5th Ed. Saunders Elsevier, Philadelphia, 2006, 367–8.

23. Myers J, Kaykha A, George S, et al. Fitness versus physical activity patterns in predicting mortality in men. Am J Med 2004; 117:912–918.

24. Froelicher VF. Screening with the exercise test: time for a guideline change? Eur Heart J. doi:10.1093/eurheartj/ehi303.

25. Froelicher VF and Myers J. Exercise and the Heart, 5th Ed. Saunders Elsevier, Philadelphia, 2006, preface, ix.

26. Pearson TA, Mensah GA, et al. Markers of Inflammation and Cardiovascular Disease, Application to Clinical and Public Health practice, A statement for Healthcare professionals from the Centers for Disease Control and Prevention and the American Heart Association. Circulation 2003; 107:499–511.

27. Wang TF, Gona P Larson MG, et al. Multiple biomarkers for the prediction of first major cardiovascular events and death. N Eng J Med 2006; 355:2631–9.

28. Ware JH, The limitations of risk factors as prognostic tools. N Eng J Med 2006; 355: 2615–7.

29. Sigal, RJ, Kenny GP, Wasserman, DH, et al. Physical Activity/Exercise and Type 2 Diabetes; A Consensus Statement from the American Diabetes Association. Diabetes Care 2006; 29: 1433–1438.

30. Greenland P and Graziano JM. Selecting Asymptomatic Patients for coronary computed tomography or electrocardiographic exercise testing. N Engl J Med 2003; 349: 465–73.

Chapter 12
Promoting Therapeutic Lifestyle Change and the Primary Prevention of Coronary Artery Disease

George D. Harris

Cardiovascular disease (CVD) is the leading cause of death in the United States claiming 927,448 American lives in 2002 [1] with coronary heart disease (CHD) as the single largest component. There were 494,382 coronary heart disease deaths in 2002, including 179,514 deaths from myocardial infarctions. Two significant populations contributing to the prevalence of CVD are those with hypertension and diabetes mellitus. There are similar multiple metabolic components and hemodynamic abnormalities that play a significant role in both chronic diseases [2].

The mortality from CVD in men has been well established and continues to be a concern. However, there is increasing concern and emphasis now being made on the significant effect CVD is having on the female population. Heart disease, stroke and other cardiovascular diseases kill nearly half a million women in the United States every year—more than the next five causes of death combined and representing nearly twice as many deaths as all forms of cancer, including breast cancer [1]. Therefore, the prevention of CVD is a significant public health concern and more emphasis is being placed on primary prevention [3] which intends both to prevent and modify risk factors and to prevent the development of chronic diseases.

Atherosclerosis begins in childhood and progresses in adolescence and early adulthood, to cause CHD in middle age or older individuals [4]. There are certain risk factors known to predict the incidence of CHD in adults which are associated with advanced atherosclerotic lesions. The major risk factors include hypertension, diabetes mellitus, hyperlipidemia, sedentary lifestyle and smoking. The Framingham Study showed that cigarette smoking, high blood pressure, dyslipidemia and diabetes mellitus, significantly and independently increased the risk of CHD.

Tobacco use, poor dietary habits and physical inactivity (three health behaviors) are associated with increased risk of CVD and account for the largest and second largest number of preventable deaths each year [5].

Aging, obesity and stress also contribute to atherosclerosis. A significant number of these risk factors—the decision to use tobacco products, the control of blood

G.D. Harris (✉)

Department of Community and Family Medicine, University of Missouri-Kansas City, School of Medicine, Truman Medical Center—Lakewood, Kansas City, MO 64139 USA

e-mail: george.harris@tmcmed.org

C.H. Evans, R.D. White (eds.), *Exercise Testing for Primary Care and Sports Medicine Physicians,* DOI 10.1007/978-0-387-76597-6_12

pressure, control of lipids, diabetes, level of physical activity and obesity all involve lifestyle practices.

Between the years of 1980–90, there was a dramatic decline in CHD of over 50% due to reducing the major risk factors; the remaining decline was due to improved treatment of clinically apparent disease [6]. Lifestyle modification and the pharmacotherapeutic management of hypertension, hyperlipidemia and diabetes mellitus are now recommended for primary and secondary prevention of CHD in adults [7].

Primary Prevention

Primary prevention of CHD intends to prevent and modify risk factors as well as prevent the development of chronic diseases. The majority of the causes of cardiovascular disease are known and modifiable. Modifiable, healthy choices such as consuming a prudent diet, exercising regularly, maintaining a healthy weight and not smoking constitute a low-risk lifestyle for coronary heart disease (CHD). This lifestyle has the potential to reduce coronary heart disease risk by improving lipids, glucose metabolism and blood pressure. In addition, this same lifestyle choice also can reduce vascular inflammation, homocysteine levels and the occurrence of arrhythmias.

Two short-term trials on diet, physical activity and weight loss have demonstrated substantial reduction in coronary risk factors and coronary events [8, 9]. Chiuve et al. revealed that a low-risk lifestyle may be an effective strategy to lower the risk of coronary heart disease among middle-aged and older men and even among men already reducing cardiovascular risk by taking antihypertensive and lipid-lowering medications [10]. Tobacco use, poor dietary habits and physical inactivity together account for almost one-quarter (23%) of all preventable deaths in the United States [5].

The American Heart Association (AHA) Position Paper states that a CVD risk factor assessment in adults should begin at age 20 years. At least every 2 years a visit to the physician should occur with the measurement of blood pressure, body mass index, waist circumference and pulse (to screen for atrial fibrillation) recorded. The patient's smoking status, diet, alcohol intake and physical activity should be assessed at every routine evaluation. At least every 5 years, a fasting serum lipoprotein profile (or total and HDL cholesterol if fasting is unavailable) and fasting blood glucose should be measured. If the patient is at risk for hyperlipidemia and diabetes, respectively, then testing should be done every 2 years [11].

For patients over age 40 years or for those patients with more than two risk factors, a 10-year risk of CHD assessment should be performed with a multiple risk score. The risk factors used in global risk assessment include age, sex, smoking status, systolic (and sometimes diastolic) blood pressure, total cholesterol, LDL- and HDL-cholesterol. Individuals with diabetes or 10-year risk >20% can be considered at a level of risk similar to a patient with established cardiovascular disease (CHD risk equivalent) [11].

The most widely used scale used for factor reduction in the primary prevention of CHD is the Framingham Risk Scoring System, which predicts the likelihood of developing CHD over a 10-year timeframe in individuals who do not already have established coronary artery disease [12].

Asymptomatic adults should have an assessment of individual risk according to the AHA guidelines. As indicated, specific and individualized lifestyle interventions and when appropriate, specific pharmacological medications, such as aspirin and lipid-lowering drugs, should be implemented. Using the Framingham Risk Score an estimated risk of clinical cardiovascular events can be made. For individuals with an estimated 10-year risk greater than 20%, aggressive interventions are appropriate. For those at intermediate risk (10–20%), testing for high risk but asymptomatic atherosclerosis with high-sensitivity C-reactive protein (CRP), stress testing, electron-beam-computed tomography, measurement of ankle-brachial index or ultrasound to measure carotid intima-media thickness (CIMT) may be indicated [13, 14]. Low-risk (<10%) individuals should receive conservative management focusing on lifestyle interventions.

The various recommendations for the primary prevention of coronary artery disease (CAD) can be itemized into eight main categories. These include (1) tobacco use cessation; (2) losing weight or achieving ideal body weight; (3) ingesting appropriate calories of carbohydrates, omega-3 fatty acids, and proteins in the daily diet; (4) daily aerobic exercise; (5) screening and aggressively treating hypertension; (6) screening and aggressively treating dyslipidemias; (7) screening and aggressively treating diabetes mellitus; and (8) promoting mental wellness.

Other recommendations to consider based on gender and age include (1) short-term estrogen supplementation for women to relieve menopausal symptoms; (2) daily low-dose aspirin therapy for men over 40 and women over 50; otherwise, low-dose (75–160 mg per day) aspirin is recommended for those individuals with a 10-year CHD risk of 10% or greater; and (3) assessment for CAD risk factors with risk stratification for exercise treadmill testing, stress echocardiogram or nuclear stress testing.

Specific Lifestyle Interventions

Tobacco Use Cessation

Cigarette smoking is the leading preventable cause of death from all causes in the United States. It is the single most prevalent modifiable risk factor for the development of coronary heart disease. The prevalence of smoking has now leveled off to about 25% of the overall population in the United States but has actually grown in certain populations, especially women, adolescents and young adults. Multiple observational studies have shown that smokeless tobacco and low-tar cigarettes do not reduce the risk of CHD. Tobacco decreases high-density lipoprotein (HDL) cholesterol, decreases coronary flow and causes spasm of the coronary arteries [15].

The United States Preventive Services Task Force (USPSTF) recommends that physicians view tobacco use as a chronic disease with remissions and relapses and view a patient's relapse as a disease stage instead of a treatment failure. The USP-STF further recommends using a treatment model approach where every patient is assessed for tobacco use and receives an intervention based on that use [16]. Each physician should develop a plan with the patient to stop smoking, initiate counseling and pharmacologic therapy, if indicated. In addition, patients should avoid exposure to secondhand smoke at work and at home.

Smoking cessation together with aspirin therapy has been shown to reduce CVD in diabetic patients. Unless there is a contraindication, patients with metabolic syndrome, pre-diabetes or diabetes mellitus should be offered 81 mg of aspirin per day [2].

Nicotine replacement therapy and several medications (bupropion SR, clonidine, and nortriptyline) have been found to be successful in smoking cessation treatments. The use of nicotine gum, patch, spray and inhaler has lead to abstinence rates of 18–31% [16].

Body Weight

Overweight and obesity have become an epidemic problem in the United States and approximately 64% of the population has one of these two conditions [17]. Obesity is a major risk factor for CAD. The First Law of Thermodynamics (Net energy = Amount ingested-amount metabolized) and a sedentary lifestyle illustrate the reason for our present obesity epidemic [2].

It is predicted that in 30 years over 95% of the US population will be obese if present trends continue. To curb this tendency, children and adolescents who are at increased risk for obesity must be identified. In addition, encouraging physical education as well as removing of high carbohydrate, high caloric foods and drinks from the school system is mandatory.

Counseling on the necessity for weight loss through proper nutrition including the restriction of calories and daily exercise are the recommendations for each patient. The initial goal should be a reduction of body weight by 10% during the first year of therapy with a long-term goal of achieving and maintaining a body mass index (BMI) between 18.5 and 24.9.

Medical Nutrition Therapy

Medical nutrition therapy focuses on caloric intake and selected food groups [2]. The USPSTF states that there is evidence that medium- to high-intensity counseling interventions by specialists (e.g., nutritionists, dietitians) can produce medium or large changes in average daily intake of saturated fat, fiber, fruits and vegetables for adult patients with hyperlipidemia or other known risk factors for cardiovascular or other diet-related chronic disease ("B"). Medium- to high-intensity counseling was defined as multiple contacts, generally more than six visits, each lasting more than 30 minutes [18].

Several of the modifiable risk factors of CVDs are influenced by diet. These include obesity and waist circumference, hypertension, dyslipidemias and blood glucose regulation. There is medical evidence supporting that emerging risk factors such as elevated plasma homocysteine, C-reactive protein, oxidative stress and certain hemostatic factors are also influenced by diet [19].

The China Study, a research project expanded over 20 years, provided an extensive survey of disease and lifestyle factors in rural China and Taiwan (in over 100 villages). T. Colin Campbell and his research partners produced over 8,000 statistically significant correlations between varying diets of the Chinese communities studied and the differences in rates of diseases [20]. Campbell stated individuals who consumed plant-based foods were the healthiest and avoided chronic diseases (significant heart disease and many cancers). He recommends not consuming any animal meats or fats. Given the fact that the Western diet is high in fat and animal meats and low in fruits and vegetables, Campbell et al. studies examined how small alterations in diet content can have significant impact on the mortality rates of people [20]. This concept is easily demonstrated when an individual from a Far East country such as China whose basic diet is fish and vegetables moves to the United States and accepts the Western diet. There is significant change in lean body weight and mass, lipid levels and the development of the metabolic syndrome, all increasing the risk of CHD and CVD. Replacing saturated fat in the diet with unsaturated fat has been shown to be more effective in reducing serum cholesterol than just lowering fat [21]. In populations with relatively low fat intake, a moderate increase of total dietary fat intake may be a risk factor for CVD [22].

Saturated and trans fats (e.g., margarine, vegetable shortenings, foods containing partially hydrogenated vegetable oil) are the most atherogenic. The monounsaturated (e.g., olive oil, canola oil, peanut oil, peanut butter, most nuts) and polyunsaturated (e.g., omega 3's-fish oil, flaxseed; Omega 6's-corn safflower, soybean oils; walnuts) fats are associated with decreased CVD risk. Initiating a larger monounsaturated fat intake can reduce triglycerides and raise HDL cholesterol.

The American Heart Association (AHA) recommendations do not completely eliminate animal meats or fats from our diet. The AHA recommends a daily intake of ≤30% total dietary fat, with <10% of the fat being saturated and a cholesterol consumption of ≤300 mg daily [23]. For individuals with established risk factors for CVD, the AHA recommends ≤200 mg cholesterol per day and ≤20% total dietary fat, with <7% of that saturated fat (e.g., cheese, butter, fatty meats) [23].

A recommended daily intake of carbohydrates should be about 50–60% of the total calories with emphasis on whole grains, fruits and vegetables (5+ serving per day). Combining a variety of less-processed foods with a diet high in vegetables, legumes, fruits, whole grains, nuts, fish and lean sources of dairy products is recommended. USDA guidelines also recommend consumption of at least two servings of fruit daily and of at least three daily servings of vegetables, with at least one-third being dark green or orange vegetables.

The type of carbohydrate may have effect on the CVD risk. For example, foods having a high glycemic index (GI), raise blood glucose rapidly upon ingestion and are implicated in increasing CVD risk more than those with a lower GI [24]. Consumption of whole grains has been shown to reduce risk factors for metabolic syndrome, CVD and type 2 diabetes mellitus and improved plasma lipid profiles [25] due to their vitamins, minerals, antioxidants, phytochemicals, lignans and dietary fibers acting synergistically in their protective effects.

The recommended daily fiber intake should be 20–30 g per day. Daily recommended protein intake should represent approximately 15% of the total calories. In addition, salt (sodium chloride) intake should be less than 6 g/day (equivalent of 2,400 mg of sodium per day) and the individual should limit alcohol intake to no more than 1 drink per day. A hypertensive patient should to follow the DASH (Dietary Approaches to Stop Hypertension) diet.

Aerobic Exercise

There is clear scientific evidence linking regular physical activity to significant cardiovascular risk reduction [26]. Aerobic exercise results in decreased myocardial oxygen demands in the physically active and fit individual for the same level of external work performed by a sedentary individual. This is demonstrated by a decrease in the product of the heart rate × systolic blood pressure, reducing the likelihood of myocardial ischemia.

Regular aerobic physical activity results in improved exercise performance and improved maximal cardiac output and peripheral oxygen extraction. These effects lead to a reduction of cardiovascular and coronary artery disease mortality in physically active and fit individuals. Exercise seems to be most cardioprotective when done daily and in moderation.

A meta-analysis of 30 cohort studies involving over two million person-years of observation demonstrated a nearly linear decline in the risk of CAD with increasing levels of physical activity [27].

A volume of moderate-intensity aerobic physical activity of 1,000 kcal/week yields a reduction in risk of all-cause and cardiovascular mortality of 20–30%, with higher volumes of physical activity providing potentially greater health benefits [28, 29]. Participating in 30 minutes or more of moderate-intensity aerobic physical activity 5–7 days per week achieves 1,000 kcal/week energy expenditure. Moderate-intensity aerobic activity is exercise performed at 40–60% of maximal oxygen uptake (VO_{2max}) and/or 50–70% of maximal predicted heart rate (equivalent to a perceived exertion score of 11–13 in the 6–20 Borg scale) [29]. Examples of aerobic physical activity include brisk walking, climbing stairs, jogging, bicycling, swimming or an aerobic class. Vigorous physical activity is anything greater than 60% VO_{2max} or 70% maximal predicted heart rate.

The intensity of the exercise is relative to the individual's age, physical condition and degree of physical fitness. Brisk walking may not meet the criteria for moderate physical activity for a person of college age and yet, may be considered a vigorous activity for an individual over age 65 [30]. Therefore, the exercise prescription should be individualized and relative to the patient's capabilities and limitations. It is not known whether a total volume expended in shorter and more frequent bouts has different effects on mortality rates then the same volume expended in longer, less frequent sessions [31].

In addition to decreasing cardiovascular risks, increased physical activity and cardiorespiratory fitness have been correlated with increased physical self-esteem and psychological well-being [32, 33], enhanced vigor and energy [34] and higher ratings of life satisfaction [35].

However, there is evidence suggesting a difference between men and women for the dose–response relationship between exercise intensity and risk for CHD or mortality [30]. The Women's Health Study [36] revealed that (1) walking 1–1.5 hours per week was associated with a 51% reduction in risk for CHD but walking more than 2 hours per week conferred no greater reduction in risk; (2) more vigorous activity was not associated with a lower risk for CHD; and (3) the relationship between walking pace and risk for CHD did not demonstrate a linear trend. In addition, two other studies (Blair et al. [37] and Sherman et al. [38]) demonstrated that all-cause mortality rates in women did not differ across the range of physical activity levels and that there was no association between physical activity level and mortality in women, respectively. Thus, risk reduction associated with physical activity appears variable depending on the study population [30].

Both physical activity and fitness are strong predictors of all-cause mortality. However, physical fitness seems to be a stronger predictor of mortality than activity level since physical fitness has demonstrated an even stronger negative association with CHD and mortality, with a 17–20% reduction in mortality for every 1-MET increase in fitness [30]. Therefore, the American College of Sports Medicine recommends vigorous physical activity to facilitate increases in cardiorespiratory fitness. However, it should be noted that even moderate physical activity, performed regularly, results in an increase in fitness and should be recommended to the individual patient [30].

All of this evidence leads to prescribing an exercise prescription specific to the individual based on aged, gender and physical limitations. The American College of Preventive Medicine takes the position that primary care physicians should incorporate physical activity counseling into routine patient visits. An effective approach can be established with a few basic strategies (providing brief provider training, creating an office support system, writing tailored exercise prescriptions, and using a variety of healthcare team members) and lead to increasing physical activity for healthy adult patients [39].

Hypertension Management

The 1999–2002 National Health and Nutrition Examination Survey (NHANES) showed that about 65 million Americans had high blood pressure in 2002 representing a 30% increase over the previous survey from 1988 to 1994.

Demonstrating that the prevalence of hypertension in the United States continues to increase with more than one-third of American adults now having hypertension [40].

The goal of blood pressure (BP) management is to reach a BP of less than 140/90 mmHg for those individuals with a history of hypertension, a goal of less than of 120/80 mmHg for the non-hypertensive patient and less than 130/80 mmHg for patients with renal disease and diabetes mellitus.

Weight loss has been shown to decrease systolic and diastolic blood pressure as well as LDL-cholesterol and lipid levels in obese diabetic patients [41, 42].

In addition to the healthy lifestyle changes of weight loss, proper nutritional intake including sodium consumption <2,400 mg per day, and daily exercise, one may need to initiate medications to achieve adequate BP goals.

Dyslipidemia

The US Male Health Professional Follow-Up Study, the Multiple Risk Factor Intervention Trial (MRFIT), and the Nurses' Health Study all have demonstrated the association between elevated blood cholesterol and increased risk of coronary artery disease. Other trials have demonstrated that lowering the LDL-cholesterol levels below 70 mg% may further reduce the risk of cardiovascular events in individuals with established CHD [43]. According to the most recent National Cholesterol Education Program (NCEP) guidelines, HDL levels lower than 40 mg/dL are considered an independent risk factor for CHD [7].

Proper management should include daily exercise, weight loss, proper nutritional intake and, if indicated, pharmacologic therapy to reach NCEP guidelines. The goal of therapy is a LDL-cholesterol less than 160 mg%, if there is less than one risk factor; less than 100 mg% if there are two or more risk factors and a 10-year CHD risk less than 20%; and less than 70 mg% if there are two or more risk factors and a 10-year CHD risk greater than 20% or if the individual has diabetes mellitus.

Pharmacotherapy includes the use of fibrates, statins and niacin. Fibrates are recommended for the treatment of elevated triglycerides and low HDL-cholesterol levels. Statins are recommended for elevated LDL-cholesterol levels and are known to be beneficial for the primary prevention of cardiovascular events in patients younger than 65 years who have hyperlipidemia. This class of drugs may increase the risk of myositis and rhabdomyolysis. Niacin raises high-density lipoprotein cholesterol (HDL-C) levels, lowers triglyceride, low-density lipoprotein cholesterol (LDL-C) and lipoprotein(a) levels and reduces atherogenic small, dense LDL particles [44]. Dietary niacin (vitamin B3 or nicotinic acid) should not be used as a substitute for prescription niacin (e.g., Niaspan, Niacor, Slo-Niacin) because of its potentially serious side effects. Prescribing an aspirin (325 mg) 30 minutes prior to dose of prescription niacin may reduce its associated flushing. Niacin may cause an elevation in glucose levels so caution its use in patients with diabetes.

Diabetes Management

A lack of physical activity and excessive eating can initiate and propagate type 2 diabetes mellitus. Multiple studies have demonstrated a strong relationship between excess weight and the risk of developing type 2 diabetes mellitus. With the incidence and prevalence of obesity rising significantly in the United States, the frequency of diabetes has risen in most age-groups and ethnicities [45].

In high-risk individuals with impaired glucose tolerance or impaired fasting glucose, lifestyle modification (diet and exercise) can decrease the likelihood of developing type 2 diabetes. The effectiveness of this approach has been demonstrated to be superior than initiating metformin therapy [46].

For patients with existing diabetes mellitus, the initial steps of management should also be proper nutritional therapy, weight loss and daily exercise to achieve a normal range plasma glucose level and A1C less than 7%. Exercise as part of a weight-loss regimen not only helps maintain weight loss but also prevents weight being regained.

Boule et al. demonstrated in patients with type 2 diabetes the effects of structured regimens of physical activity for 8 weeks or longer can improve A1C independent of changes in body mass as well as further improvement in A1C as the intensity of exercise is increased [47,48].

In addition to controlling one's weight and daily aerobic exercise, smoking cessation, blood pressure control, instituting a low saturated fat and low cholesterol diet are highly recommended. A diet restricted to 1,100 kcal/day has been shown to decrease fasting blood glucose of obese patients with diabetes and even in those without diabetes in as few as 4 days due to a decreased hepatic glucose output. With continued calorie restriction, a further decline in the fasting glucose levels of obese diabetic subjects was noted along with significant improvement in insulin sensitivity. The average weight loss was only 6 kg to attain the results [45].

Lifestyle modification sometimes falls short in achieving adequate glucose control. At that point, one initiates pharmacotherapy with a sulfonylurea, biguanide (metformin) or insulin with the addition of a thiazolidinedione (TZD) or one of the other agents, if not instituted previously. For patients with type 1 diabetes oral agents are not indicated, and insulin (basal and bolus dosing) is implemented.

As far as which oral agent to supplement lifestyle changes should be initiated, there are advantages and disadvantages to all of them. Metformin therapy can cause nausea, vomiting, anorexia and diarrhea. However, most patients taking metformin lose weight mainly due to loss of body fat mass and the weight loss during its initiation occurs even without a change in energy expenditure [49]. There are three disadvantages to using a sulfonyurea: the risk of hypoglycemia, the risk of weight gain and a contraindication in patients with sulfa allergies. Patients using a thiazolidinedione require hepatic monitoring due to its potential hepatotoxicity. TZDs tend to cause increase in body weight and redistribution of adipose tissue from visceral to subcutaneous sites and cause or worsen peripheral edema. They also can precipitate or worsen congestive heart failure. A recent meta-analysis suggests that patients using a thiazolidinedione (rosiglitazone) may have an increase in the risk of myocardial infarction and death from cardiovascular causes [50]. However, further studies regarding the safety and efficacy of thiazolidinediones in the setting of cardiac disease are needed.

Mental Wellness and Behavorial Management

Body image and physical activity level can have significant effects on an individual's overall sense of wellness. Physical activity aids in successful weight and can help manage mood, including depression and anxiety [34] as well as help prevent the weight gain that may accompany smoking cessation. Weight loss and adequate sleep can improve emotional and mental wellness. Addressing any underlying depression or anxiety disorder may improve mental wellness and allow for behavior change.

A collaborative, patient-centered approach on goals, specific strategies, and barriers to change can assist the physician and the patient in learning specific behavioral skills as well as provide support to initiate and maintain change. Arranging and expecting follow-up through visits, phone calls, mail or email demonstrate commitment and lead to meaningful behavior changes. Understanding specific cultural, religious and/or psychosocial barriers can dampen the stress and frustration for both parties and set more realistic goals.

There are four evidence-based models that can be used for facilitating lifestyle change: (1) the transtheoretical model, (2) brief motivational model, (3) patient-centered patient education model, and (4) the five A's contract [51].

The transtheoretical model describes the stages an individual passes when making a change in a health behavior. It has five stages: precontemplation, contemplation, preparation, action and maintenance. This model was initially developed for smoking cessation but can be adapted for most health behaviors.

The brief motivational model has five general principles: express empathy, develop discrepancy, avoid argumentation, roll with resistance and support self-efficacy.

The patient-centered patient education model has five domains of assessment and interventions: cognitive domain, attitudinal domain, instrumental domain, behavioral domain and social domain.

The five A's contract consists of assess, advise, agree, assist and arrange [51]. Behavioral counseling interventions can be effective but multiple barriers (skepticism of their effectiveness, lack or limited training in these techniques, and time required) limit their use [51].

Conclusion

Coronary heart disease (CHD) is the leading cause of death in the United States and remains more common among men than women. However, the mortality related to CHD and the percentage of sudden deaths related to CHD without previous symptoms are higher among women. Lifestyle and dietary changes have been demonstrated to reduce the clinical effect of CHD.

A healthy lifestyle can be an effective, non-pharmacological approach to reducing coronary heart disease and plays an important role in the primary prevention of CHD. Conversely, a sedentary lifestyle and low cardiorespiratory fitness increases the risk of cardiovascular disease (CVD) with the same impact as the presence of smoking, high blood pressure or elevated cholesterol levels [52]. Tobacco use, poor dietary habits and physical inactivity (three health behaviors) are associated with increased risk of CVD and account for the largest and second largest number of preventable deaths each year [5].

Primary prevention of CHD intends to prevent and modify risk factors as well as prevent the development of chronic diseases (hypertension, diabetes, dyslipidemias). As obesity, hypertension, dyslipidemia, type 2 diabetes mellitus, tobacco use and sedentary lifestyle become more prevalent in the pre-teen and adolescent, physicians need to be directing more attention to the promotion and maintenance of a healthy lifestyle in these age groups to reduce the risk of premature cardiovascular disease as an adult.

Presently, there are ongoing trials studying the ability of intensive lifestyle interventions to decrease the rate of cardiovascular disease events in type 2 diabetes [53]. Continued evaluation of primary benefits of intensive lifestyle interventions in individuals with two or more co-morbidities (hypertension, dyslipidemia and diabetes mellitus) lies ahead.

The primary prevention process needs to identify the patient early, stratify their individual risk factors, initiate an exercise program, provide nutritional education, emphasize smoking cessation and attain weight-loss goals. These measures will impact the prevention and progression of CAD and decrease a patient's overall morbidity and mortality from cardiovascular disease [2].

References

1. American Heart Association's Heart Disease and Stroke Statistics – 2005 Update. http://www.americanheart.org/downloadable/heart/1105390918119HDSStats2005Update.pdf
2. Harris GD, White RD. Lifestyle modifications for the prevention and treatment of cardiovascular disease: an evidence-based approach. Missouri Medicine 2004:101(3): 222–226.
3. Thompson PD, Buchner D, Pina IL, et al. Exercise and physical activity in the prevention and treatment of atherosclerotic cardiovascular disease. A statement from the Council on Clinical Cardiology (Subcommittee on Exercise, Rehabilitation, and Prevention) and the Council on Nutrition, Physical Activity, and Metabolism (Subcommittee on Physical Activity). Circulation 2003;107:3109–3116.
4. McGill HC and McMahan CA. Starting earlier to prevent heart disease. JAMA 2003;290:2320–2322.
5. McGinnis JM, Foege WH. Actual causes of death in the United States. JAMA 1993;270: 2207–2212.
6. Hunlink MG, Goldman L, Tosteson AN, et al. The recent decline in mortality from coronary heart disease, 1980–1990: the effect of secular trends in risk factors and treatment. JAMA 1997;277:535–542.
7. Expert Panel on the Detection, Evaluation, and Treatment of High Blood Cholesterol in Adults. Executive Summary of the third report of the National Cholesterol Education Program

(NCEP) Expert Panel on the Detection, Evaluation, and Treatment of High Blood Cholesterol in Adults (Adult Treatment Panel III). JAMA 2001;285:2486–2497.

8. de Lorgeril M, Salen P, Martin JL, et al. Mediterranean diet, traditional risk factors, and the rate of cardiovascular complications after myocardial infarction: final report of the Lyon Diet Heart Study. Circulation 1999;99:779–785.

9. Appel LJ, Champagne CM, Harsha DW, et al. Effects of comprehensive lifestyle modification on blood pressure control: main results of the PREMIER clinical trial. JAMA 2003;289: 2083–2093.

10. Chiuve SE, McCullough ML, Sacks FM, et al. Healthy lifestyle factors in the primary prevention of coronary heart disease and among men: benefits among users and nonusers of lipid-lowering and antihypertensive medications. Circulation 2006;114;160–167.

11. Pearson TA, Blair SN, Daniels SR, et al. AHA Scientific Statement. AHA guidelines for primary prevention of cardiovascular disease and stroke: 2002 Update: Consensus panel guide to comprehensive risk reduction for adult patients without coronary or other atherosclerotic vascular diseases. Circulation 2002;106:388–391.

12. Wilson PWF, D'Agostino R, Levy D, Belanger A, Silbershatz H, Kannel W. Prediction of coronary heart disease using risk factor categories. Circulation 1998;97:1837–1847.

13. Greenland P, Smith SC Jr, Grundy SM. Improving coronary heart disease risk assessment in asymptomatic people: role of traditional risk factors and noninvasive cardiovascular tests. Circulation 2001;104:1863–1867.

14. Lauer MS. Primary prevention of atherosclerotic cardiovascular disease. The high public burden of low individual risk. JAMA 2007;297:1376–1378.

15. Negri E, Franzosi MG, LaVecchia C, et al. Tar yield of cigarettes and risk of acute myocardial infarction. BMJ 1993;306:1567.

16. Fiore MC, Bailey WC, Cohen SJ, et al. Treating Tobacco Use and Dependence. Clinical Practice Guidelines Rockville (MD): US Department of Health and Human Services. US Public Health Service, 2000.

17. Eckel R. Obesity and heart disease: a statement for the healthcare professionals from the Nutrition Committee, American Heart Association. Circulation 1997;96:3248–3250.

18. U.S. Preventive Services Task Force. Behavioral counseling in primary care to promote a healthy diet: recommendations and rationale. Am J Prev Med 2003;24:93–100.

19. DeCaterina RD, Zampolli A, Del Turco S, et al. Nutritional mechanisms that influence cardiovascular disease. Am J Clin Nutr 2006;83(suppl):421S–426S.

20. Campbell TC and Campbell TM. The China Study 2005. Chicago, Illnois: BenBella Books, Inc. Dallas, Texas and Independent Publishers Group.

21. Krauss RM, Eckel RH, Howard B, et al. AHA dietary guidelines: revision 2000: a statement for healthcare professionals from the nutrition committee of the American Heart Association. Circulation 2000;102:2284–2299.

22. Hu FB, Manson JE, Willett WC. Types of dietary fat and risk of coronary heart disease: a critical review. J Am Coll Nutr 2001;20:5–19.

23. Suh I, Oh KW, Lee KH, et al. Moderate dietary fat consumption as a risk factor for ischemic heart disease in a population with a low fat intake: a case-control study in Korean men. Am J Clin Nutr 2001;73:722–727.

24. Leeds AR. Glycemic index and heart disease. Am J Clin Nutr 2002;76(suppl):286S–289S.

25. McKeown NM, Meigs JB, Liu S, Saltzman E, Wilson PW, Jaques PF. Carbohydrate nutrition, insulin resistance, and the prevalence of the metabolic syndrome in the Framingham Offspring Cohort. Diabetes Care 2004;27:538–546.

26. US Dept. of Health and Human Services. Physical activity and health: a report of the Surgeon General. Atlanta, GA: US Department of Health and Human Services, Centers for Disease Control and Prevention, National Center for Chronic Disease Prevention and Health Promotion, 1996.

27. Williams PT. Physical fitness and activity as separate heart disease risk factors: a meta-analysis. Med Sci Sports Exer 2001;33:754–761.

28. Myers J. Exercise and cardiovascular health. Circulation 2003;107:e2–e5.
29. American College of Sports Medicine. Guidelines for Exercise Testing and Prescription, 6th ed. Baltimore, MD: Lippincott Williams & Wilkins, 2000.
30. Zoeller RF. Physical activity and fitness in the prevention of coronary artery disease and its associated risk factors. American Journal of Lifestyle Medicine 2007;1:29–33.
31. Giannuzzi P, Mezzani A, Saner H, et al. Position Paper. Physical activity for primary and secondary prevention. Position paper of the Working Group on Cardiac Rehabilitation and Exercise Physiology of the European Society of Cardiology. Eur J Cardiovasc Prev Rehabil 2003;10(5):319–327.
32. Norris R, Carroll D, Cochrane R. The effects of aerobic and anaerobic training on fitness, blood pressure and psychological stress and well-being. J Psychosom Res 1990;34: 367–375.
33. North TC, McCullagh P, Tran ZV. Effect of exercise on depression. Exerc Sport Sci Rev 1990;18:379–415.
34. Moses J, Steptoe A, Matthews A, Edwards S. The effects of exercise training on mental well-being in the normal population: a controlled study. J Psychosom Res 1989;3:47–61.
35. King A, Taylor CB, Haskell W, Debusk RF. Influence of regular aerobic exercise on psychological health: a randomized, controlled trial of health in middle-aged adults. Health Psychol. 1989;8:305–324.
36. Lee IM, Rexrode KM, Cook NR, Manson JE, Buring JE. Physical activity and coronary heart disease in women: is "no pain, no gain" passé? JAMA 2001;285:1447–1454.
37. Blair SN, Kohl HW, Barlow CE. Physical activity, physical fitness, and all-cause mortality in women: do women need to be active? J Am Coll Nutr 1993;12:368–371.
38. Sherman SE, D'Agostino RB, Cobb JL, Kannel WB. Physical activity and mortality in women in the Framingham Heart Study. Am Heart J 1994;128:879–884.
39. Jacobson DM, Strohecker L, Compton MT, Katz KL. Physical activity counseling in the adult primary care setting position statement of the American College of Preventive Medicine. Am J Prev Med 2005;29(2):158–162.
40. National Institutes of Health, National Heart, Lung and Blood Institute. Fact Book Fiscal Year 2003. Bethesda, MD: National Institutes of Health, 2004.
41. Amatruda JM, Richeson JF, Welle SL, et al. The safety and efficacy of a controlled low-energy ('very-low-calorie') diet in the treatment of non-insulin-dependent diabetes and obesity. Arch Intern Med 1988;148:873–877.
42. Anderson JW, Brinkman-Kaplan V, Hamilton CC, et al. Food-containing hypocaloric diets are as effective as liquid-supplement diets for obese individuals with NIDDM. Diabetes Care 1994;17:602–604.
43. Wiviott SD, deLemos JA, Cannon CP, et al. A tale of two trials: a comparison of the post-acute coronary syndrome lipid-lowering trials A to Z and PROVE IT–TIMI 22. Circulation 2006;113:1406–1414.
44. Guyton JR. Extended-release niacin for modifying the lipoprotein profile. Expert Opin Pharmacother 2004 Jun;5(6):1385–1398.
45. Fowler MJ. Diabetes treatment, part 1: Diet and exercise. Clinical Diabetes 2007;25(3): 105–109.
46. Knowler WC, Barrett-Connor E, Fowler SE, et al. Reduction in the incidence of type 2 diabetes with lifestyle intervention or metformin. N Engl J Med 2002;346:393–403.
47. Sigal RJ, Kenny GP, Wasserman DH, et al. Physical activity/exercise and type 2 diabetes: a consensus statement from the American Diabetes Association. Diabetes Care 2006;29: 1433–1438.
48. Boule NG, Haddad E, Kenny GP, et al. Effects of exercise on glycemic control and body mass in type 2 diabetes mellitus: a meta-analysis of controlled clinical trials. JAMA 2001;286: 1218–1227.
49. Stumvoll M, Nurjhan N, Perriello G, et al. Metabolic effects of metformin in non-insulin-dependent diabetes mellitus. N Engl J Med 1995;333:550–554.

50. Nissen SE, Wolski K. Effect of rosiglitazone on the risk of myocardial infarction and death from cardiovascular causes. N Engl J Med 2007;356:2457–2471.
51. Egede LE. Counseling interventions for primary prevention of coronary heart disease in individuals with type-2 diabetes. Comp Therapy 2004;30(3):141–147.
52. Tanasescu M, Leitzmann M, Rimm E, Willett W, Stamfer M, Hu F. Exercise type and intensity in relation to coronary heart disease in men. JAMA 2002;288:1994–2000.
53. Espeland M. Reduction in weight and cardiovascular disease risk factors in individuals with type 2 diabetes: one-year results of the Look AHEAD trial. Diabetes Care 2007;30: 1374–1383.

Chapter 13
Exercise Testing After Bypass or Percutaneous Coronary Intervention

Grant Fowler and Michael Altman

Coronary artery bypass graft (CABG) surgery continues to be performed for patients with coronary artery disease (CAD), especially those with symptomatic multi-vessel disease and diabetes. Percutaneous coronary intervention (PCI) is not only used to treat patients with symptoms from CAD, but has also become the treatment of choice for patients with destabilized coronary plaque, whether they present with acute myocardial infarction (ST or non-ST elevation MI) or unstable angina. PCI is also being used for multi-vessel CAD. Consequently, clinicians now manage a larger number of patients who have undergone PCI. Whether the revascularization has been accomplished by CABG or PCI, primary care clinicians often have to decide if the result remains functional (i.e., graft or stent remains patent) and whether a test is needed to optimize prognosis. While certain clinicians always combine an imaging test with an exercise ECG test (ET) to evaluate these patients, other experts support the use of ET alone. This chapter explores the options for these patients.

Management of Patients After Bypass or Percutaneous Coronary Intervention

Although the frequency of coronary artery bypass graft (CABG) surgery has decreased, primary care clinicians continue to manage a large number of patients with coronary artery disease (CAD) whose status is post-CABG. With the advent of drug-eluting stents and the expansion of their use to acute myocardial infarction (ST or non-ST elevation MI) and unstable angina, primary care clinicians are also caring for more patients whose status is post-percutaneous coronary intervention (PCI). In addition, PCI is being used for multi-vessel CAD for patients who, until recently, would have undergone CABG. Whether the revascularization has been accomplished by CABG or PCI, primary care clinicians often have to decide if the

G. Fowler (✉)

Department of Family and Community Medicine, The University of Texas Health Science Center Houston, Houston, TX 77030 USA

e-mail: grant.c.fowler@uth.tmc.edu

C.H. Evans, R.D. White (eds.), *Exercise Testing for Primary Care and Sports Medicine Physicians,* DOI 10.1007/978-0-387-76597-6_13

result remains functional (i.e., graft or stent remains patent) or whether the patient needs a re-intervention. Examples include the primary care clinician evaluating such a patient prior to noncardiac surgery or in the interim between their annual exam with the cardiologist. Other examples include the primary care clinician working in the emergency department or as a hospitalist managing a revascularized patient when he or she presents with a chest pain syndrome. In these and other situations, primary care clinicians must be adept at deciding which test to perform to assure adequate coronary perfusion and to maximize patient outcomes.

It should be noted that the medical literature basically reports two different phases or timeframes of evaluation post-revascularization, whether by CABG or PCI, and each phase has a different goal. In the early phase, usually within the first 6 months to a year following revascularization, the goal of testing is to evaluate the immediate results of revascularization. In other words, the goal is to *diagnose* graft failure or PCI restenosis. Such a diagnosis may be critical in high-risk patients (Table 13.1). In the second or late phase, since the patient is more than 6 months post-revascularization, the goal of testing is to hopefully evaluate stable CAD. In addition to diagnosing graft failure/PCI restenosis or CAD progression, testing during this phase may also prognose future events.

Which Revascularization?

Since the late 1980s, there have been at least nine randomized trials (BARI, CABRI, RITA-1, EAST, GABI, Toulouse, MASS, Lausanne, ERACI) [1–8] comparing PCI with CABG in patients with angina. Most were smaller studies, but BARI (the Bypass Angioplasty Revascularization Investigation) included 1,829 patients [1], CABRI (Coronary Angioplasty versus Bypass Revascularization Investigation) 1,054 patients [2], and RITA-1 (first Randomized Intervention Treatment of Angina trial) 1,011 patients [3]. Although these trials differ slightly in their design and in the sort of patients who were included, the findings have all been remarkably consistent. At almost any point after initial treatment, whether the patient was treated with

Table 13.1 High-risk patients post-revascularization (CABG or PCI)

Decreased left ventricular function
Multi-vessel CAD
Proximal left anterior descending (LAD) CAD
Previous sudden cardiac death
Diabetes
Hazardous occupations
Suboptimal results from the revascularization
Saphenous vein interventions*
Congestive heart failure*

*Although not listed as high risk in American College of Cardiology/American Heart Association (ACC/AHA) guidelines, patients with these conditions have worse long-term outcomes post-revascularization compared to other patients.

CABG or PCI, the rates of death or non-fatal MI are essentially the same. However, at the time of these trials, patients undergoing PCI usually received percutaneous transluminal coronary angioplasty (PTCA). Consequently the re-intervention rate was much higher among patients initially treated with PCI than for those undergoing CABG. In recent years, there have been several additional trials (ERACI II [9], ARTS [10], SoS [11]) using stents for PCI and comparing outcomes with CABG. While the re-intervention rate with PCI remains higher than that for CABG, it has been significantly reduced with the use of stents. Mortality and non-fatal MI rates have again remained basically the same whether the patient is treated with PCI or CABG. One major benefit of these trials is the opportunity to observe which tests the experts deemed necessary to follow patients during the trials and the timing of these tests. Another benefit is the ability to observe the outcomes of patients based upon the results of testing during the trials.

[Author note: Since there are very similar outcomes, whether the revascularization is performed by CABG or PCI, "post-revascularization" will refer generically to patients having undergone either procedure for the remainder of this chapter.]

Which Test?

Controversy surrounds the choice of test to assure adequate coronary perfusion and optimal prognosis after CABG or PCI. This controversy is about which is the "best" test to assess these patients. While some clinicians only evaluate patients who have recurrent chest pain after revascularization, other clinicians always obtain an exercise test (with or without imaging by radionuclide or ultrasound/echocardiography) prior to revascularization followed by an elective test, using the same modality, post-revascularization. This is just an example of the complexity of deciding between the options available.

Although the most recent (2002) American College of Cardiology (ACC)/ American Heart Association (AHA) guidelines on ET do not recommend pre- and post-procedure testing for all revascularized patients, they do recommend *documentation of ischemia* pre-procedure (prior to an intervention) [12]. There is good evidence supporting use of ET to document ischemia, whether prior to the initial revascularization or before a re-intervention. However, if the decision to revascularize or perform a re-intervention will be based upon the site and extent of ischemia, the ET is less desirable than an imaging test (Table 13.2).

If Imaging Is Used, Which Type?

Realizing exercise radionuclide perfusion imaging and exercise echocardiography are using different parameters to define ischemia, one would not expect 100% concordance between the two techniques (see also Chapter 7, Nuclear Imaging with Exercise Testing, and Chapter 8, Stress Echocardiography). However, since the early 1980s, there has been a consistent number of reports of similar sensitivities

Table 13.2 ACC/AHA guidelines and evidence supporting use of ET

In the patient prior to revascularization (or prior to a pe-intervention)	
ET should be performed to demonstrate proof of ischemia before revascularization (and this includes re-intervention)	Indication: class I. Level of evidence: B
ET should not be performed for localization of ischemia for determining site of intervention	Indication: class III. Level of evidence: A
In the asymptomatic patient post-revascularization	
ET should not be performed for routine monitoring of asymptomatic patients after PCI or CABG without specific indications	Indication: class III. Level of evidence: B

(70–80%) and specificities (80–90%) for these two techniques for diagnosis of CAD. Regarding post-revascularized patients, two recent large meta-analyses compared these techniques for diagnosis of restenosis within the first year post-PCI [13,14]. Another large meta-analysis did the same for patients post-CABG although some of these studies followed patients for many years [20]. All tests were followed by angiography for confirmation. Based on very similar sensitivities, specificities and accuracies for diagnosis of CAD, regardless of the technique used, the choice of imaging post-revascularization will likely depend on clinician experience and other local factors such as availability and expertise. (This is discussed under the section on the symptomatic patient post-revascularization.)

Exercise ECG Testing Post-Revascularization

Perhaps the most compelling data regarding use of ET post-revascularization were produced during the BARI trial [15]. These data not only enable us to evaluate the use of ET post-revascularization for multi-vessel CAD (regardless of whether CABG or PCI was utilized) but also help us to evaluate the ACC/AHA guidelines for the use of ET post-revascularization [16].

During the BARI trial, a symptom-limited ET was mandated by protocol at years 1, 3, and 5 post-revascularization [15]. At years 1, 3, and 5, 1,388, 1,208, and 1,097 patients, respectively, underwent ET. Overall, only 9% developed angina when taking the ET, consistent with the "protocol-not symptom driven" indication for testing. The risk of 2 year mortality after taking the ET increased from 1.5 to 3.5% and then decreased to 3.3% at years 1, 3, and 5, respectively. The combined risk of mortality and MI in the 2 years following ET ranged from 3.6 to 4.6 to 5% at the year 1, 3, and 5, respectively. Overall, patients taking an ET during the first 3 years of the study had a very low risk of mortality or MI leading the authors to conclude that their study supported ACC/AHA guidelines which do not recommend routine testing for 3–5 years following successful revascularization. They also speculated that imaging by exercise radionuclide or echocardiography would not have been helpful because such a low-risk population would likely have produced a large percentage of false-positive results. Consequently, only a fraction of those with a significant perfusion or echocardiographic defect would have had a subsequent event.

The authors did note that ST depression on the 1-year test was associated with re-interventions. This is probably due to restenosis or graft reocclusion or failure which has the highest likelihood of occurrence in the first year. Otherwise, when exercise parameters (e.g., heart rate >85% of 220-age, systolic blood pressure >130 mmHg, stage 3 Bruce, ST-segment depression) were evaluated in an attempt to predict survival or MI, they did not improve the model over the basic ET until the 2 years following the 5-year test. Specifically, exercising to Bruce stage 3, heart rate >85%, and DTS > −6 were associated with an improved 5-year survival in the multivariate analysis, but only Bruce stage 3 was an independent predictor. Decreased exercise duration was also associated with increased risk of MI after the 3-year test.

Who to Test Post-Revascularization?

Obviously patients who become symptomatic post-revascularization need to be evaluated and this is discussed in the latter part of this article. However, the majority of patients primary care clinicians manage post-revascularization will be asymptomatic. Interestingly, in the asymptomatic population, *not taking the ET* in the BARI trial was a stronger predictor of mortality than results of the ET [15]. At years 1, 3, and 5, 310 (18%), 424 (26%), and 474 (31%), respectively, did not take the ET. Overall, non-exercisers had a 3- to 10-fold increased risk of mortality compared to exercisers. The mortality for non-exercisers was 3.9% in the year following the scheduled test and 25.9% at 5 years compared with a 0.4% 1-year mortality and an 8.1% 5-year mortality in those taking the ET. What was striking about this data was that diabetic non-exercisers who had undergone CABG had a 30% 5-year mortality rate, and even more striking was that diabetic non-exercisers who had undergone PTCA had a 52.4% 5-year risk of mortality. While this is subgroup analysis and the total number of diabetics and diabetic non-exercisers was small (365 diabetics total, 87 diabetic non-exercisers at year 1), the results are nonetheless quite impressive. Overall, while no relation was found between the reason for not taking the ET (e.g., patient refusal, orthopedic reasons, peripheral vascular disease, other) and survival, there was the suggestion that orthopedic limitation decreased the 5-year survival (66.7 versus 74.1%).

Since the vast majority of patients in the BARI trial who were tested remained asymptomatic, combining these data with ACC/AHA guidelines suggests an algorithm for testing asymptomatic patients post-revascularization (Fig. 13.1). Clearly patients needing a cardiac rehabilitation program or reassurance to begin an exercise program should undergo an ET. In addition, since the BARI investigators did not separate high-risk individuals from the remainder of the group, a step was included in this algorithm to incorporate ACC/AHA guidelines for high-risk patients. According to ACC/AHA guidelines, in addition to testing prior to a cardiac rehabilitation program [12], ET can be considered in selected, high-risk patients

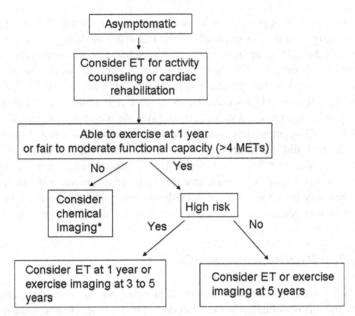

Fig. 13.1 Algorithm for testing the asymptomatic patient post-revascularization. *Especially those with prior MI, renal insufficiency

(see Table 13.1) post-PTCA within the first month post-procedure for detection of restenosis. Also, in selected, high-risk individuals (Table 13.1), whether the revascularization was performed by CABG or PCI, ET can be considered for periodic monitoring for restenosis, graft occlusion, or disease progression. Exercise imaging is an option at 3–5 years for these individuals. At this time, there is no evidence to suggest how often (the periodicity) such patients should be tested post-revascularization (Table 13.3).

We have long known that patients with CAD and poor functional or exercise capacity (<4 METs) are high risk for cardiovascular events [17], and this may correlate with what BARI investigators found to be non-exercisers. We have also known that an abnormal chemical imaging study can be predictive of an adverse outcome in patients who are at high risk for CAD and unable to exercise [18]. Therefore, similar to ACC/AHA guidelines for assessing perioperative cardiac risk (Table 13.4), a recommendation for assessing non-exercisers or those with a poor exercise capacity (especially those with additional intermediate-risk predictors [Table 13.4] such as prior MI or renal insufficiency) has been included in the algorithm (Fig. 13.1).

With growing evidence that silent ischemia worsens the prognosis in the revascularized patient, it should be noted that many clinicians monitor the high-risk group (see Table 13.1) more closely in the first 6 months to a year post-revascularization, even if they remain asymptomatic. This is a common timeframe for CABG grafts to fail (especially if venous conduits were used), and for restenosis to occur post-PCI.

Table 13.3 ACC/AHA guidelines and evidence supporting use of ET or imaging in the asymptomatic patient post-revascularization

A reasonable use for ET in the post-revascularization patient is after discharge for activity counseling and/or exercise training as part of a cardiac rehabilitation program	Indication: class IIa
While the evidence is less well established, ET may be considered for the detection of restenosis within the first months after PTCA in selected high-risk (Table 13.1) asymptomatic patients	Indication: class IIb. Level of evidence: B
Likewise, while the evidence is less well established, ET may be considered for periodic testing for restenosis, graft occlusion, or disease progression in selected, high-risk (Table 13.1) asymptomatic individuals post-revascularization	Indication: class IIb. Level of evidence: B
Myocardial imaging* may be considered for the evaluation of selected, high-risk (Table 13.1) asymptomatic patients 3–5 years post-revascularization, whether they were revascularized by CABG or PCI. If they are able to exercise, this imaging* can follow an exercise protocol. If unable to exercise, a chemical imaging* test can be performed (chemical = adenosine or dipyridamole infusion, dobutamine or arbutamine infusion in those contraindicated)**	Indication: class IIb. Level of evidence: B

*While imaging in the guidelines refers to myocardial single photon emission computerized tomography (SPECT) perfusion imaging, based upon three large meta-analyses as explained in the text of this article, exercise or chemical echocardiography has been found to have about the same sensitivity, specificity, and accuracy for diagnosis of restenosis/reocclusion or graft failure post-revascularization.

**Although not stated in the guidelines, an option for chemical myocardial SPECT perfusion imaging is chemical echocardiography (chemical = dobutamine or arbutamine infusion, adenosine or dipyridamole infusion in those contraindicated).

Consequently, during this time, cardiologists are often uncomfortable clearing such patients for major surgery without some form of testing. The algorithm (Fig. 13.1) therefore addresses the concerns of these clinicians.

For all other patients not previously evaluated, there may be value of an ET and/or an imaging test at 5 years. In the BARI trial [15], while decreased exercise capacity on the ET at 3 years was associated with an increased risk of future MI, at 5 years, decreased exercise capacity as well as additional abnormal physiologic results (high-risk Duke Treadmill Score (DTS), chronotropic incompetence) on the ET was

Table 13.4 Shortcut to determine indicators for noninvasive testing (2 of 3 must be present) before noncardiac surgery

Poor functional or exercise capacity by questionnaire or specific questioning (<4 METs, or inability to climb one flight of stairs)
High-risk surgical procedure
Intermediate clinical risk predictors are present (Canadian class I or II angina, prior MI by ECG or history, CHF, diabetes, renal insufficiency)

predictive of increased mortality. By defining extent of ischemia, an imaging test at this point may further stratify patients into low, intermediate, or high risk which in turn could be used to determine future management and testing.

Which Test Did the Experts Use?

In the majority of the nine trials comparing outcomes of CABG versus PCI, and in particular, the three largest trials (BARI, CABRI, RITA-1) [1–3], ET was performed during the first 6 months to a year to monitor patients. (Obviously the investigators trusted ET for monitoring patients post-revascularization.) Likewise, if one looks at the re-intervention rate over time curves for these nine trials, most re-interventions occurred during the first year. In the BARI trial, ST-segment depression on the 1-year test was associated with re-interventions [1]. Therefore, in the algorithm (Fig. 13.1) for the asymptomatic patient post-revascularization, clinicians may appreciate that the year 1 point seems to be a good time to not only assess whether the patient is able to exercise and/or to assess their functional or exercise capacity, but it also seems to be a good time to consider an ET or exercise imaging, especially in high-risk (Table 13.1) patients.

Granted, revascularized patients are by definition at higher risk than those with stable CAD; however, at some point many approach the same level of risk. The latest guidelines (2002) from AHA/ACC for risk stratification in the patient with stable CAD indicate that an ET is a reasonable test in patients with a normal resting ECG and who are able to exercise [12]. In part, these guidelines are based on the simplicity, lower cost, and widespread familiarity with the performance and interpretation of the standard ET. Also, when imaging has been studied in patients divided into risk groups based on the DTS, few patients (<5%) who have a low-risk treadmill score (≤ 1% annual cardiac mortality rate) will be identified as high risk after imaging, and thus the cost of identifying these patients argues against routine imaging. Those patients identified as high risk (≥3% per year annual cardiac mortality) based on the DTS should probably be referred directly for cardiac catheterization and a possible intervention. Only those patients with an intermediate DTS (>1% and <3%) seem to benefit from an imaging study in order to further differentiate low-risk patients from those who might benefit from an intervention. In other words, a step-like progression of testing is reasonable. Granted, the DTS was originally based on a cohort of patients who have not had cardiac surgery, however, data from later trials have confirmed that the DTS is helpful in post-revascularized patients [1, 15].

What would seem to argue against a step-like progression of testing in the revascularized patients is that all patients combined in the BARI trial had about a 2% average annual cardiac mortality rate for the first 5 years of the study [15]. At first glance, therefore, all revascularized patients appear to be at intermediate risk and likely to benefit from an imaging study. Again, however, the ability to differentiate between low- and high-risk (Table 13.1) patients post-revascularization in the BARI trial is lacking. While those able to exercise had <1.7% annual mortality risk, which would also be intermediate, perhaps those with normal left ventricular function, no involvement of the proximal LAD and no history of sudden cardiac death would have had <1% annual mortality and possibly be good candidates for ET (at least for the first 5 years post-revascularization). Therefore, ET would seem to be a reasonable test on a periodic basis in these individuals.

Which Test Prior to Noncardiac Surgery in the Revascularized Patient?

In the most recent (2002) ACC/AHA guideline update for perioperative cardiovascular evaluation for noncardiac surgery, other than a resting ECG, further cardiac workup is generally not deemed necessary if the patient has undergone complete revascularization in the last 5 years and the clinical status has remained stable without recurrent signs or symptoms of ischemia (see also Chapter 10, Exercise Testing as Applied to the Preoperative Patient) [12]. All other patients with a favorable result from a recent (<2 years) thorough coronary evaluation (e.g., angiogram, ET, imaging, exercise imaging) are also deemed low risk for surgery if there has been no change in symptoms since their evaluation. (This can apply to patients who are more than 5 years post-revascularization).

Table 13.4 lists a shortcut of indicators for noninvasive testing prior to noncardiac surgery, which may be helpful in patients >5 years post-revascularization. In the guidelines (Table 13.5), there is support for recommending an ET or chemical imaging for the patient when a subjective evaluation of exercise capacity would be unreliable.

In general, coronary revascularization before noncardiac surgery to enable the patient to get through the noncardiac procedure is not deemed appropriate except for a small subset of patients at very high risk. The guidelines also suggest that perioperative testing should be limited to circumstances in which the results will affect patient treatment and outcomes. Overall, the ACC/AHA guidelines recommend a conservative approach to the use of expensive tests and treatments [12].

Table 13.5 ACC/AHA guidelines for testing the revascularized patient before noncardiac surgery

A resting ECG in patients with prior coronary revascularization	Indication: class IIb
ET or chemical testing for evaluation of exercise capacity when subjective assessment is unreliable	Indication: class IIa
ET or chemical testing for detection of restenosis in high-risk asymptomatic subjects within the initial months post-PCI	Indication: class IIb
If the patient has been completely revascularized in the past 5 years, no further testing is deemed necessary if the clinical status has remained stable without recurrent signs or symptoms of ischemia	Indication: class III
All other patients with a favorable result from a recent (<2 years) thorough coronary evaluation (angiogram, ET, imaging, exercise imaging) are deemed low risk for surgery if there has been no change in symptoms since their evaluation (this can apply to patients more than 5 years post-revascularization)	Indication: class III
Coronary angiography is not recommended in asymptomatic patients post-revascularization with a good exercise capacity (≥ 7 METs)	Indication: class III

Asymptomatic Versus Symptomatic

One factor determining the choice of testing in the revascularized patient is whether or not they have developed symptoms. Other factors include the timeframe following revascularization, the evidence supporting the use of each test, whether the site of ischemia needs to be localized for re-intervention, and local experience, availability, and expertise with the various tests.

Recurrent chest pain after revascularization is common. Ten to 20% of patients in the first month post-PTCA experience chest pain or ischemic-type symptoms, and the frequency increases to from 20 to 40% of patients by 6 months [13]. However, due to the low incidence of restenosis in the first 2 months post-PTCA, which would increase the risk of false-positive results, there appears to be little value in noninvasive testing during that timeframe. Therefore, the management decision during the first 2 months of the patient who becomes symptomatic is usually made by the cardiologist. Atypical chest pain is common in the patient post-CABG, and an ET can be used to help distinguish between cardiac and noncardiac causes if the patient is able to exercise (which is usually >2 months post-CABG). Even if the patient develops ischemic-type symptoms, an ET can be useful for documenting ischemia; however, an imaging study will help determine the site of ischemia as well as the extent of ischemia. Figure 13.2 provides an algorithm for testing the symptomatic patient.

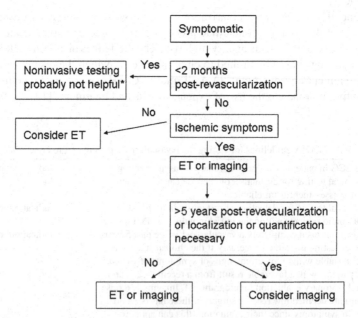

Fig. 13.2 Algorithm for testing the symptomatic patient. *CT angiography may be useful ≥ 16 slice post-CABG, ≥ 64 slice post-PCI

Symptomatic Patients

For many years, coronary angiography was considered the gold standard for not only diagnosing CAD but also assuring adequate coronary perfusion in revascularized patients (Table 13.6). Clearly it has been perceived as the gold standard in revascularized patients who have symptoms compatible with ischemia. However, while coronary angiography will provide the diagnosis of graft failure/PCI restenosis, it offers little toward determining the prognosis. Despite it being an invasive procedure, angiography provides little information regarding the patient's total atherosclerotic plaque burden within the vessel walls or plaque stability, and therefore, it provides incomplete information regarding the patient's prognosis or need for revascularization.

This has been confirmed in a study of 503 patients over a mean of 4.4 years where angiography was compared with exercise radionuclide imaging in patients with suspected CAD. In this study, while radionuclide imaging independently predicted adverse events, angiography provided no additional prognostic data [19]. When this prognostic data from imaging is combined with the additional prognostic data provided by exercise variables such as heart rate in recovery, exercise capacity, and chronotropic response to exercise, it becomes obvious why certain experts consider exercise imaging to be the more appropriate gold standard for risk-stratifying patients with CAD. However, the unanswered question is whether imaging is always needed to adequately risk stratify a patient. Using an ET alone, the DTS and algorithm have provided clinicians excellent tools for prognosing patients with CAD. In addition to DTS, ET also determines heart rate in recovery, functional capacity, and chronotropic response to exercise, all important prognostic markers.

Table 13.6 ACC/AHA guidelines and evidence supporting use of exercise testing in the symptomatic patient post-revascularization

ET should be performed to evaluate patients with recurrent symptoms suggesting ischemia after revascularization	Indication: class I, level of evidence: B
Atypical chest pain is common in patients after CABG, and an ET can be used to help distinguish between cardiac and noncardiac causes	Indication: class I, level of evidence: B
However, many experts suggest that imaging studies may be more desirable than ET in these patients since imaging studies help determine the site and extent of ischemia for positive tests	Indication: class IIb, level of evidence: B

Evidence Supporting Use of Imaging Studies in Symptomatic Patients Post-Revascularization

Evidence supporting the use of imaging studies in the symptomatic patient post-revascularization is found in three large meta-analyses. Most recently, 30 studies of symptomatic patients being tested post-PTCA from 1980 through 2001 were combined into a meta-analysis [13]. ET (14 studies, although 3 utilized dobutamine as a "chemical" study to replace exercise) was compared with radionuclide (6 exercise, 3 chemical studies) and echocardiographic (7 studies, of which 2 were chemical and one used atrial pacing) imaging for sensitivity and specificity with angiography being used as the gold standard. Radionuclide imaging (sensitivity 83%, specificity 79%, positive predictive value (PPV) 80%, negative predictive value (NPV) 85%) was found to be comparable to echocardiography (sensitivity 82%, specificity 86%, PPV 88%, NPV 79%) for diagnosing restenosis. Both were slightly superior to ET (sensitivity 54%, specificity 70%, PPV 64%, NPV 61%). While none of the tests were accurate in the first month post-PTCA, mainly because of a high risk of false positives, the usual time for development of symptoms was about 6 months.

These results were similar to those of an earlier meta-analysis [14] of studies between 1975 and 2000 testing patients post-PTCA. Due to slightly different selection criteria and timeframes, this meta-analysis included fewer studies than the prior. While asymptomatic and symptomatic patients were included in this study, the vast majority of patients were symptomatic. When exercise radionuclide (5 studies) was compared with echocardiographic (4 studies, of which 3 were chemical) imaging and ET (10 studies), radionuclide imaging (sensitivity 87%, specificity 78%) was again found to be fairly comparable to echocardiography (sensitivity 63%, specificity 87%) for diagnosing restenosis. Both were superior to ET (sensitivity 46%, specificity 77%).

In post-CABG patients, a recent meta-analysis [20] of studies between 1977 and 1998 compared ET (14 studies) with radionuclide (11 studies, of which 2 were chemical studies) and echocardiographic (6 studies, of which 3 were chemical studies) imaging for diagnosis of graft stenosis or CAD progression. Radionuclide (sensitivity 68%, specificity 84%) was found to have a similar ability to echocardiography (sensitivity 86%, specificity 90%) for diagnosis of graft failure or progression of CAD. Again, both were superior to ET (sensitivity 45%, specificity 82%).

Interestingly, in patients in whom an ET could not be used (e.g., ECG abnormalities, digoxin use), and therefore a DTS could not be calculated, a large prospective study (7,163 patients) at the Cleveland Clinic followed patients for 6.7 years, and radionuclide imaging was found to have no better ability than exercise capacity or heart rate in recovery for risk-stratifying non-revascularized patients. However, in the revascularized patients (2,932 patients), radionuclide imaging was found to be a better predictor of risk, even in the patient with a poor exercise capacity or an abnormal heart rate in recovery or both [21].

Coronary Artery Bypass Graft

The anatomic basis for ischemia is particularly heterogeneous as well as its implications for morbidity and mortality in patients post-CABG. Overall, about 10–15% of grafts fail within the first 6 months post-CABG [22], and this is usually the result of peri-anastomotic graft stenosis. After 12 months, while progression of CAD in the native arteries is not uncommon, saphenous vein graft attrition or obstruction due to an atherosclerotic lesion is more frequently the cause for ischemia and/or the development of symptoms. Since saphenous vein graft atherosclerotic lesions are particularly unstable and prone to rapid progression and thrombotic occlusion [23–26], most experts have a low threshold to perform an angiographic evaluation and intervention when patients develop signs or symptoms of ischemia more than 5 years post-CABG. Fortunately, arterial graft conduits (e.g., internal mammary artery) seem to have much better durability with reports of full patency >20 years post-CABG.

Exercise ECG Testing Post-CABG

Some authors believe that 90% of patients can be converted to a normal ET post-CABG, especially if strict criteria are used to determine a positive test (i.e., only flat or downsloping ST segments used to define a positive test which minimizes the number of false positives). The presumption is that all vessels are reperfused post-CABG, and therefore the ST-segment depression on the ET should return to normal. However, there is a wide range of results found in the literature with one study reporting only 30% of ETs improving to normal following multi-vessel CABG [27]. What we do know is that the conversion of a markedly positive test preoperatively to a negative postoperative test does correlate with successful revascularization.

We also know that the ET post-CABG can be interpreted more reliability when the preoperative ET is available. Therefore, having the preoperative ET for comparison is valuable because a significant number of patients with complete revascularization will continue to have ST-segment depression (30% in one study). It may be reassuring if such ST-segment depression has improved. Since ST-segment depression is common post-CABG, Ellestad suspects that it is not as reliable as preoperative ST-segment depression for predicting the presence of ischemia [28]. Conversely, many post-CABG patients with failed grafts will have a normal ST response on ET.

Limitations following a CABG include the fact that patients are often not able to perform a symptom-limited ET for weeks or months following the procedure, during which time the highest rate of early graft occlusion is reported [29]. Other limitations for ET post-CABG are the frequent abnormalities on the resting ECG which are occasionally of a magnitude to make ET a relative contraindication. If an imaging test is not combined with ET, more reliance must also be placed on patient symptoms, hemodynamic response to exercise, and functional or exercise capacity.

Additional Studies of Exercise Testing Post-CABG

In one recent prospective, cohort study of routine versus selective ET in 408 patients within the first 12 months post-CABG, patients undergoing routine ET underwent fewer follow-up cardiac catheterizations. Clinical events, including unstable angina, MI, and death were less common among patients who underwent routine ET versus selective ET (indicated due to symptoms). However, the authors concluded that since routine ET in the first year post-CABG is associated with so few events, such a strategy is probably not warranted [30].

In a classic study from the 1980s, patients with incomplete revascularizations post-CABG were studied with ET in Germany [31]. Serial ETs were performed in 435 patients, 1–6 years post-CABG, and compared with coronary angiography 2–12 months post-CABG. Revascularization was complete in 182 patients, sufficient in 176 patients, and incomplete in 57 patients. In another 20 patients, all the grafts were occluded. Exercise capacity improved by 50% at 1 year in patients with complete and sufficient revascularization and had still improved by 30% at 5 years. Surprisingly, it was also improved in patients with incomplete revascularization or with all grafts occluded. However, perhaps this should not be so surprising because Ellestad tells us that >90% of patients post-CABG lose their angina, even those with incomplete revascularization [28].

From a study in Houston in the 1970s [32], 20% of patients with a normal ET post-CABG converted to an abnormal test within 23 months. Many of those patients had graft failure or progression of CAD. Ellestad found that onset of angina at a lower workload or lower double product usually led to the discovery of progressive ischemia [28]. With better medical management of CAD, grafts post-CABG hopefully will last much longer these days. Nevertheless, it is important to know what to expect with subsequent ETs post-CABG.

Prognostic Studies of Radionuclide Imaging Post-CABG

Many studies of a small number of patients have evaluated the use of exercise radionuclide imaging in patients that are status post-CABG. Results of these studies run the gamut from it being "far superior to ET" [33] to it being merely a useful test for determining whether CABG has protected the myocardium and prevented enlargement of the ischemic areas [34]. Perhaps the main benefit of these smaller studies was the resulting question of whether exercise imaging could predict prognosis and consequently affect choice of therapy following revascularization [35].

Most of the larger prognostic studies using radionuclide imaging post-CABG were done more than 5 years post-revascularization, and they not only help clinicians prognose patients but they also help risk-stratify patients. From those studies, using cardiac death as the end point, the largest study to date (1,544 patients) by Zellweger et al. found that moderately severe to severe abnormalities on radionuclide imaging done from 2 to 11 years post-CABG predicted a significantly higher (3.1%) annual risk of death than mildly abnormal or normal scans (0.7%) [36]. In concordance with ACC/AHA guidelines, the annual risk of cardiac death was rather low (1.3%) in patients ≤ 5 years post-CABG [12]. In another large study performed at the Cleveland Clinic (873 patients), patients with radionuclide (thallium) perfusion defects and poor to fair (impaired) exercise capacity (<7 METs) were at increased risk of subsequent death and non-fatal MI, even if symptom free [37].

Using cardiac death or acute MI as end points, two additional studies, of 294 and 255 patients performed at 5 years or more post-CABG, found that adding radionuclide imaging not only increased the prognostic accuracy three-fold over ET, but multi-vessel perfusion defects and lung uptake of thallium were also independent predictors of events [38, 39].

In the only large study of radionuclide imaging done within 2 years of CABG (411 patients, a mean of 11 months post-CABG, 55% symptomatic), an abnormal radionuclide test was strongly predictive of events with perfusion defect extent being the best predictor of outcome. Exercise duration and age were also predictive of overall mortality, and exercise angina score was predictive of cardiac death or MI. Originally this study led experts to question whether waiting 5 years post-CABG to scan patients as suggested by ACC/AHA guidelines was aggressive enough. However, these experts now agree with the national guidelines [40].

Other Tests Post-CABG

In a study of 50 patients post-CABG [41], contrast-enhanced multi-detector (16-slice) CT angiography had excellent sensitivity (92.8%), specificity (100%), positive predictive value (100%), and negative predictive value (85.8%) for graft patency when compared with coronary angiography. From this same reference, a pooled analysis of eight studies involving 932 grafts confirmed a 97% accuracy for the detection of graft patency by multi-detector CT. Obviously, multi-detector CT angiography stands out as an excellent alternative to coronary angiography for documentation of graft patency. With even higher resolution, 64-slice and 128-slice CT angiographies are being studied, and accuracy should improve. Although insurance companies often consider this test experimental and refuse to pay for it, and it is not available to all patients and clinicians, many experts are considering this option, certainly in high-risk individuals (Table 13.1).

From a small study of 106 patients in Italy post-CABG, chemical echocardiography (using dipyridamole) combined with Doppler evaluation of the actual bypass grafts produced a sensitivity of 93%, specificity of 93%, and accuracy of 93% for identification of restenosis when compared with angiography [42].

Comments

Most patients do not develop symptoms in the first 5 years post-CABG. However, during this time period, there may be benefit of monitoring the high-risk (Table 13.1) asymptomatic patient more closely. An ET seems to be a reasonable test for monitoring patients that can exercise. At some point, it is probably worth adding an imaging study, probably by 5 years post-revascularization.

At the 5-year point, if a patient has a good exercise capacity ($\geq$ 7 METs) and a normal imaging study, they should have a low risk of events (1% per year) and should benefit most from medical management. Patients with a good exercise capacity but with intermediate risk based upon their imaging test should have more intensive medical management and possible angiography. Patients with poor exercise capacity (<4 METs) and high-risk imaging results should probably receive the most aggressive medical management and coronary angiography. It should be noted that these recommendations are not based on randomized trial data, so, other than recognizing increased risk, it is unclear whether the use of testing in this manner and responding accordingly actually decreases risk.

Percutaneous Coronary Intervention

The advent of drug-eluting stents (2003) has rapidly revolutionized interventional cardiology, basically replacing bare-metal stents which in turn had replaced PTCA for treatment of symptomatic CAD. At their peak, in early 2007, more than 85% of PCIs were performed with drug-eluting stents. (This percentage has decreased since late 2007, and bare-metal stents have made a rebound.) Meanwhile, increasingly complex and riskier lesions and multi-vessel CAD are being treated with PCI. In fact, in the setting of an acute MI, given the option of treating multiple vessels with stenting or the sentinel vessel only, from a study of 125 patients, outcomes seem to be better if multiple vessels are stented [43].

This is in contrast to the patient with stable CAD. In a recent trial of 2,287 patients followed for a median of 4.6 years, PCI did not reduce the risk of death, MI, or other cardiovascular complications when compared with optimal medical management [44]. Optimal medical management has also been proven effective in high-risk patients compared to PCI. In a study of 2,166 high-risk patients who failed to undergo initial PCI for acute MI, compared to medical therapy, even later PCI for a totally occluded artery did not reduce the risk of death, reinfarction, or heart failure during 4 years of follow-up [45]. To be included in this study, patients had total occlusion of the infarct-related artery and met the criteria for high risk with either an ejection fraction <50% or a proximal occlusion. Instinctively, most of these patients would receive a stent if angiography was performed; however, outcomes from medical management matched interventional management which may lead clinicians to question the value of angiography.

That said, the concern for patients post-PCI is restenosis because when it occurs with a drug-eluting stent it results in MI in 60–70% of patients and death in 45%. Meta-analyses done in 2005 found no difference between the two types of commercially available drug-eluting stents regarding the incidence of stent thrombosis [46–48]. In fact, the overall incidence of stent thrombosis was <1% for either bare-metal stents or drug-eluting stents in these studies. However, more recent evidence has shown that the incidence of very late stent thrombosis (>1 year after placement of the stent) is approximately 0.5% for drug-eluting stents compared with no events for bare-metal stents. Since the original randomized trials excluded patients at high risk (e.g., acute MI, anatomically risky lesions such as long lesions or those near bifurcations), the long-term "real-world" risk may be higher than 0.5%.

In an attempt to aggressively diagnose restenosis post-PCI in high-risk patients (e.g., multi-vessel CAD, diabetes, ejection fraction <35%, proximal LAD lesion), 41 patients undergoing routine testing with maximal ET combined with radionuclide imaging at 1.5 and 6 months were compared with 43 patients undergoing testing only for a clinical indication. All patients underwent maximal ET at 9 months. While cardiac events, cardiac procedures, angina index and quality of life were not significantly different between the groups, exercise capacity was significantly increased in the group that underwent routine testing (10.3 versus 8.6 METs) [49]. Perhaps there is value to not only reassuring patients of the safety of exercise post-revascularization, but also demonstrating how to exercise on a treadmill, twice, during the immediate follow-up.

Additional Studies of Exercise Testing Post-PCI

In a study of 731 patients randomized to PCI for treatment of ST elevation acute MI who underwent symptom-limited maximal ET prior to discharge post-PCI, while exercise capacity was a strong prognostic predictor of death or reinfarction, there was not a significant relationship between ST-segment depression on the ET and outcome [50].

In a study of 211 patients tested with ET at 1–3 years post-PTCA, the DTS score was found to be predictive of both hard and soft cardiovascular events during a median follow-up of 7.3 years [51].

Prognostic Studies Using Radionuclide Imaging Post-PCI

In a study of 370 patients at least 1 month post-stenting, the presence of ischemia on radionuclide imaging predicted almost twice the risk of death or MI (17%) over 30 months compared with the absence of ischemia (9%), whether or not the patient had symptoms [52]. In two other studies (152 and 356 patients [36], respectively) performed 5–6 months post-PCI using end points of death, MI or revascularization, ischemia on radionuclide imaging significantly increased the risk of events (41 and 20%, respectively).

In a study of 206 patients 12–18 months post-PCI, absence of ischemia on radionuclide imaging predicted an 89% event-free survival compared with 27% if there was evidence of ischemia [53]. Likewise, when 346 patients were evaluated with radionuclide imaging 12–18 months post-PCI, during the follow-up of about 3 years, patients with no evidence of ischemia on imaging were 98% event free (defined by MI or cardiac death) [54]. In contrast, patients with ischemia on radionuclide imaging had a 12% risk of an event over this same time period.

So while it may be difficult to decide when to scan patients post-PCI, there appears to be benefit to screening all patients. However, the results of the literature are somewhat mixed because in a study of 791 patients, of which 462 underwent PCI with stenting, there was no difference in rates of death, MI, unstable angina, angiography, or revascularization between those undergoing routine functional testing and those only undergoing testing for clinically driven symptoms [55].

Diabetics have a higher risk of restenosis following PCI, and if they develop ischemia it is frequently asymptomatic (silent). However, one study of 61 diabetics found no benefit to routine functional testing in diabetics post-PCI and followed for 9 months [56].

Other Tests Post-PCI

Although artifact from stents has previously been a challenge, in a study of 95 patients in Italy, 64-slice CT angiography had a sensitivity of 93% and a negative predictive value of 99% for >50% stent restenosis or occlusion when compared with coronary angiography [57].

From a small study of 105 patients in Japan post-PCI for LAD lesions, Doppler evaluation of grafts following chemical perfusion (adenosine) provided sensitivity (91%), specificity (88%), and accuracy (89%) which should be comparable to radionuclide imaging for identification of 50–100% restenosis, especially since exercise imaging with radionuclide SPECT was used to confirm the restenosis [58].

After dobutamine infusion, perfusion imaging utilizing contrast echocardiography was performed in 56 patients about 2 years post-PCI. Restenosis was detected in 41 coronary arteries with a sensitivity of 73%, a specificity of 75%, and an accuracy of 74% when compared with coronary angiography [59].

Comments

Most cardiologists agree that ET is an adequate test to screen a patient prior to a cardiac rehabilitation program immediately following PCI, including a patient where the PCI was performed for acute MI. Other than these patients, since no large studies have proven that any type of testing post-stenting accurately predicts MI or death, many experts do not recommend any type of screening or testing unless the patient develops symptoms or signs of ischemia. In fact, this is given a Class IIB recommendation by the ACC/AHA guidelines since the prognostic benefit of controlling silent ischemia remains to be proved [12].

Since medical management appears equal to PCI (from a mortality and cardiovascular event perspective) for patients with stable CAD, it will be very difficult to prove any benefit of evaluating such a patient on a routine basis unless they have developed symptoms or signs of ischemia. However, many experts recommend periodic testing of patients post-PCI who are at high risk (Table 13.1), and it is also probably prudent to evaluate such patients prior to surgery.

It may also be rational to screen patients with additional intermediate-risk factors such as prior MI or renal insufficiency (Table 13.2) on a periodic basis. Those with a good exercise capacity ($>= 7$ METs) and a low-risk DTS would have a low risk of events. A periodic imaging test would also seem beneficial for confirming low risk, certainly by 5 years post-revascularization. For patients with an intermediate DTS, an imaging test should help further risk stratify the patient. For those unable to exercise, a chemical imaging test would seem beneficial.

Cost

Compared with ET, using Medicare Relative Value Unit (RVU) data from 2000, the cost of exercise echocardiography is at least 2 times higher, exercise radionuclide imaging 6 times higher, and coronary angiography 22 times higher [60]. However, it should be kept in mind that the lower cost of ET does not always result in a lower cost of patient care because the cost of additional testing and interventions may be higher due to the lower accuracy of ET.

Summary

The goal of evaluating the post-revascularized patient early, within the first 6 months to a year, is to evaluate the immediate results of revascularization. This is when CABG grafts or PCI are most likely to fail. Among the experts, the majority of the trials comparing CABG versus PCI for revascularization utilized ET during this timeframe to monitor their patients. Even if ACC/AHA guidelines do not recommend evaluating all patients immediately post-revascularization, or for 3–5 year unless they have symptoms, it certainly makes sense to evaluate high-risk patients (Table 13.1), or patients unable to exercise or with a poor exercise capacity (<4 METs), especially if they are about to undergo surgery. Eventually, the multi-slice CT angiogram (16-slice or higher for CABG, 64-slice or higher for PCI) may be recognized as the procedure of choice for early evaluation of patients post-revascularization. Combining an ET with a multi-slice angiogram would provide additional physiologic data which may be important for determining prognosis (e.g., exercise capacity, heart rate in recovery, systolic blood pressure response to exercise).

Whether CABG or PCI is utilized for revascularization, outcomes are comparable other than for diabetics who may do better with CABG. Ten year follow-up data from BARI were recently published revealing no difference in mortality, MI, or angina whether CABG or PTCA was performed for multi-vessel CAD [15]. The average overall mortality rate remained fairly low (2.8%) considering these patients have multi-vessel CAD. While it has not been studied prospectively, following an algorithm such as Fig. 13.1 (based largely upon ACC/AHA guidelines) may lower mortality even further.

Based on the BARI data, in asymptomatic patients post-revascularization, there may be value in testing non-exercisers with a chemical imaging study. This would probably also apply to patients with a poor exercise capacity (<4 METs). There also seems to be value in testing high-risk (Table 13.1) patients on a periodic basis, although there is no data to define the periodicity of testing. ET is capable of documenting ischemia in these patients, while exercise imaging is needed if it is important to define location and extent of ischemia. At 5 years post-revascularization, there is probably value to performing an exercise imaging test. In the absence of a change in clinical status, the results of this test (low, intermediate or high risk) can then play a role in individual recommendations for future testing.

In the patient who develops signs or symptoms of ischemia post-revascularization, an ET can be used to document ischemia. Local experience, expertise, and availability will likely determine whether an imaging test, or which, will be added to the ET. Three large meta-analyses have found exercise radionuclide and exercise echocardiography to have very similar sensitivities, specificities, and predictive accuracies for diagnosing restenosis or graft failure post-revascularization [13, 14].

What remains to be seen is the impact of improvements in medical management of CAD combined with increased use of stents, minimally invasive cardiac surgery, and use of arterial conduits for CABG. However, with the low mortality rates from the BARI trial, what is clear is that primary care clinicians will be caring for an increasing number of older patients post-revascularization for multi-vessel disease [15].

References

1. BARI Investigators: Comparison of coronary bypass surgery with angioplasty in patients with multivessel disease. N Engl J Med. 1996 Jul 25;335(4):217–25
2. Kurbaan AS, Bowker TJ, Ilsley CD, Rickards AF. Impact of postangioplasty restenosis on comparisons of outcome between angioplasty and bypass grafting. Coronary Angioplasty versus Bypass Revascularisation Investigation (CABRI) Investigators. Am J Cardiol. 1998 Aug 1;82(3):272–76
3. Henderson RA, Pocock SJ, Sharp SJ, Nanchahal K, Sculpher MJ, Buxton MJ, Hampton JR. Long-term results of RITA-1 trial: clinical and cost comparisons of coronary angioplasty and coronary-artery bypass grafting. Randomised Intervention Treatment of Angina. Lancet 1998 Oct 31;352(9138):1419–25
4. King SB 3rd, Barnhart HX, Kosinski AS, et al. Angioplasty or surgery for multivessel coronary artery disease: comparison of eligible registry and randomized patients in the EAST trial and influence of treatment selection on outcomes. Emory Angioplasty versus Surgery Trial Investigators. Am J Cardiol. 1997 Jun 1;79(11):1453–9
5. Rupprecht HJ, Hamm C, Ischinger T, Dietz U, Reimers J, Meyer J. Angiographic follow-up results of a randomized study on angioplasty versus bypass surgery (GABI trial). GABI Study Group. Eur Heart J. 1996 Aug;17(8):1192–8
6. Carrié D, Elbaz M, Puel J, Fourcade J, Karouny E, Fournial G, Galinier M. Five-year outcome after coronary angioplasty versus bypass surgery in multivessel coronary artery disease: results from the French Monocentric Study. Circulation 1997 Nov 4;96(9 Suppl):II-1–6
7. Urban P, Stauffer JC, Bleed D, Khatchatrian N, Amann W, Bertel O, van den Brand M, Danchin N, Kaufmann U, Meier B, Machecourt J, Pfisterer M. A randomized evaluation of early revascularization to treat shock complicating acute myocardial infarction. The (Swiss) Multicenter Trial of Angioplasty for Shock-(S)MASH. Eur Heart J. 1999 Jul;20(14):1030–8
8. Dagres N, Erbel R. [Comparison between PTCA and bypass operation. Results of large randomized studies]. Med Klin (Munich). 1998 Jan 15;93(1):22–6, 58

9. Rodriguez AE, Baldi J, Fernández Pereira C, Navia J, Rodriguez Alemparte M, Delacasa A, Vigo F, Vogel D, O'Neill W, Palacios IF, ERACI II Investigators. Five-year follow-up of the Argentine randomized trial of coronary angioplasty with stenting versus coronary bypass surgery in patients with multiple vessel disease (ERACI II). J Am Coll Cardiol. 2005 Aug 16;46(4):582–8

10. Serruys PW, Ong AT, van Herwerden LA, Sousa JE, Jatene A, Bonnier JJ, Schönberger JP, Buller N, Bonser R, Disco C, Backx B, Hugenholtz PG, Firth BG, Unger F. Five-year outcomes after coronary stenting versus bypass surgery for the treatment of multivessel disease: the final analysis of the Arterial Revascularization Therapies Study (ARTS) randomized trial. J Am Coll Cardiol. 2005 Aug 16;46(4):575–81

11. Zhang Z, Mahoney EM, Spertus JA, Booth J, Nugara F, Kolm P, Stables RH, Weintraub WS. The impact of age on outcomes after coronary artery bypass surgery versus stent-assisted percutaneous coronary intervention: one-year results from the Stent or Surgery (SoS) trial. Am Heart J. 2006 Dec;152(6):1153–60

12. Eagle KA, Berger PB, Calkins H, et al. American College of Cardiology/American Heart Association Task Force on Practice Guidelines (Committee to Update the 1996 Guidelines on Perioperative Cardiovascular Evaluation for Noncardiac Surgery). ACC/AHA guideline update for perioperative cardiovascular evaluation for noncardiac surgery—executive summary a report of the American College of Cardiology/American Heart Association Task Force on Practice Guidelines (Committee to Update the 1996 Guidelines on Perioperative Cardiovascular Evaluation for Noncardiac Surgery). Circulation 2002 Mar 12;105(10):1257–67

13. Dori G, Denekamp Y, Fishman S, Bitterman H. Exercise stress testing, myocardial perfusion imaging and stress echocardiography for detecting restenosis after successful percutaneous transluminal coronary angioplasty: a review of performance. J Intern Med. 2003 Mar;253(3):253–62

14. Garzon PP, Eisenberg MJ. Functional testing for the detection of restenosis after percutaneous transluminal coronary angioplasty: a meta-analysis. Can J Cardiol. 2001 Jan;17(1):41–8

15. BARI Investigators. The final 10-year follow-up results from the BARI randomized trial. J Am Coll Cardiol. 2007 Apr 17;49(15):1600–6. Epub 2007 Apr 2

16. Krone RJ, Hardison RM, Chaitman BR, Gibbons RJ, Sopko G, Bach R, Detre KM. Risk stratification after successful coronary revascularization: the lack of a role for routine exercise testing. J Am Coll Cardiol. 2001 Jul;38(1):136–42

17. Snader CE, Marwick TH, Pashkow FJ, Harvey SA, Thomas JD, Lauer MS. Importance of estimated functional capacity as a predictor of all-cause mortality among patients referred for exercise thallium single-photon emission computed tomography: report of 3,400 patients from a single center. J Am Coll Cardiol. 1997 Sep;30(3):641–8

18. Stratmann HG, Tamesis BR, Younis LT, Wittry MD, Miller DD. Prognostic value of dipyridamole technetium-99m sestamibi myocardial tomography in patients with stable chest pain who are unable to exercise. Am J Cardiol. 1994 Apr 1;73(9):647–52

19. Pollock SG, Abbott RD, Boucher CA, Beller GA, Kaul S. Independent and incremental prognostic value of tests performed in hierarchical order to evaluate patients with suspected coronary artery disease. Validation of models based on these tests. Circulation 1992 Jan;85(1): 237–48

20. Chin AS, Goldman LE, Eisenberg MJ. Functional testing after coronary artery bypass graft surgery: a meta-analysis. Can J Cardiol. 2003 Jun;19(7):802–8

21. Diaz LA, Brunken RC, Blackstone EH, Snader CE, Lauer MS. Independent contribution of myocardial perfusion defects to exercise capacity and heart rate recovery for prediction of all-cause mortality in patients with known or suspected coronary heart disease. J Am Coll Cardiol. 2001 May;37(6):1558–64

22. Froelicher VF. Miscellaneous applications of exercise testing. In Exercise and the Heart (5th edition), Froelicher VF, Myers J (eds.). Philadelphia: Elsevier, 2006

23. Waller BF, Rothbaum DA, Gorfinkel HJ, Ulbright TM, Linnemeier TJ, Berger SM. Morphologic observations after percutaneous transluminal balloon angioplasty of early and late aortocoronary saphenous vein bypass grafts. J Am Coll Cardiol. 1984 Oct;4(4):784–92

24. Neitzel GF, Barboriak JJ, Pintar K, Qureshi I. Atherosclerosis in aortocoronary bypass grafts. Morphologic study and risk factor analysis 6 to 12 years after surgery. Arteriosclerosis 1986 Nov–Dec;6(6):594–600

25. Walts AE, Fishbein MC, Sustaita H, Matloff JM. Ruptured atheromatous plaques in saphenous vein coronary artery bypass grafts: a mechanism of acute, thrombotic, late graft occlusion. Circulation 1982 Jan;65(1):197–201

26. Tilli FV, Kaplan BM, Safian RD, et al. Angioscopic plaque friability: a new risk factor for procedural complications following saphenous vein graft interventions (abstract). J Am Coll Cardiol. 1996;27(Suppl A):364A

27. Sommerhaug RG, Wolfe SF, Reid DA, Lindsey DE. Improved stress test results after multiple coronary grafting. Am J Surg. 1985 May;149(5):583–6

28. Ellestad MH. Stress testing after surgical intervention and coronary angioplasty. In Stress Testing: Principals and Practice (5th edition), Ellestad MH (ed.). New York: Oxford, 2003

29. Grondin CM, Campeau L, Thornton JC, Engle JC, Cross FS, Schreiber H. Coronary artery bypass grafting with saphenous vein. Circulation 1989 Jun;79(6 Pt 2):I24–9

30. ROSETTA-CABG Registry, Eisenberg MJ, Wou K, Nguyen H, Duerr R, Del Core M, Fourchy D, et al. Lack of benefit for routine functional testing early after coronary artery bypass graft surgery: results from the ROSETTA-CABG Registry. J Invasive Cardiol. 2006 Apr;18(4): 147–52

31. Gohlke H, Gohlke-Bärwolf C, Samek L, Stürzenofecker P, Schmuziger M, Roskamm H. Serial exercise testing up to 6 years after coronary bypass surgery: behavior of exercise parameters in groups with different degrees of revascularization determined by postoperative angiography. Am J Cardiol. 1983 May 1;51(8):1301–6

32. Guttin J. Longitudinal evaluation of patients after coronary artery bypass by serial treadmill testing. Am J Cardiol. 1975 35:142

33. Lakkis NM, Mahmarian JJ, Verani MS. Exercise thallium-201 single photon emission computed tomography for evaluation of coronary artery bypass graft patency. Am J Cardiol. 1995 Jul 15;76(3):107–11

34. Sakamoto Y, Takakura H, Saitoh F, Ohnishi K, Shiratori K, Takagi K, Ikei H, Kurosawa H. Assessment of coronary artery bypass surgery by exercise thallium imaging. Ann Thorac Cardiovasc Surg. 1999 Dec;5(6):387–90

35. Shapira I, Heller I, Kornizky Y, Topilsky M, Isakov A. The value of stress thallium-201 single photon emission CT imaging as a predictor of outcome and long-term prognosis after CABG. J Med. 2001;32(5–6):271–82

36. Zellweger MJ, Lewin HC, Lai S, Dubois EA, Friedman JD, Germano G, Kang X, Sharir T, Berman DS. When to stress patients after coronary artery bypass surgery? Risk stratification in patients early and late post-CABG using stress myocardial perfusion SPECT: implications of appropriate clinical strategies. J Am Coll Cardiol. 2001 Jan;37(1):144–52

37. Lauer MS, Ellis S. Is routine functional testing after coronary bypass surgery worthwhile? J Invasive Cardiol. 2006 Apr;18(4):153–4

38. Kawachi Y, Nakashima A, Toshima Y, Komesu I, Kimura S, Arinaga K. Risk stratification analysis of operative mortality in coronary artery bypass surgery. Jpn J Thorac Cardiovasc Surg. 2001 Sep;49(9):557–63

39. Nallamothu N, Johnson JH, Bagheri B, et al. Utility of stress single-photon emission computed tomography (SPECT) perfusion imaging in predicting outcome after coronary artery bypass grafting. Am J Cardiol. 1997 Dec 15;80(12):1517–21

40. Miller TD, Christian TF, Hodge DO, Mullan BP, Gibbons RJ. Prognostic value of exercise thallium-201 imaging performed within 2 years of coronary artery bypass graft surgery. J Am Coll Cardiol. 1998 Mar 15;31(4):848–54

41. Houslay ES, Lawton T, Sengupta A, Uren NG, McKillop G, Newby DE. Non-invasive assessment of coronary artery bypass graft patency using 16-slice computed tomography angiography. J Cardiothorac Surg. 2007 Jun 5;2:27

42. Chirillo F, Bruni A, De Leo A, Olivari Z, Franceschini-Grisolia E, Totis O, Stritoni P. Usefulness of dipyridamole stress echocardiography for predicting graft patency after coronary artery bypass grafting. Am J Cardiol. 2004 Jan 1;93(1):24–30

43. Qarawani D, Nahir M, Abboud M, et al. Culprit only versus complete coronary revascularization during primary PCI. Int J Cardiol. 2008 Jan 24;123(3):288–92

44. Boden WE, O'Rourke RA, Teo KK, et al., COURAGE Trial Research Group. Optimal medical therapy with or without PCI for stable coronary disease. N Engl J Med. 2007 Apr 12;356(15):1503–16. Epub 2007 Mar 26

45. Hochman JS, Lamas GA, Buller CE, et al., Occluded Artery Trial Investigators. Coronary intervention for persistent occlusion after myocardial infarction. N Engl J Med. 2006 Dec 7;355(23):2395–407. Epub 2006 Nov 14

46. Moreno R, Fernandez C, Hernandez R, Alfonso F, Angiolillo DJ, Sabate M, Escaned J, Banuelos C, Fernandez-Ortiz A, Macaya C. Drug-eluting stent thrombosis: results from a pooled analysis including 10 randomized studies. J Am Coll Cardiol. 2005 Mar 15;45(6): 954–9

47. Bavry AA, Kumbhani DJ, Helton TJ, Bhatt DL. Risk of thrombosis with the use of sirolimus-eluting stents for percutaneous coronary intervention (from registry and clinical trial data). Am J Cardiol. 2005 Jun 15;95(12):1469–72

48. Bavry AA, Kumbhani DJ, Helton TJ, Bhatt DL. What is the risk of stent thrombosis associated with the use of paclitaxel-eluting stents for percutaneous coronary intervention? a meta-analysis. J Am Coll Cardiol. 2005 Mar 15;45(6):941–6

49. Eisenberg MJ, Wilson B, Lauzon C, Huynh T, Eisenhauer M, Mak KH, Blankenship JC, Doucet M, Pilote L, ADORE II Investigators. Routine functional testing after percutaneous coronary intervention: results of the aggressive diagnosis of restenosis in high-risk patients (ADORE II) trial. Acta Cardiol. 2007 Apr;62(2):143–50

50. Valeur N, Clemmensen P, Saunamaki K, Grande P, DANAMI-2 Investigators. The prognostic value of pre-discharge exercise testing after myocardial infarction treated with either primary PCI or fibrinolysis: a DANAMI-2 sub-study. Eur Heart J. 2005 Jan;26(2):119–27. Epub 2004 Dec 6

51. Ho KT, Miller TD, Holmes DR, Hodge DO, Gibbons RJ. Long-term prognostic value of Duke treadmill score and exercise thallium-201 imaging performed one to three years after percutaneous transluminal coronary angioplasty. Am J Cardiol. 1999 Dec 1;84(11):1323–7

52. Rajagopal V, Lauer MS. Nuclear imaging in patients with a history of coronary revascularization. In Clinical Nuclear Cardiology: State of the Art and Future Directions (3rd edition), Zaret BL, Beller GA (eds.). Philadelphia: Elsevier, 2004

53. Acampa W, Petretta M, Florimonte L, Mattera A, Cuocolo A. Prognostic value of exercise cardiac tomography performed late after percutaneous coronary intervention in symptomatic and symptom-free patients. Am J Cardiol. 2003 Feb 1;91(3):259–63

54. Acampa W, Evangelista L, Petretta M, Liuzzi R, Cuocolo A. Usefulness of stress cardiac single-photon emission computed tomographic imaging late after percutaneous coronary intervention for assessing cardiac events and time to such events. Am J Cardiol. 2007 Aug 1;100(3):436–41. Epub 2007 Jun 13

55. Mak KH, Eisenberg MJ, Tsang J, Okrainiec K, Huynh T, Brown DL, ROSETTA Investigators. Clinical impact of functional testing strategy among stented and non-stented patients: insights from the ROSETTA Registry. Int J Cardiol. 2004 Jun;95(2–3):321–7

56. Saririan M, Cugno S, Blankenship J, Huynh T, Sedlis S, Starling M, Pilote L, Wilson B, Eisenberg MJ. Routine versus selective functional testing after percutaneous coronary intervention in patients with diabetes mellitus. J Invasive Cardiol. 2005 Jan;17(1):25–9

57. Cademartiri F, Palumbo A, Maffei E, La Grutta L, Runza G, Pugliese F, Midiri M, Mollet NR, Meijboom WB, Menozzi A, Vignali L, Reverberi C, Ardissino D, Krestin GP. Radiol Med (Torino). Diagnostic accuracy of 64-slice CT in the assessment of coronary stents. 2007 Jun;112(4):526–37. Epub 2007 Jun 11

58. Hirata K, Watanabe H, Otsuka R, et al. Noninvasive diagnosis of restenosis by transthoracic Doppler echocardiography after percutaneous coronary intervention: comparison with exercise TI-SPECT. J Am Soc Echocardiogr. 2006 Feb;19(2):165–71

59. Elhendy A, Tsutsui JM, O'Leary EL, Xie F, Majeed F, Porter TR. Evaluation of restenosis and extent of coronary artery disease in patients with previous percutaneous coronary interventions by dobutamine stress real-time myocardial contrast perfusion imaging. Heart 2006 Oct;92(10):1480–3. Epub 2006 Apr 10

60. Gibbons RJ, Balady GJ, Bricker JT, et al. ACC/AHA 2002 guideline update for exercise testing: summary article: a report of the American College of Cardiology/American Heart Association Task Force on Practice Guidelines (Committee to Update the 1997 Exercise Testing Guidelines). Circulation 2002 Oct 1;106(14):1883–92

Chapter 14
Legal Aspects of Graded Exercise Testing

**David L. Herbert, William G. Herbert, Russell D. White,
and Victor F. Froelicher**

Graded exercise testing (ET) is performed by family physicians, internists and cardiologists. Currently, only about 13% of family physicians and 29% of internists perform this procedure in the cardiac evaluation of patients [1, 2]. A survey of the graduates of one family medicine residency program found a decrease in the percent of graduates performing exercise testing from 14.9% in the graduation years of 1975–1983 to 5.3% in the graduation years of 1994–2003 [3]. While the American Board of Internal Medicine requires its members to do this procedure, the number of internists performing exercise testing continues to decline.

This procedure is useful in the diagnosis of coronary artery disease as well as in determining prognosis of these patients at the primary care level. Multiple recommendations for the evaluation of patients for coronary artery disease include stress testing (exercise or pharmaceutical) with and without simultaneous imaging. Several authors have found that those patients in the low-risk group can be followed with medical intervention and risk-factor reduction while those patients at higher risk should be referred for further evaluation and consideration for interventional therapy [4, 5].

There is an accumulation of case law concerning the proper evaluation of patients with possible coronary artery disease, the timely response to symptomatic patients following exercise testing and the appropriate follow-up of those individuals identified as high risk. Questions have arisen concerning the training and credentialing of primary care physicians in exercise testing as well as the credentialing and privileging of physicians in both the in-patient and out-patient clinical settings. In this chapter case law concerning the evaluation of patients presenting with either chest pain or symptoms of coronary artery disease will be reviewed. The appropriate training and education of primary physicians along with subsequent credentialing and privileging are discussed.

D.L. Herbert (✉)
David L. Herbert and Associates, LLC, 4580 Stephen Circle NW, Canton, OH 44718 USA
e-mail: herblegal@aol.com

C.H. Evans, R.D. White (eds.), *Exercise Testing for Primary Care and Sports Medicine Physicians*, DOI 10.1007/978-0-387-76597-6_14
© Springer Science+Business Media, LLC 2009

Body of Law

Even though it seems clear that graded exercise testing procedures are associated with a low incidence of serious cardiovascular injuries or deaths among selected patients undergoing diagnostic procedures, a body of law has developed over the last 30 years in response to these considerations. Over that same time, the health profession has undergone notable malpractice crises which have resulted in health-care and legal reforms designed to stem these problems. Relevant responsive efforts have included tort and medical malpractice reform, health-care standards development, risk management programs and apology or "I'm sorry" type campaigns. The latter of these developments has focused on quick medical acknowledgment of untoward results, combined with the adoption of legal protections for such physician expressions for bad results, as well as other similar educational steps and other programs.

This section explores that body of law surrounding exercising testing (ET) and analyzes what risk management suggestions may flow out of that analysis. However, it is no substitution for individualized risk management or professional and legal advice which all practitioners need to seek out and apply as they properly carry out their responsibilities and duties.

Perhaps one of the first cases to have substantial visibility arose in 1981 in the case of *Tart v. McGann* (1982, 2nd Cir.), 697 F.2d 75. While it is one of a significant number of other subsequent litigations, the case was very important to the subject since it dealt specifically with the ET process, those professional standards in existence at the time, and invoked specific statements within the litigation [6].

In this case, the plaintiff, Mr. Tart, was an airline pilot in his early forties who was undergoing an annual physical examination for applicable commercial pilot's licensing requirements. During the last stage of a physician-performed graded exercise stress test, he contended he was unduly stressed and requested that the test be stopped. Shortly after completion of his test, Tart suffered a myocardial infarction (MI) and ultimately lost his commercial pilot's license. He subsequently instituted suit against the physicians involved with the procedure contending that they were negligent.

During the case certain expert testimony was offered. It included the following, which highlights how such key issues in these cases are developed and used for trial.

Establishing Qualification for Testimony

Q. Dr. . . . you have had occasion to examine Mr. William Tart, I believe?
A. Yes, sir, I have.
Q. Could you tell us, Doctor, something about your medical background, please?

In response, the expert summarized his training which included a Master's degree in physiology, three-and-a-half years of postgraduate work at Harvard Medical School in the Department of Cardiology and serving on the faculty at Harvard. Later at Columbia-Presbyterian Medical Center he was in charge of the heart station. Subsequently, he had risen to full professor at New York University. He testified to writing over 250 articles and four books while contributing to an additional six books.

He then testified to the purpose of exercise stress testing and testified that the 42-year-old patient in question achieved a maximum heart rate of 185 beats per minute while exercising on the Bruce protocol at 16% grade and at 4.2 miles per hour. His opinion was that the maximum heart rate of 185 per minute "was too much".

Laying a Foundation for Testimony

Q. Is a part of your job, Doctor, to give electrocardiograph[ic] examinations?
A. Yes, it is.

He then delineated his 35-year history of performing such tests and confirmed he was performing such tests currently. He outlined various protocols including the Naughton, Modified Balke–Naughton and the Bruce protocols as well as the classic Master Two-Step test.

Q. Have you been doing that for many years?
A. Longer than I care to remember. About 35 years.
Q. At the present time, do you do the stress or exercise test for your patients?
A. Yes, sir. I was the one to do that at University Hospital, New York University Medical Center
Q. What is the point of [a] ... treadmill test?
A. There are about three or four reasons for a treadmill test. First of all, it is used to detect heart disease. Secondly, it is used in formulating a prescription for cardiac rehabilitation from the treadmill test. Thirdly, it is designed to give you a measurement of the heart's limit of work activity so, therefore, you can write a prescription as to whether the person can do a certain job. Fourthly, it is designed to give you measurements of progress in cardiac rehabilitation. Fifthly, we sometimes do it to give the person a measure of well-being and confidence. That's a psychological effect.
Q. Now, Doctor, in terms of the stress test itself, could you explain to the jury the equipment and procedures involved in completing the stress test in this case.

He then proceeded to describe how an exercise test is done, which parameters are monitored and what the results indicate when completed.

Opinion Testimony

Q. Do you have an opinion [based upon a reasonable degree of medical cer-
tainty as to whether or not it was proper under the facts and circumstances of
this case, and drawing upon your own education, training and background],
to bring Mr. Tart to that point [as you have described]?

A. Yes, I do.

Q. What is your opinion?

A. I think it was too much.

He then proceeded to elucidate several parameters including the patient's feelings or symptoms, blood pressure and heart rate measurements every three minutes,
serial electrocardiogram (ECG) recordings, and careful monitoring for ST-segment
depression. He then commented on the patient's tiredness and excessive perspiration
and felt that continuation of the stress test was improper treatment. In summary,
he felt the rapidity with which the heart was stressed, the extent by which it was
stressed, was a definite contributing factor to his myocardial infarction or heart
attack [7].

Differences in Professional Standards

In the course of any expert's presentation of testimony amounting to the expression
of opinion, proof of compliance with or adherence to the most prominent professional standards or practices will quite clearly provide a basis for a defense of that
individual and the professional course of practice followed therein. This becomes
extremely complicated in certain cases where there are no clear-cut standards or
guidelines. Moreover, problems frequently develop where standards within a given
profession are neither uniform nor consistent, or where different professional standards of practice are set differently by diverse professional organizations. As a result
of the different professional standards of practice for this field, a number of confusing problems may arise [8].

Standards of practice for exercise testing have been developed by such groups
as the American Heart Association (AHA), the American Medical Association
(AMA), the American College of Sports Medicine (ACSM), the American College
of Cardiology (ACC) and the American Association of Cardiovascular and Pulmonary Rehabilitation (AACPR). These standards are frequently updated and new
standards are always forthcoming and evolving [9, 10].

Thus, there are potentially several sets of standards aside from statutory or administrative standards which could be utilized in any trial of a negligence or malpractice claim against a physician as a basis to judge a defendant's conduct. Any
overt or implied differences in these standards can greatly and adversely affect
the expert testimony presented in a negligence or malpractice case in ways that
can either strengthen or weaken a particular position. For example, differences
in standards can give rise to claims of negligence on the part of a professional

rendering services in the course of an exercise program when he/she selects and follows one set of standards over another set of perhaps equally authoritative standards [11, 12].

Malpractice/Negligence Claims Illustrated

In the *Tart* case, the expert testimony presented at trial probably affected the jury's perception of the facts presented in the case. However, only one set of professional guidelines – those of the AHA – were utilized in the course of examination and cross-examination of the experts. Under cross-examination by the defendant's counsel, the plaintiff's expert was asked questions regarding these standards. The expert witness was queried whether he agreed with the statement that the criteria for whether or not a patient who suffered a heart attack has a maximal or submaximal test is not based on a numerical heart rate but is based on other data as follows:

> [A] maximal test is a test that takes a patient, whether he be sedentary or a crack athlete, to a level where he cannot go any higher and a submaximal test is anything below that in varying steps and does not depend on numerical heart rate.

In this case, certain individual experts testified for both the plaintiff and the defendant on the question of the defendant's adherence or lack thereof to certain professional standards. Questions centered upon the propriety of using the Bruce protocol performed upon the plaintiff. The focal point of the trial involved questions regarding the alleged failure of the defendants to terminate the testing procedure in the presence of certain alleged clinical indications [13–15]. The jury focused its attention upon the question of when the test should have been terminated based upon all the facts and circumstances existing at the time the patient completed stage four and began to enter stage five of the test. At that point, the procedure was terminated, with the patient having attained a heart rate of 185 beats per minute and a performance level of 4.2 miles per hour and 16% grade. Tart's peak functional capacity was calculated at 12 METs, with normal responses throughout the entire test and during the post-exercise monitoring period. However, approximately one-half hour after the test was completed, the patient began to experience chest pains and he suffered a myocardial infarction. In the course of deliberations the jury asked a question of the court as to whether or not a subject's facial expressions could be considered as the equivalent to a request to stop a particular test. The trial judge instructed the jury that mere facial expressions of fatigue could not be equated with a request to stop the test. The jury shortly thereafter returned a defendant's verdict, but on appeal the Court of Appeals stated:

> A better response to the jury's question would have been something like the following: 'The expression of fatigue may be regarded as a request to stop, or it may not be; it is a question of fact for you [the jury] to determine. In other words, whether a doctor in the position of Dr. Mooney should reasonably have regarded Mr. Tart's expression of [facial] fatigue as a request to stop is a question for you, the jury, to determine in light of all of the circumstances, including Mr. Tart's condition, the duration of the test, the stage of the test, his previous medical history, and Dr. Mooney's acquaintance with that condition and history.' [16]

Based in part upon the trial court's answer to the jury's question, the Court of Appeals determined the outcome of the trial to be erroneous; thus, the case was reversed and remanded and went through a second jury trial which also resulted in a defendant's verdict (although due to a pre-verdict agreement between the plaintiff and the defendant the plaintiff received $50,000.) [9] Even though the first jury's question involved a great many potential sub-issues, one question clearly centered upon the physician's duty to stop a given stress test on the basis of alleged patient discomfort as evidenced by facial expressions that might have reflected discomfort or fatigue.

But no professional would probably testify that he or she would terminate a stress test upon the basis of facial expressions of discomfort alone when there is more objective information available from an exercise test. The jury in *Tart v. McGann* was apparently concerned about the defendant's independent judgment to terminate a test upon the basis of all pertinent information, even in the absence of Mr. Tart's overt request to stop.

A 1985 case from Missouri, *Hedgecorth v. United States*, dealt with the importance of the risk disclosure process associated with the ET procedure [17]. The plaintiff in this case contended that he suffered a stroke or other cardiovascular accident in 1980 while undergoing a physician prescribed and monitored diagnostic exercise stress test at a Veteran's Administration Medical Center (VAMC). The plaintiff's relevant medical history included myocardial infarctions in 1978 and 1979, post-Ml angina pain, a 1979 cardiac catheterization procedure which revealed severely occluded coronary arteries, a 1979 five-vessel coronary bypass graft operation and an exercise test that induced premature ventricular contractions (PVC's) without evidence of myocardial ischemia, which was administered in the post-surgical period. Prior to the exercise test in question, the plaintiff had undergone a graded exercise test performed for the Social Security Administration (SSA) in reference to a disability application. Later that same month, however, the plaintiff returned to the VAMC for follow-up treatment for his coronary condition and some minimal effort was made by the VAMC physicians to obtain the results of the earlier SSA-sponsored exercise test. Those test results were not obtained as of March 20, 1980, and as a consequence, the VAMC physicians scheduled the exercise test in question to be performed on March 31, 1980. It was during this test that the plaintiff contended that he suffered a stroke or some other cardiovascular event. The court later found that inadequate efforts had been put forth by the VAMC physicians to secure the test results from the March 3, 1980, exercise test.

Prior to the administration of the second exercise test, the VAMC physician met with the plaintiff and orally informed him of some of the dangers associated with taking such a test but did not inform the patient that stroke was one of the dangers. While a written informed consent was obtained and signed by the plaintiff, it did not list any dangers or side effects that could result from such testing.

Once the testing procedure began in the cardiology section of the VAMC under the supervision of a physician and a technician, the plaintiff complained of a loss of vision in his left eye and chest pain approximately 5.2 minutes into the test. As a consequence the test was terminated. Suit was later instituted by the patient claiming malpractice in the performance of the stress testing procedure.

The court examined all of the evidence offered by the plaintiff including expert testimony which consisted of the testimony of an ophthalmologist and an emergency medicine specialist and agreed with the plaintiff in concluding: "Under the facts and circumstances of this case the giving of the stress test was both negligent and the proximate cause of plaintiff's injuries" [18, 19]. The court based its conclusion upon two separate findings. First, as to the decision to administer a stress test when the results of another, recently conducted test were available, the court stated: "[A] patient should not be given a stress test if there are available adequate results from a prior stress test given less than one month prior to the subsequent test. Because of the dangers associated in giving the stress test, the results from the immediately preceding stress test should be used by the ordinary careful and prudent physician in lieu of retesting the patient" [19]. Second, as to the informed consent process, the court concluded: "The credible medical evidence presented at trial demonstrates that giving the (VAMC conducted) stress test to the plaintiff . . . was a deviation from the appropriate standard of care. The purpose of a stress test is, as the name implies, to place a stress on the heart through physical exercise and thereby derive information concerning the heart's condition. Because of the nature of the test certain dangers accompany its administration. These dangers include the possibility that the patient will suffer a stroke. The patient should be warned that a stroke could result from the administration of the test, and the plaintiff was not warned of this danger. Thus, plaintiff . . . did not take the test with informed consent of its dangers" [19].

The court in accessing the plaintiff's case found: "As a direct result of the negligent acts and omissions of the defendants, the plaintiff . . . suffered an infarct in the right occipital lobe of his brain. This stroke directly caused plaintiff . . ., total and permanent disability" [20]. The plaintiff was awarded $750,000 in damages for his injuries and his wife was awarded $75,000 for her loss of consortium, companionship and services.

Although the *Hedgecorth* decision is not binding precedent outside the Eastern District of Missouri, the court's ruling has some rather broad and far-reaching implications. Normally, a physician or other provider is required in the informed consent process to disclose all risks which are *material* to the procedure about to be performed upon the patient. Materiality is generally equated with *probable, anticipated* or *likely* occurrences which might arise. The law does not generally require a disclosure of improbable, remote or unlikely risks or occurrences, which can possibly arise during a procedure.

While early publications of the AHA and the ACSM did not list the possibility of stroke within their risk disclosure items as stated in their sample informed consent forms, one of ACSM's later publications did include an informed consent form which listed such a possibility within the proffered list of risks related to the procedure [20–28].

Even though clear statistical evidence of the risk of stroke occurrence during exercise testing procedures is not readily apparent, it is very clear that the risk of stroke is very minimal, even unlikely. It is not even listed in the classic risk studies or literature dealing with stress testing risks [29]. Given this minimal risk of occurrence, the *Hedgecorth* ruling is extremely troublesome from several perspectives. First, it may be prudent to disclose the risk of stroke during the informed consent process; if so, should the risk of blindness due to stroke also be disclosed, or risks of total or partial, temporary or permanent paralysis or a host of other possible consequences due to stroke? Secondly, is it now also necessary to disclose other remote, possible risks which could occur during such a procedure? If so, which ones? Thirdly, if remote risks must be disclosed, how are the risks to be disclosed, differentiated from all conceivable risks which will not be disclosed?

As a practical matter, what disclosure course is minimally prudent to conduct in light of the *Hedgecorth* opinion? First, it may be prudent to include "risk of stroke" and "risk of blindness" due to stroke disclosures in the risk disclosure section of the informed consent form. However, the inclusion of such remote risks, especially the possibility of blindness due to stroke, without inclusion of all other remote possibilities may bring "failure to disclose" challenges related to any number of other remote risks that proximately caused an untoward event and thus lead to a *Hedgecorth*-type suit. Secondly, it may be minimally prudent conduct to review orally with the patient those risks which are associated with the procedure and just simply list in the informed consent form the fact that the risks were disclosed and make an accompanying note in the chart that a discussion as to the risks took place. Then, however in the event of some untoward event and suit, the proof as to whether or not a risk disclosure was made will depend upon what the trier of fact believes after hearing individualized testimony. Thirdly, it may be prudent to include a "catch all" type provision within each informed consent form which provides in general terms that there are other risks of injury, along with the risk of death.

Material risks associated with any procedure must be disclosed if there is to be any valid consent to support a defense to battery or negligence/malpractice claims based upon a failure to obtain an informed consent. Traditionally, the courts have ruled that the more remote and unlikely the risk, the less a need for disclosure. However, there are well-known risks associated with exercise testing and exercise training which should be disclosed. This certainly includes the risk of death. While the previously mentioned statements of the AHA, the ACSM and the AACVPR now all provide for the delineated risk of "death" within the proffered informed consent documents therein located, the form originally proffered by the AACVPR did not so specifically provide, instead characterizing this risk as the possibility of a "fatal" or "non-fatal" heart attack. Such word choices rather than the word choice of "death" may be somewhat paternalistic at best and potentially confusing and of real little meaning to many patients, including those without sufficient education [30]. Such word choices for the informed consent risk disclosure process have the potential to render the entire process invalid in the event of patient confusion [29].

At least one case has specifically dealt with this issue. In the case of *Smogor v. Enke*, the patient suffered a heart attack in 1971 [31]. In August of 1984, he suffered pain and went to an emergency room with complaints of chest pain. The emergency room physician performed certain tests including an ECG and scheduled an appointment for the patient to see his family physician the next day. During that appointment with the family physician, a stress test was scheduled to be performed by a cardiologist for the following day. On that day, a stress test was performed and was preceded by completion of another resting (pre-exercise) ECG. By the last stage of the test the patient experienced pain and it was stopped. He was hospitalized due to worsening cardiac symptoms and unfortunately died the following day.

The patient's family subsequently brought suit against the family physician and the cardiologist asserting that the physicians were negligent. The plaintiff contended that the cardiologist "failed to inform [the patient] . . . of the risks of the stress test or obtain . . . [the patient's] informed consent to undergo the test" [31]. The plaintiffs also contended that both physicians were negligent due to insufficient communication with the patient prior to the test, that the taking of medical history information was insufficient and that the cardiologist failed to compare his pre-test ECG with the one which had been performed 2 days earlier.

At time of trial, the jury returned a verdict for the defendants. The plaintiffs appealed contending that the jury's verdict was against the "great weight of the evidence." On appeal the appellate court reviewed the facts and the plaintiff's allegations of trial court error. In reference to the informed consent process the court held, "[the patient] did sign a consent form that explicitly informed him of the risk of death" [31]. Thus the court found that there was no error related to that aspect of the informed consent process and the verdict in favor of the defendant physicians was affirmed.

In light of findings like those reported in this case, as well as those of prior decisions (*Hedgecorth v. United States*), consent forms for these programs should be reviewed by program counsel [32]. In some cases, consideration must be given to broadening the risk disclosure process in light of relevant case law and judicial pronouncements.

In the course of rendering its decision in *Smogor v. Enke* case, *supra*, the court also examined the risk disclosure and information exchange process of the informed consent procedure. The court found that the physician delegated the information disclosure process to a technician and approved that process finding that it violated no requirement of law to do so. Moreover, a delegation of certain aspects of the procedure does not allow a delegation of responsibility for the process. Thus, where the patient asks questions about a procedure, or seeks more information about risks, alternatives to the procedure or benefits to be expected, these questions may need to be addressed by a physician as opposed to a technician. Any technician who attempts to answer such concerns might well run afoul of unauthorized practice of medicine statutes while also laying the groundwork for a judicial declaration voiding a "tainted" informed consent process. This may also create a basis upon which to hold the provider liable for any untoward occurrence which arises during or following the procedure. In some states, however, such a delegation may be permissible [33].

In a 1992 case, *Hoem v. Zia*, the decedent underwent a physical examination in March of 1988. An ECG test was performed as part of his examination, which reportedly was clinically negative. Later that year he had complained to his family doctor of chest pain and shortness of breath.

Subsequently the decedent went to the defendant pulmonologist who had treated him some 4 years earlier. The pulmonologist administered certain tests to assess lung problems and scheduled the decedent to undergo a cardiopulmonary stress test. While the pulmonologist was out of town on the test date, his partner administered a cycle ergometer ECG-monitored test that was designed to assess signs of myocardial ischemia, heart rate and blood pressure, pulmonary/respiratory function and aerobic capacity. Reportedly, the decedent did not complain of any chest pain during the test.

Two weeks later the pulmonologist's partner prepared a test report which resulted in him recommending that the decedent see a cardiologist for a "blockage" which was discovered during the test. Allegedly he complained of radiating pain in his chest the weekend before the appointment. Subsequently, the decedent collapsed while walking up a flight of stairs to his office. Despite prompt Emergency Medical Services (EMS) response, he died.

Suit was subsequently brought against the pulmonologist, his partner and others. The plaintiff's cardiologist testified that the ergometer ECG "revealed certain heart problems that indicated [the decedent] had recently suffered a 'silent heart attack'" and that if the partner had prepared an immediate assessment report following the test "he should have noticed this fact from the test results." The expert also testified that the pulmonologist's partner failed to recognize the urgency of the decedent's condition and his need for immediate cardiac care and consultation.

The defendant's expert, the cardiologist to whom they had referred the decedent, testified that the decedent's condition did not present an urgent medical condition and that the care recommended by the pulmonologist and his partner was appropriate. In addition, the defendant providers utilized a pulmonologist to testify that while a cardiologist might have noticed subtle, life-threatening heart problems in the test results, the standard of care for pulmonologists did not mandate the discovery and assessment of such subtleties.

A defense verdict was ultimately rendered and the plaintiffs appealed citing numerous errors. Subsequently, the appellate court reversed the trial court's verdict and remanded the case for a new trial.

This case points up some highly relevant issues and should serve as a graphic illustration of what could happen in litigation dealing with the negligent administration of ETs. If the issues in this case had indeed focused on claimed negligence in the performance of the test as opposed to claimed negligence in the independent and prompt analysis and reporting of test results, an expert's lack of experience with the procedure would indeed be fertile grounds for cross-examination and attack. Professionals would be well advised to consider the potential issues which can arise in the administration of stress testing.

There has been considerable interest in the advantages and consequences of assigning ET supervisory responsibilities to non-physicians [34]. Some commentators have examined the medico-legal risks when ETs are performed without the direct supervision of a physician, as well as how professional conduct for such actions of the non-physician may be judged in court when litigation does occur [35–38]. One author has suggested a framework of assessment techniques and administrative practices to maximize the utility of testing and yet reduce the chances of untoward events when decisions are made to supervise with a physician surrogate [39].

The trend in health care to delegate procedures to non-physician providers is likely to increase. It is essential that they adopt approaches relative to policies and procedures, delegation of duties, supervision of staff and documentation that will keep the quality of care high and the risks of litigation as low as possible. State statutes governing the practice of medicine and allied health-care professions should be examined to illustrate how practice laws may affect decisions on the delegation of physician authority for ET supervision.

Exercise testing provided in the context of some health service, e.g., diagnosis or prescription of exercise to improve some function or symptom related to disease or deficit, would appear to be problematic in certain jurisdictions where such authority is limited to the authorized scope of practice of a physician. Physicians often delegate the supervision of clinical exercise tests to their surrogates through the "physician standing order" process. The most typical example is the Registered Nurse with appropriate training and current competencies in Advanced Cardiac Life Support (ACLS) who may act on behalf of the physician in providing emergency care when untoward cardiac events occur in conjunction with a ET. Of course, questions about the legal authority for such arrangements all too often arise, "after the fact," when personal injury has occurred in conjunction with the exercise test. Consequently, if it is established in a case that the physician's standard of care is applicable, then there is a potential for the surrogate to be exposed to a higher standard of care and to criminal charges for practicing medicine without a license.

Contemporary Standards of Care

When legal questions arise concerning the applicable standard of care in particular cases, the courts establish this, in part, through an examination of contemporary standards of care that are promulgated by health-care provider associations. Recent published guidelines and recommendations on exercise testing from professional societies provide some insight as to what might be considered the contemporary standard in this area of health-care service.

Other Case Law Involving Exercise Testing in the Health-Care Setting

Other types of issues have emerged in the administration of ETs. The following cases span a period of 1975–2006 and all involve alleged failures or deficiencies related to test administration [40]. Physician defendants were identified in all of these cases. Some involved alleged failures in preliminary screenings of the patients, whereas other cases involved alleged failures in post-exercise monitoring or post-acute surveillance, or involved follow-up care stemming from alleged failures in some aspect of ET interpretation. Selected cases follow:

1. *Michael Corbett v. Virginia Mason Hospital*, King County (WA) Superior Court Case No. 92-2-28260-7. A physical therapist (PT) administered a physical capacity evaluation test and the plaintiff alleged that the PT was negligent in proceeding with the test after it was determined that his blood pressure was elevated. Following the physical test and after lunch, the patient needed stabilization in hospital emergency room. Later, this was followed by coronary artery bypass graft surgery [41].

2. *Gage v. Long*, Case No. 579-025 (Orange County, CA, Superior Court, Settled 1991). The decedent underwent exercise testing at an emergency facility. The procedure failed to uncover heart disease which was determined to be the cause of death [42].

3. *Estate of Guy O. Gangi, deceased v. Dr. Carl E. Berkowitz*, Cook County (IL) Circuit Court, Case No. 88L-1 3066. A man died one hour after stress testing and the family claimed more monitoring should have been done [43].

4. *Kolodny v. United States*, Civil Case No. M-74-108, United States District Court, Maryland, 1975. Legal action was based upon alleged negligent acts or omissions related to exercise testing procedures [44].

5. *Crook v. Funk*, 447 S.E.2d 60 (Ga.App. 1994). Patient died within hours after a physician administered a diagnostic treadmill test. Allegations of negligence toward the attending physician were made, as well as against the physician who supervised the ET and other defendants. Part of the claim centered upon an alleged failure to properly evaluate the patient's condition, including failure to diagnose a pre-existing aneurysm. The trial court dismissed the plaintiff's claim, but the appeals court reversed the ruling and the case was returned to a lower court for trial [45].

6. *Raymond Dolney and Nancy Dolney v. E.A. DeChellis*, Trumbull County (OH) Court of Common Pleas, Case No. 91CV1279. A man suffered a heart attack 3 months after an exercise stress test. The plaintiff claimed failure to diagnose problems. The defendant claimed the plaintiff did not return for follow-up, as requested [46].

7. *Hoem v. Zia*, 606 N.E.2d 818 (Ill. App. 4 Dist. 1992). The plaintiff alleged that a pulmonologist failed to detect a contraindication to exercise and that subsequently such test proximately caused a fatal heart attack [47].

8. *Bobby Carpenter, Ph.D. v. Arlington Memorial Hospital*, Tarrant County (TX) District Court, Case No. 48-1127236-90. A man with a history of heart disease alleged that a physician failed to assess and treat symptoms. The man suffered a myocardial infarction. The court found in favor of the defendant hospital, after a confidential settlement with physician was reached [48].

9. *Ronald and Christine Bonnes v. R.P. Feidner, M.D. and John U. Lanman, M.D.*, 622 N.E.2d 197 (Ind. App. 3 Dist. 1993). The plaintiffs alleged failure to monitor patient after a normal submaximal stress test, which resulted in a defense verdict [49, 50].

10. *Lynda Kelly as Administrator of the Estate of John Kelly v. George Berk, M.D. and Peter Mercurio, M.D.*, Westchester County (NY) Supreme Court, Index No. 10564/90. This was a claim of wrongful death blamed on an alleged failure of the physician to treat reappearing ventricular tachycardia following an exercise stress test [51].
11. *Taylor v. Mobil Corp.*, 444 S.E2d 705 (Va. 1994). This was an alleged wrongful death that followed advice given by a physician to a patient for continuing exercise on a home treadmill. The physician had, previous to the untoward event, supervised and evaluated the patient's ET. A plaintiffs' verdict in this case resulted in a jury award of $4 million [52].
12. *Guida v. Lesser*, 2003 Ga.App.LEXIS 1297. This case involved the death of a patient following alleged negligence in performing an ET [53].

Recommendations

All of these cases suggest that legal challenges associated with the provision of exercise testing services may often involve tangential health-care issues other than administration of the procedure itself. The aforementioned cases provide several examples of these issues such as screening for contraindications, rendering a diagnosis based on test findings, follow-up surveillance and use of the test results to plan subsequent care. Thus, it may be helpful for organizations and professionals to establish policies and practices to limit their legal exposure when using physician surrogates to supervise ETs. These might, at least, include tests done for patients with evidence of disease risk or a prior diagnosis of disease, those performed explicitly for diagnostic purposes or those in which the findings are clinically equivocal or positive.

Conclusion

Physicians, other professionals and agencies increasingly will seek to develop protocols for immediate supervision of exercise tests by non-physicians. The following list of key concerns may assist professionals in their focused discussions about these matters with local legal counsel and institutional risk managers while taking into account these legal concerns notes and reviewed herein:

- Independent supervision of ETs by non-licensed providers may be inconsistent with some state statutes governing the practice of medicine.
- Professional guidelines give considerable direction as to the standard of care relative to supervision of exercise tests in the health-care and health-fitness settings, but a lack of uniformity causes legal uncertainty.
- The physician standing order mechanism for delegating ET-related duties may have uncertain legal validity in some clinical contexts, facilities and states.

Medico-legal risks of ET monitoring by non-physicians will be lowered by providing immediate physician back-up, adhering to contemporary professional guidelines and securing patient informed consent that clearly informs the patient of the specific supervisory and back-up arrangements that are used when the test is performed [54].

Training and Education of Physicians

The training and education of physicians in exercise testing varies widely. Some residency training programs include exercise testing as part of a specific cardiology experience or as an elective rotation. If this is a 4-week experience, the resident physician is given the opportunity to both observe and then conduct, under supervision, several formal tests. With additional didactic study and review of exercise physiology the resident physician should obtain adequate training to supervise and conduct exercise testing. During this experience the physician should conduct 25–50 such tests and be familiar with both normal as well as abnormal responses. In addition, the physician should be familiar with the critical signs and symptoms of significant coronary artery disease uncovered with exercise testing. There is not a "magic" number to determine clinical competency in exercise testing. After the observation of 10–20 tests followed by the personal management of an additional 10–20 examinations the physician should feel comfortable with conducting exercise testing utilizing correct pre-test evaluation, selecting an appropriate exercise protocol, evaluating for signs and symptoms of significant heart disease with exercise and determining appropriate cessation of the test. Procedural testing skills and decision-making should increase with further experience. During this training period patients identified in the pre-test screening as high risk can be referred to those physicians with more experience, and questionable or unsure results in those studied can be reviewed with a colleague skilled in exercise testing. The American College of Cardiology and the American Heart Association recommend that physicians perform 50 procedures during their period of training to achieve competency in exercise testing [54]. This Task Force included members from the American Academy of Family Physicians, the American College of Physicians and the American College of Sports Medicine.

This Task Force further divided training into categories of (1) supervision of stress testing, (2) interpretation of stress testing or (3) both and recommended 50 tests for physicians who supervised and interpreted stress tests. While physicians and organizations focus on the "number" of tests performed, many times the exercise tests that were considered but never ordered are also critical. Careful pre-test screening often identifies patients in whom an exercise test is not indicated or may be harmful to the patient. In certain cases an alternative test (e.g., pharmacological stress imaging) is indicated or immediate cardiology consultation is recommended. Thus, the number of patients who were appropriately screened and then *not* tested may be as important as the number of tests actually completed.

The method of obtaining experience varies. For residents-in-training this experience can be obtained during a clinical rotation. During this time the resident physician should assume the primary role for conducting tests. For those physicians in clinical practice one should first master the didactic information that is offered in organized courses. Then one can accumulate clinical cases by observing a trained colleague perform the tests. Later, the trainee can assume the primary role with the trained colleague serving as observer until satisfactory numbers are achieved.

Credentialing and Privileging

Many hospital facilities require 50 tests before granting privileges. If a physician has been performing stress testing previously, the facility may require documentation of a minimum of 150 previous tests with a minimum of 25 tests per year "to maintain competence" [54]. Or a facility may assign a credentialed physician to proctor a staff physician applying for privileges. With approval from the proctor privileges are granted without documentation of a minimum number of tests. Following initial credentialing physicians should perform a minimum of 25 tests per year to maintain competency. Many times persons other than licensed physicians (nurse practitioners, physician assistants, exercise physiologists) complete exercise stress tests following prescribed protocols. The American College of Cardiology and the American Heart Association have recommended that non-physician providers be certified by the American College of Sports Medicine [54].

Finally, testing facilities, medical centers and insurance companies may require Advanced Cardiac Life Support (ACLS) certification for all persons performing exercise tests. This is a reasonable requirement since rare, but serious, complications including arrhythmias, acute chest pain, hypotension, myocardial infarction or stroke do occur.

Summary

Physicians who perform stress tests must be properly trained. This training may be a formal process during the residency education or via workshops, didactic sessions and experience during the post-residency period. An awareness of the legal case law concerning stress testing is important and examples have been discussed. Credentialing is based on either (1) formal training, (2) clinical experience or (3) a proctoring program with a credentialed physician. Complications with stress testing do occur but the occurrence is rare. Many institutions require ACLS certification.

References

1. http://wwwlaafp.org/online/en/home/aboutus/specialty/facts/64.html
2. Wigton RS, Alguire P. The declining number and variety of procedures done by general internists: A resurvey of members of the American College of Physicians. Ann Intern Med 2007;146:355–60.

3. Ringdahl E, Delzell JE, Kruse RL. Changing practice patterns of Family Medicine graduates: A comparison of alumni surveys from 1998–2004. J Am Board Fam Med 2006;19:404–12.

4. Mark DB, Hlatky MA, Harrell FE Jr, et al. Exercise Treadmill Score for predicting prognosis in coronary artery disease. Ann Intern Med 1987;106:793–800.

5. Morrow K, Morris CK, Froelicher VF, et al. Prediction of cardiovascular disease in men undergoing noninvasive evaluation for coronary artery disease. Ann Intern Med 1993;118:689–95.

6. Herbert DL, Herbert WG. Legal Aspects of Preventive, Rehabilitative and Recreational Exercise Programs, 4th edition. Canton, Ohio: PRC Publishing, Inc., 2002.

7. Edelman PS. The Case of *Tart v. McGann*: Legal Implications Associated with Exercise Stress Testing. The Exercise Standards and Malpractice Reporter 1987;1:24–6.

8. Herbert DL, Herbert WG. The practice and unauthorized practice of medicine and other allied health professions. In: Herbert DL, Herbert WG, editors. Legal Aspects of Preventive, Rehabilitative and Recreational Exercise Programs. Canton, Ohio: PRC Publishing, Inc., 2002; 113–44.

9. Herbert DL. New Cardiac Rehabilitation Guidelines to be Developed. The Exercise Standards and Malpractice Reporter 1993;7:15.

10. Herbert DL. Standards of care for health and fitness facilities are ever evolving. ACSM's Health and Fitness J 2000;4:18–20.

11. *Gonzales v. Roth*, et al., Case No. 90CV1570, District Court, City and County of Denver, Colorado, 1991.

12. American College of Sports Medicine. Guidelines for Exercise Testing and Prescription, 3rd edition. Philadelphia: Lea & Febiger, 1986.

13. *Rosenberg v. Equitable Life Assurance Society of the United States*, 564 N.Y.S.2d.387 (A.D. 1 Dept. 1991), reversed in, *Rosenberg v. Equitable Life Assurance Soc.*, 584 N.Y.S.2d. (Ct.App.1992).

14. *Harvey v. Stanley*, 803 S.W.2d.721 (Tex.App.-Fort Worth 1990).

15. *Melito v. Genesee Hospital*, 561 N.Y.S.2d.951 (A.D.4 Dept. 1990).

16. *Tart v. McGann*, 697 F.2d. 75,77 (2d.Cir.1982).

17. Herbert DL. Informed Consent and New Disclosure Responsibilities for Exercise Stress Testing: The Case of *Hedgecorth v. United States*. The Exercise Standards and Malpractice Reporter 1987;1:30–2.

18. Herbert DL. Who Will Judge Your Professional Conduct in Court? The Exercise Standards and Malpractice Reporter 1987;1:14–6.

19. Hedgecorth V. United States, 618 F. Supp. 627(Dist.Co., E.D.Mo.) at 631–632.

20. American Heart Association. The Exercise Standards Book: 1978:12.

21. American Heart Association. Exercise Testing and Training of Individuals with Heart Disease or At High Risk for Its Development: A Handbook for Physicians. 1975; 52.

22. American College of Sports Medicine. Guidelines for Exercise Testing and Prescription, 3rd edition. Philadelphia: Lea & Febiger, 1986; 145–6.

23. American Heart Association, Greater Los Angeles Affiliate, Guidelines For Cardiac Rehabilitation Centers (revised Second Edition:71, 1982).

24. American College of Sports Medicine. Guidelines for Exercise Testing and Prescription, 6th edition. Philadelphia: Lippincott, Williams &Wilkins, 2000; 53.

25. Fletcher GF, Balady G, Froelicher VF, et al. Exercise Standards. A statement for healthcare professionals from the American Heart Association. Writing Group. Circulation 1995;91:580–615.

26. Fletcher GF, Froelicher VF, Hartley LH, et al. Exercise Standards. A statement for health professionals from the American Heart Association. Circulation 1990;82:2286–322.

27. American Association of Cardiovascular and Pulmonary Rehabilitation. Guidelines for Cardiac Rehabilitation Programs. Champaign, IL, Human Kinetics, 1991.

28. Herbert DL. Sample informed consent forms from the AHA, AACVRP and the ACSM. The Exercise Standards and Malpractice Reporter 1991;5:7–8.

29. Herbert DL. Word choices for informed consent documents may render process invalid. The Exercise Standards and Malpractice Reporter 1992;6:43–4.

30. *Hidding v. Williams*, 578 S.2d 1192 (La.Ct. Appeals, Fifth Cir. 1991)
31. Herbert DL. Exercise stress testing lawsuit results in defense verdict. The Exercise Standards and Malpractice Reporter 1990;4:23–4.
32. Herbert DL. Informed consent and new disclosure responsibilities for exercise stress testing: The Case of *Hedgecorth v. United States*. The Exercise Standards and Malpractice Reporter 1987;1:30–2.
33. Herbert DL. Nurse can act as physician's agent in obtaining informed consent. The Exercise Standards and Malpractice Reporter 1989;3:81.
34. Debusk RF. Exercise test supervision: Time for reassessment. The Exercise Standards and Malpractice Reporter 1988;2:65–70.
35. Herbert DL. Medico-legal concerns and risk management suggestions for medical directors of exercise rehabilitation programs. The Exercise Standards and Malpractice Reporter 1989;3:44–8.
36. Herbert DL. Are nutritionists engaged in the unauthorized practice of medicine? The Exercise Standards and Malpractice Reporter 1988;2:76–8.
37. Herbert DL. Is physician supervision of exercise stress testing required? The Exercise Standards and Malpractice Reporter 1988;2:6–7.
38. Herbert DL. Who will judge your professional conduct in court? The Exercise Standards and Malpractice Reporter 1987;1:14–6.
39. Ribisl PM. Uncertainties regarding medical supervision and maximal graded exercise testing prior to exercise training. The Exercise Standards and Malpractice Reporter 1987;1:6–7.
40. Westlaw data base search was conducted using search terms: "exercise testing", "treadmill testing" or "GXT".
41. *Michael Corbett v. Virginia Mason Hospital*, King County (WA) Superior Court Case No. 92-2-28260-7. The Exercise Standards and Malpractice Reporter 1995;9:30.
42. *Gage v. Long*, Case No. 579-025 (Orange County, CA, Superior Court). The Exercise Standards and Malpractice Reporter 1992;6:73.
43. *Estate of Guy O. Gangi, deceased v. Dr. Carl E. Berkowitz*, Cook County (IL) Circuit Court, Case No. 88L-1 3066. The Exercise Standards and Malpractice Reporter (Herbert DL) 1994;8:44.
44. *Kolodny v. United States*, Civil Case No. M-74-108, United States District Court, Maryland, 1975. The Exercise Standards and Malpractice Reporter 1988;2:6.
45. *Crook v. Funk*, 447 S.E.2d 60 (Ga.App. 1994). The Exercise Standards and Malpractice Reporter 1995;9:24–5.
46. *Raymond Dolney and Nancy Dolney v. E.A. DeChellis*, Trumbull County (OH) Court of Common Pleas, Case No. 91CV1279. The Exercise Standards and Malpractice Reporter 1994;8:27.
47. *Hoem v. Zia*, 606 N.E.2d 818 (Ill. App. 4 Dist. 1992). The Exercise Standards and Malpractice Reporter 1993;7:17.
48. *Bobby Carpenter, Ph.D. v. Arlington Memorial Hospital*, Tarrant County (TX) District Court, Case No. 48-1127236-90. The Exercise Standards and Malpractice Reporter 1994;8:93.
49. *Ronald and Christine Bonnes v. R.P. Feidner, M.D. and John U. Lanman, M.D.*, 622 N.E.2d 197 (Ind. App. 3 Dist. 1993). The Exercise Standards and Malpractice Reporter 1994;8:29.
50. Herbert DL. The Exercise Standards and Malpractice Reporter 1994;8:94.
51. *Lynda Kelly as Administrator of the Estate of John Kelly v. George Berk, M.D. and Peter Mercurio, M.D.*, Westchester County (NY) Supreme Court, Index No. 10564/90. The Exercise Standards and Malpractice Reporter 1993;7:73.
52. *Taylor v. Mobil Corp.*, 444 S.E2d 705 (Va. 1994). The Exercise Standards and Malpractice Reporter 1995;9:25.
53. *Guida v. Lesser*, 2003 Ga.App.LEXIS 1297. The Exercise Standards and Malpractice Reporter 2004; 18: 39–40.
54. Rodgers GP, Ayanian JZ, Balady G, et al. American College of Cardiology/American Heart Association Clinical Competence Statement on Stress Testing. Circulation 2000;102: 1726–38.

Part III
Sports Medicine Applications
of Exercise Testing

Chapter 15
Measuring Physical Fitness

Steven C. Masley

What Is Physical Fitness

Physical fitness refers to good health or physical condition as a result of exercise and proper nutrition. Generally, health-enhancing aspects of physical fitness can be divided into three categories:

1. Aerobic fitness (cardiorespiratory capacity)
2. Strength
3. Flexibility

Aerobic fitness is the ability of the cardiovascular and respiratory systems to supply oxygen to large muscle groups over extended time. Examples of aerobic activities include running, cycling, and swimming. Strength is the ability to move a one effort force against resistance, while muscular endurance is the ability to repeat a motion against resistance multiple times. Lifting a maximum weight once is a measure of strength, while doing as many push-ups or sit-ups as possible is a measure of muscular endurance. Flexibility is the ability to stretch muscles and joints. A static stretch is stretching a muscle group to the point of mild discomfort for 10–30 s. An expanded list of fitness components which are more related to athletic performance and less so to health would include power, agility, balance, reaction time, speed, and coordination.

What Are the Benefits of Fitness?

Aerobic Exercise

The beneficial attributes to aerobic fitness training are extensive and include reductions in cardiovascular events for the general population and for cardiac

S.C. Masley (✉)
University of South Florida, Tampa; Masley Optimal Health Center, St. Petersburg, FL, USA
e-mail: steven@drmasley.com

C.H. Evans, R.D. White (eds.), *Exercise Testing for Primary Care and Sports Medicine Physicians*, DOI 10.1007/978-0-387-76597-6_15
© Springer Science+Business Media, LLC 2009

rehabilitation following myocardial infarction, improved blood pressure, a rise in HDL cholesterol level, a reduced risk for Alzheimer's disease, and a reduced risk for diabetes. Simple walking has been shown to prevent and treat type 2 diabetes [1, 2]. Aerobic exercise is also associated with a decreased risk for depression, osteoporosis, and anxiety. Aerobic activity may also be associated with enhanced cognitive performance.

Research has shown that regular physical activity may slow some aspects of aging [3]. In one study conducted on a group of aging runners, those who maintained their lean body mass through physical activity lived longer and healthier. One of the mechanisms for benefit involves C-reactive protein (CRP), a substance the liver creates in response to body-wide production of inflammatory compounds. High CRP levels are strongly associated with an increased risk for strokes, heart attacks, and sudden cardiac death. Regular exercise lowers CRP levels and decreases the risk of a heart attack or stroke by up to 40%.

Indeed, of all the options for preventing and treating cardiovascular disease, the single most effective choice is exercise. People who work out regularly have 40% fewer heart attacks, strokes, and cases of sudden cardiac death.

Strength Training

Strength training has been shown to decrease fall and fracture risk and minimize loss in bone density [4, 5]. It has further been shown to fortify joint muscle strength and provide enhanced stability with motion, which is an effective way to minimize arthritis progression [6]. Not surprisingly, strength training is also associated with diminished musculoskeletal pain, such as low back pain. Even with advancing years, studies have shown that patients can restore 75% of muscle mass lost over 10 years with a short 12-week exercise program [7].

Exercise Enhances Weight Control

Both aerobic activity and strength training are essential components for weight loss and long-term weight control. Exercise helps with weight loss in several ways:

- It burns calories.
- It increases sympathetic nervous system tone.
- Increases resting metabolic rate.

Daily exercise also helps prevent weight regain. This concept is reinforced by research conducted by the National Weight Control Registry, which studies successful weight loss and long-term weight control. Americans who have lost at least 10% of their body weight and kept it off for a year have registered and documented their activity level and diet. Research to date shows that the single best predictor of long-term weight loss is activity. Generally, those who succeed walk at least

3–4 miles a day or use exercise machines to burn at least 2,000–2,500 cal every week. People who exercise at least 5 days but often 6–7 days a week had the best success [8].

In another study, conducted at the Division of Preventive and Nutritional Medicine in Michigan [9], researchers compared weight regain with the distances their research subjects – previously obese people – walked. Those who had lost weight only to regain it again walked less than 16 miles a week. Those who kept the weight off walked on average more than 16 miles spread over more than 5 days a week.

Strength training is also associated with weight loss. One pound of muscle burns 35–40 cal a day. Adding lean muscle mass through a strength training program has been shown to reduce fat mass. On average, increasing muscle mass by 1 lb burns an *extra* 12,000 cal a year. As eating 3,500 extra calories is associated with gaining 1 lb of fat mass, adding 1 lb of lean mass should result in losing 3.5 lb of fat over 1 year.

Stretching

In contrast to aerobic and strength training, which have been shown to result in well-documented benefits, stretching is commonly believed to enhance athletic and dance performance, as well as martial art-related skill. Yet we lack clinical outcome studies showing clinical benefits from stretching.

Measuring Physical Fitness

With normal aging, there is a linear decrease in aerobic fitness, muscle mass, and gains in fat mass over time. Even in master senior athletes, aerobic capacity drops by 1% per year [3], muscle mass decreases by 1% per year, and fat mass rises by 1% per year. Physicians can and should measure all three components of physical fitness (aerobic fitness, strength, and flexibility) as part of a comprehensive health assessment.

Testing Aerobic Fitness

Aerobic fitness is the epitome of feeling and staying healthy. There are several ways to measure aerobic fitness, including submaximal tests, 1-min heart rate recovery, MET level, and VO_2max. The good news is that patients can improve upon their fitness with changes in lifestyle.

Optimally fitness testing would be performed with a physician during ECG stress testing. A second option in a low-risk, healthy individual would be following a stress test while working out at the gym with an exercise physiologist or trainer.

When measuring fitness, the more significant medical problems that exist, the more important that testing should be with a physician.

Yet physician-monitored stress testing adds both expense and inconvenience for many people. An alternative that has been adopted by the American College of Sports Medicine for exercise trainer use is submaximal testing [10] Submaximal testing has a person exercise at a specific workload and their achieved heart rate is extrapolated to estimate VO_2max and maximum heart rate. Many forms of submaximal testing are used, including step tests and the YMCA cycle ergometer test. Although as a one-time test, submaximal testing shows significant variability and limitations in predicting true VO_2max levels. Yet the best use of submaximal testing would be to follow people serially over time, similar to other commonly collected vital signs, empowering people to improve their peak fitness score.

Another useful measure of fitness and also a strong predictor of cardiac risk is to measure how quickly the heart rate drops after peak exercise at 1 and 2 min. After achieving peak heart rate, exertion levels should drop to either resting or walking without incline at not more than 1 mile per hour. An athletic heart rate drop at 1 min usually exceeds 30–40 beats, less than a 25 beat drop would be considered abnormal, less than a 22 beat drop is associated with a moderate increased risk for a cardiovascular event, and less than a 12 beat drop signifies a marked increase risk for a cardiac event over the subsequent 5 years. At 2 min, the heart rate should drop by at least 45 beats. In several studies assessing the predictive value of various measures during an exercise stress tests to predict the risk of future cardiovascular events in people between the ages of 30 and 80 with or without heart disease, the 1- or 2-min heart rate recovery was judged to be the best outcome measure, when compared with blood pressure response, exercise time and MET level achieved, and ECG findings [11–13].

METS

METS is a term that describes how much energy is used while performing a particular activity, as in *MET*-abolic energy burning rate. The usual measurement for your overall exertion level is called your "MET level achieved." One MET of energy is what is burned lying completely still in bed. While running on a treadmill machine at a 14% elevation at 3.4 miles per hour, this would reach 8.0–8.3 METS during the first minute (Table 15.1).

Most people should comfortably achieve at least 10 METS on a standard treadmill fitness test. Twelve METS is a good level of fitness, and 13.5 METS is excellent. Truly athletic participants from their thirties through their sixties may reach 15–18 METS.

For every single MET increase in fitness, the risk of a heart attack, stroke, or sudden death drops by 12.5%. If patients can increase their fitness level by 2 METS (from 8 to 10) they decrease their cardiac event risk by 25%.

Table 15.1 MET levels for various jobs and activities

Occupation	METS	Activities	METS
Receptionist	1.0–2.0	Walking with a suitcase	7
Housekeeper	1.5–4.0	Cleaning floors	4
Farm worker	3.5–7.5	Cooking	3
Construction worker	4.0–8.5	Gardening	4
Miner	4.0–9.0	Push a power mower	5
Mail carrier	2.5–5.0	Sexual intercourse	5
Medical professional	1.5–3.5	Making the bed	5–6

Adapted with permission from Masley S, *Ten Years Younger*, Random House, 2005.

Table 15.2 Approximate MET score based on walking or running on a treadmill at a specific speed and elevation

Minutes completed	Speed (mph)	Elevation (% grade)	MET level men	MET level women
1	1.7	10	3.2	3.1
2	1.7	10	4.0	3.9
3	1.7	10	4.9	4.7
4	2.5	12	5.7	5.4
5	2.5	12	6.6	6.2
6	2.5	12	7.4	7.0
7	3.4	14	8.3	8.0
8	3.4	14	9.1	8.6
9	3.4	14	10.0	9.4
10	4.2	16*	10.7	10.1
11	4.2	16*	11.6	10.9
12	4.2	16*	12.5	11.7
13	5.0	18*	13.3	12.5
14	5.0	18*	14.1	13.2
15	5.0	18*	15.0	14.1

*If the treadmill does not go beyond 15% elevation, at 10 min adjust the incline to 15% and increase the speed to 4.4 miles per hour and at 13 min maintain the 15% incline and increase the speed to 5.4 MPH.
Adapted with permission from Masley S, *Ten Years Younger*, Random House 2005.

To assess a MET level, Table 15.2 below gives an approximate MET score based on walking or running on a treadmill at a specific speed and elevation. These are increased every 3 min. To calculate a score, read the number of METS achieved at the end of each minute you complete. The standard Bruce protocol starts at 1.7 miles per hour with a 10% elevation. Every 3 min it increases about 1 mile per hour and by 2% in elevation.

VO₂max

The gold standard for aerobic fitness testing is measuring VO_2max. This computes the volume of oxygen burned during peak exercise. VO_2max is reported as the volume of oxygen burned per minute per kilogram of body weight. Every cell has

Table 15.3 VO$_2$ max testing for men and women

Men: Aerobic capacity (ml/kg/min)				
Percentile	20–29	30–39	40–49	50–59	60+
90	51.4	50.4	48.2	45.3	42.5
80	48.2	46.8	44.1	41.0	38.1
70	46.8	44.6	41.8	38.5	35.3
60	44.2	42.4	41.8	38.5	35.3
50	42.5	41.0	38.1	35.2	31.8
40	41.0	38.9	36.7	33.8	30.2
30	39.5	37.4	35.1	32.3	28.7
20	37.1	35.4	33.0	30.2	26.5
10	34.5	32.5	30.9	28.0	23.1
Women: Aerobic capacity (ml/kg/min)				
90	44.2	41.0	39.5	35.2	35.2
80	41.0	38.6	36.3	32.3	31.2
70	38.1	36.7	33.8	30.9	29.4
60	36.7	24.6	32.3	29.4	27.2
50	35.2	33.8	30.9	28.2	25.8
40	33.8	32.3	29.5	26.9	24.5
30	32.3	30.5	28.3	25.5	23.8
20	30.6	28.7	26.5	24.3	22.8
10	28.4	26.5	25.1	22.3	20.8

Adapted with permission from the American College of Sports Medicine's Guidelines for Exercise Testing and Prescript, 6th Edition, 2000. Data provided by the Institute for Aerobics Research, Dallas, TX, with permission from Wolters Kluwer.

mitochondria that burn oxygen to produce energy; hence, VO$_2$max assesses mitochondria capacity. With regular exercise and a healthy diet, patients can increase results significantly. Like other fitness markers, VO$_2$max usually decreases by 1% a year with aging during adult years [14].

A simple estimate of VO$_2$max is to multiply the estimated MET level achieved with treadmill testing by 3.5, although this may overestimate VO$_2$max in some patients. A more detailed estimate can be calculated from the length of time in minutes until exhaustion with the Bruce treadmill protocol using this equation: VO$_2$max $= 14.76 - (1.379 \times \text{time}) + (0.451 \times \text{time}^2) - (0.012 \times \text{time}^3)$ (see Fig. 5.11). Table 15.3 shows average VO$_2$max levels achieved for men and women. High-level-endurance athletes reach VO$_2$max levels from 65 to 95 ml/kg/min.

Strength and Endurance Testing

The ability to perform sit-ups and push-ups is an excellent indicator of muscle endurance. The American College of Sports Medicine (ACSM) has developed tables that determine strength in relation to age.

Push-Up Test

The push-up test is administered in the standard push-up position with hands shoulder-width apart, back straight, and head up. Female push-ups are performed with knees on the floor. Men must do their push-ups on their toes. The arms must transition from straight in the up position to bent to at least a 90° angle in the down position. The maximum number of push-ups performed consecutively without rest is counted as the score (Table 15.4).

Table 15.4 Push-up test by age and gender

Push-Ups	Age									
Ages	20–29		30–39		40–49		50–59		60–69	
Gender:	M	F	M	F	M	F	M	F	M	F
Age % below										
90th	41	32	32	31	25	28	24	25	24	23
80th	34	26	27	24	21	22	17	17	16	15
70th	30	22	24	21	19	18	14	13	11	12
60th	27	20	21	17	16	14	11	10	10	10
50th	24	16	19	14	13	12	10	9	9	6
40th	21	14	16	12	12	10	9	5	7	4
30th	18	11	14	10	10	7	7	3	6	2
20th	16	9	11	7	8	4	5	1	4	0
10th	11	5	8	4	5	2	4	0	2	0

Adapted with permission from the Canadian Fitness and Lifestyle Research Institute.

Sit-Up Test

You can also use sit-ups to measure muscular endurance. To do this properly, a metronome is set for 40 beats per minute, with one sit-up with each beat, or a quick one-thousand-one, one-thousand-two, to perform a little more than one sit-up a second.

Lie on the back with knees bent at 90° and arms at the sides. At rest, flat on the back with hands extended down the sides, the fingertips should be touching a tape line. Place a second tape line 3 ¼ in. (8 cm) down toward the feet if 45 years or older and 4 ¾ in. (12 cm) away if less than age 45. Fingers must touch the second tape with each and every crunch. The score measures the maximum sit-ups performed without missing a beat and without time to rest (Table 15.5).

Grip Strength

Grip is another way to estimate strength. It is easily measured with a specially designed tool. Grip strength has been well studied in middle-aged men. The stronger a man's grip, the greater the chances for longevity [15].

Table 15.5 Sit-up test by age and gender

Sit-Ups	Age									
Ages	20–29		30–39		40–49		50–59		60–69	
Gender	M	F	M	F	M	F	M	F	M	F
Age percentile										
90th	76	70	75	55	75	50	74	50	53	50
80th	76	45	75	43	69	42	60	30	33	30
70th	66	37	61	34	57	33	45	23	26	24
60th	51	29	49	27	36	27	35	20	19	19
50th	39	25	31	21	27	21	27	19	16	13
40th	26	22	24	21	23	17	21	15	9	9
30th	26	17	20	12	19	14	19	10	6	3
20th	13	12	13	10	11	5	11	0	0	0
10th	10	5	10	0	3	0	0	0	0	0

Adapted with permission from the Canadian Fitness and Lifestyle Research Institute.

Measuring Body Composition

There are several methods to assess body composition, which include measures of body mass index, body fat, and lean mass.

Body Mass Index

Body mass index (BMI) is the weight in kilograms divided by the height in meters squared (kg/m [2]). Table 15.6 shows the most common BMIs. Strong evidence shows a linearly increase in health risk from a BMI of 25–30, and above a BMI of 30, further weight gain increases the risk of morbidity and mortality logarithmically (Table 15.7). Unfortunately, BMI does not distinguish between muscle and fat mass and thus cannot distinguish health risk in either high or low muscle mass individuals.

Measuring Body Fat

There are several approaches available to measure body fat, including skin fold thickness, bioelectrical impedance, and DEXA (Table 15.8). Measuring body fat directly helps to eliminate the errors noted assessing risk with BMI alone.

Skin Fold Thickness

A technician uses calipers to gauge the thickness of skin over the triceps, sub-scapula, and abdomen near the umbilicus. Many nutritionists, exercise physiologists, physical therapists, and trainers perform skin fold thickness testing. Although this technique is not highly precise for assessing body fat percentage, it does give a rough estimate and importantly can be used to follow changes in body fat over time. For details on converting skin fold thickness into body fat percentage, see exercise testing by Nieman [16].

Table 15.6 Body mass index

Male or female – use your height and weight to identify your BMI

	Height (in.)																		
Weight (lb)	58	59	60	61	62	63	64	65	66	67	68	69	70	71	72	73	74	75	76
100	21	20	20	19	18	18	17	17	16	15	15	15	14	14	14	13			
105	22	21	21	20	19	19	18	17	17	16	16	16	15	15	14	14	13		
110	23	22	21	21	20	19	19	18	18	17	17	16	16	15	15	15	14	14	13
115	24	23	22	22	21	20	20	19	19	18	17	17	17	16	16	15	15	14	14
120	25	24	23	23	22	21	21	20	19	19	18	18	17	17	16	16	16	15	15
125	26	25	24	24	23	22	21	21	20	20	19	18	18	17	17	16	16	16	15
130	27	26	25	25	24	23	22	22	21	20	20	19	19	18	18	17	17	16	16
135	28	27	26	26	25	24	23	22	22	21	21	20	19	19	18	18	17	16	16
140	29	28	27	26	26	25	24	23	23	22	21	21	20	20	19	18	18	17	17
145	30	29	28	27	26	26	25	24	23	23	22	21	21	20	20	19	19	17	18
150	31	30	29	28	27	27	26	25	24	23	23	22	22	21	20	20	20	18	18
155	32	31	30	29	28	27	27	26	25	24	24	23	22	22	21	20	20	19	19
160	33	32	31	30	29	28	27	27	26	25	24	24	23	22	22	21	21	20	19
165	34	33	32	31	30	29	28	27	27	26	25	24	24	23	22	22	21	21	20
170	36	34	33	32	31	30	29	28	27	27	26	25	24	24	23	22	22	21	21
175	37	35	34	33	32	31	30	29	28	27	27	26	25	24	24	23	23	22	21
180	38	36	35	34	33	32	31	30	28	28	27	27	26	25	24	24	23	22	22
185	39	37	36	35	34	33	32	31	29	29	28	27	27	26	25	24	24	23	23
190	40	38	37	36	35	34	33	32	30	30	29	28	27	26	26	25	25	24	23
195	41	39	38	37	36	35	34	33	31	31	30	29	28	27	26	26	25	24	24
200	42	40	39	38	37	36	35	34	32	32	31	30	29	28	27	26	26	25	24
205	43	41	40	39	38	37	36	35	33	33	32	31	30	29	28	27	27	26	25
210	44	42	41	40	39	38	37	36	34	34	32	31	31	30	29	28	28	26	26
215	45	43	42	41	39	39	38	37	35	34	33	32	32	30	30	29	28	27	26
220	46	44	43	42	40	39	38	37	36	35	34	33	32	31	30	29	29	27	27
225	47	45	44	43	41	40	39	38	36	35	34	33	32	32	31	30	30	28	27
230	48	47	45	44	42	41	39	39	37	36	35	34	33	32	31	30	30	29	28
235	49	48	46	45	43	42	40	39	38	37	36	35	34	33	32	31	31	29	29
240	50	49	47	46	44	43	41	40	39	38	37	36	34	34	33	32	31	30	29
245	51	50	48	47	45	43	42	41	40	38	37	36	35	34	33	32	32	30	30
250	52	51	49	48	46	44	43	42	40	39	38	37	36	35	34	33	32	31	30
255	53	52	50	49	47	45	44	42	41	40	39	38	37	36	35	34	33	31	33
260	54	53	51	50	48	46	45	43	42	41	40	39	37	36	35	34	34	32	32
265	55	54	52	51	49	47	46	44	43	42	40	39	38	37	36	35	34	33	33
270	56	54	53	52	49	48	46	45	44	42	41	40	39	38	37	36	35	34	33
275			54	53	50	49	47	46	45	43	42	41	40	38	37	36	35	35	34
280			55	54	51	50	48	46	45	44	43	41	40	39	38	37	36	35	34

Adapted with permission from Masley S, *Ten Years Younger*, Random House 2005.

Bioelectrical Impedance and DEXA

Both bioelectrical impedance and DEXA determine

- lean mass (includes bone mass, organ mass, water mass, and muscle mass)
- fat mass
- percent body fat

Table 15.7 World Health Organization standard classification of obesity

	BMI	Risk illnesses
Normal BMI	18.5–24.9	Average
OVERWEIGHT:		
Pre-obese	25.0–29.9	Increased
OBESE:		
Obesity class I	30.0–34.9	Moderate
Obesity class II	35.0–39.9	Severe
Obesity class III	40 or more	Very severe

Adapted from World Health Organization, 1995, 2000, and 2004, http://www.who.int/bmi/index.jsp?introPage=intro_3.html.

Table 15.8 Body fat percentage ranges and health risks

Adult male	Under weight, moderate risk	Desired body fat	Moderate risk, over weight	High risk, overweight	Very high risk, overweight
Age 18–39	Less than 10%	10–20%	20–25%	25–30%	More than 30%
Age 40–60	Less than 10%	10–22%	22–27%	27–34%	More than 33%
Age over 60	Less than 13%	13–24%	24–29%	29–35%	More than 35%
Adult female	Under weight, moderate risk	Desired body fat	Mild to moderate risk, overweight	Moderate to high risk, overweight	Very high risk, overweight
Age 18–39	Less than 18%	18–25%	25–30%	30–39%	More than 39%
Age 40–60	Less than 20%	20–26%	26–33%	33–40%	More than 40%
Age over 60	Less than 22%	22–27%	27–35%	35–42%	More than 42%

Adapted with Permission from Masley S, *Ten Years Younger*, Random House, 2005.

Bioelectrical impedance measures the strength and speed at which a mild electrical signal travels through the body. Fat tissue conducts this signal slower than lean. High-quality machines reach a 98% precision rate. Bioelectrical impedance can be performed in gyms, physicians' offices, and health centers. If bioelectrical impedance is used in a clinical setting, for it to be clinically useful, it should be precise enough to detect a 2% change in body fat composition. For example, if a 200 lb person with a 30% body fat loses 5 lb of fat mass their fat mass decreases from 60 lb to 55 lb, corresponding to a 1.8% drop in body fat percentage. If a bioelectrical machine does not have at least 2% precision, then it cannot accurately measure a change of 5 lb of body fat. Always clarify with the manufacturer a machine's precision for use in clinical situations.

DEXA (dual energy x-ray absorptometry) can be used to assess both bone density and body fat percentage. Although much more expensive than bioelectrical impedance, the precision rate is similar, and DEXA does produce minimal radiation exposure.

Flexibility

Flexibility can be measured with a sit and reach test. Usually a specific box is used for this test. To perform the test while sitting, the arms are extended forward, fingertips even, reaching forward with feet against the box, measuring reaching capacity in centimeters. As a simpler measure of flexibility, physicians can ask patients to attempt to touch their toes with their legs straight without causing discomfort. This provides a rough estimate of patient flexibility, which can be graded as good, average, or limited.

Evidence-Based Recommendations to Enhance Physical Fitness

The American College of Sports Medicine has updated its position stand on the quantity and quality of exercise to maintain aerobic and muscular fitness (aafp.org/afp/990115ap/special.html). The revised ACSM guidelines include for the first time a recommendation for flexibility training as a component in maintaining fitness in addition to aerobic and strength training exercises. The ACSM position stand was published in the June 1998 issue of *Medicine and Science in Sports and Exercise* [17]. The following information highlights the ACSM recommendations for exercise in healthy adults (Table 15.9).

There are generally two methods to coach patients toward better fitness. One option is to recommend time intervals and intensity levels for training. The second is to challenge patients to achieve specific targets using the ACSM tables listed in this chapter. The minimal goal would be to challenge patients to reach the 50th percentile for a given activity, such as push-ups, sit-ups, or VO_2max aerobic testing. For example, a man in his forties should be able to do at least 13 push-ups, and a greater challenge would be to reach the 80th percentile of at least 21 push-ups.

Table 15.9 Physical fitness training recommendations and levels of evidence

Recommendations	Class	Level of evidence	References
Moderate aerobic exercise decreases cardiovascular events	I	A	17
Weight loss is associated with daily moderate aerobic activity	I	A	17
Strength training reduces falls and fracture risk	I	A	17
Strength training is associated with weight loss	I	A	17

Aerobic Fitness and Weight Control

To maintain aerobic fitness and weight control, aerobic exercise should be performed at least 3–5 days a week for 20–60 min at an intensity that achieves 55–90% of the maximum heart rate and 40–85% of the maximum oxygen uptake reserve. In place of one 20- to 60-min session on a given day, the recommendations state that two to six 10-min periods of aerobic activity throughout the day can be used to fulfill the requirements for the amount of exercise.

Lower-intensity exercise (55–70% of maximum achieved heart rate) is recommended for persons who are unfit. Lower-intensity exercise should be performed for 30 min or more.

Persons training at higher levels should exercise for at least 20 min. Moderate-intensity exercise (70–85% of maximum achieved heart rate) for a longer duration (30–60 min) at least 5–6 days per week is recommended for most adults.

Muscular Strength

Resistance training should be a part of a fitness program and of sufficient intensity to enhance muscular strength and endurance. One set of 8–10 exercises that work the major muscle groups should be performed 2 or 3 days a week. The guidelines advocate for most persons 8–12 repetitions (or to a near-fatigue level) of each exercise. Persons who are older or frail may benefit from 10 to 15 repetitions.

Flexibility

There are several forms of stretching. The most efficacious is known as a static stretch. This entails stretching a muscle group for 10–30 s to the point of mild discomfort. To maximize flexibility, the same stretch is performed 2–3 times. Most of the benefit from stretching follows an exercise warm-up.

Yoga is a form of stretching that utilizes prolonged static stretches, combined with deep breathing, and strength endurance activities.

Stretching should be performed at least 2–3 times per week, for most major muscle groups. Optimal exercise performance would require stretching after each exercise cessation.

Summary

All major health organizations, including the United States Surgeon General's office, recommend daily activity, although the specific recommendations may vary. Inactivity refers to achieving less than 30 min of activity daily. An optimal training regimen would include aerobic activity 5–6 days per week for at least 30–40 min, with at least one interval session per week, plus two to three strength training sessions per week. Stretching should be performed at least 2–3 times per week, and preferably following each exercise session. Enhanced physical fitness is associated with many health benefits and a prolonged health span.

References

1. Watkins LL, Sherwood A, Feinglos M, et al. Effects of exercise and weight loss on cardiac risk factors associated with syndrome X. Arch Intern Med 2003;163:1889–95.
2. Gregg EW, et al. Relationship of walking to mortality among US adults with diabetes. Arch Intern Med 2003;163:1440–2.
3. Trappe SW, Costill DL, Vukovich MD, et al. Aging among elite distance runners: a 22-year longitudinal study. J Appl Physiol 1996;314:605–13.
4. Gillick M. Pinning down frailty. J Gerontol Med Sci 2001;56A:M134–5.
5. Visser M, Kritchevsky SB, Goodpaster BH, et al. Leg muscle mass and composition in relation to lower extremity performance in men and women age 70–79: the health, aging and body composition study. J Am Geriat Soc 2002;50:897–904.
6. Nelson M. Strong Women Stay Young. New York: Bantam, 2000.
7. Roubenoff R. Sarcopenia: Effects on body composition and function. J Gerontol 2003;58A:1012–7
8. Wing RR, Hill JO. Successful weight loss maintenance. Ann Rev Nutr 2001;21:323–41.
9. Ewbank PP, Darga LL, Lucas CP, et al. Physical activity as a predictor of weight maintenance in previously obese subjects. Obesity Res 1995;3:257–62.
10. Whaley MH, ed. American College of Sports Medicine's Guidelines for Exercise Testing and Prescription, Seventh Edition, Lippincott Williams and Wilkins, Philadelphia, 2006, 70–6.
11. Aktas MK. Global risk scores and exercise testing for predicting all-cause mortality in a preventive medicine program. JAMA. 2004 Sep 22;292(12):1462–8.
12. Vivekananthan DP, Blackstone EH, Pothier CE, et al. Heart rate recovery after exercise is a predictor of mortality, independent of the angiographic severity of coronary disease. J Am Coll Cardiol 2003 Sep 3;42(5):831–8.
13. Mora S, Redberg RF, Cui Y, et al. Ability of exercise testing to predict cardiovascular and all cause death in asymptomatic women. JAMA 2003;290:1600–7.
14. Cole CR, Foody JM, Blackstone EH, et al. Heart rate recover after submaximal exercise testing as a predictor of mortality in a cardiovascularly healthy cohort. Ann Intern Med 2000;132:552–5.
15. Rantanen T, Harris T, Leveille SG, et al. Muscle strength and body mass index as long-term predictors of mortality in initially healthy men. J Gerontol A Biol Sci Med Sci. 2000;55: 168–73.
16. Nieman DC. The exercise test as a component of the total fitness evaluation. Exercise Testing, Primary Care. Volume 28, number 1, March 2001.
17. American College of Sports Medicine Position Stand and American Heart Association. Recommendations for cardiovascular screening, staffing, and emergency policies at health/fitness facilities. Med Sci Sports Exerc 1998 Jun;30(6):1009–18.

Chapter 16
Generating an Exercise Prescription from the Exercise Test

Kevin Edward Elder

Thus far we have examined the importance of exercise testing by primary care physicians and discussed the physiology behind the test, including indications and interpretation of the results. These results are used for purposes of risk stratification. The formulation of an exercise prescription is another application of the exercise test results, which will be examined here. Primary care physicians need to be prepared to recommend and structure an exercise program for many different types of patients, including the healthy as well as those with chronic medical conditions. The exercise test can be used to prescribe appropriate activity levels to these patients, including recommendations for specific exercise regimens.

Obesity and the rise of associated comorbidities including type 2 diabetes mellitus, hypertension, dyslipidemia, increased cancer risk, and metabolic syndrome are clearly of concern to physicians. Recent media outlets have begun to examine the role of diet and exercise on general health and cardiovascular disease prevention in greater detail. Movies such as "Super Size Me" (directed by Morgan Spurlock) have brought some of these issues to the public, while efforts by school boards to curb rising obesity rates in children have led to changes in school vending machines. Sixty percent of Americans are either obese or overweight [1]. Three out of every four Americans do not engage in sufficient physical activity on a regular basis [2]. Despite the rising concern among patients in regard to physical activity counseling, physicians often do not provide adequate information or guidance in regard to a specific exercise plan. Previous studies have shown that only 20–40% of preventative health care visits document physical activity counseling [3–6]. Physical activity has been listed as a leading health issue for the national public health initiative (*Healthy People 2010*). Exercise as a component of lifestyle change and its relation to the primary prevention of coronary artery disease has been examined in a prior chapter. Additional benefits of exercise are increased vagal tone, lowering of catecholamines, decrease in serum triglycerides, increase in the ratio of high-density lipoprotein (HDL) to low-density lipoprotein (LDL) cholesterol, slowing loss of bone mass, reduction in adipose tissue, increase in circulating fibrinolytic activity,

K.E. Elder (✉)
Department of Family Medicine, University of South Florida, Tampa, FL, USA
e-mail: kelder@tampabay.rr.com

C.H. Evans, R.D. White (eds.), *Exercise Testing for Primary Care and Sports Medicine Physicians*, DOI 10.1007/978-0-387-76597-6_16
© Springer Science+Business Media, LLC 2009

and an improvement in overall sense of well-being [7]. Fitness is the presumed goal of all exercise. The American College of Sports Medicine (ACSM) describes fitness as "the ability to perform moderate to vigorous levels of physical activity without undue fatigue and the capability of maintaining such ability throughout life" [8]. The formulation of an exercise prescription is an effective tool for physicians in safely providing guidelines to patients seeking to achieve fitness.

Components of an Exercise Prescription

An exercise prescription is a specific level of recommended physical activity for an individual, which has been derived in an individualized and systematic manner [9]. Objective evaluation of an individual's response to exercise, including measuring heart rate, blood pressure, rate of perceived exertion, electrocardiogram (ECG), and VO2, measured directly or estimated will provide an optimal exercise prescription [9]. Healthy people under 45 years do not require special testing to determine an exercise program; however people above the age of 45 and those of all ages with cardiac risk factors should consider stress testing prior to beginning an exercise program [7]. For healthy adults, recommendations for exercise should take into account the various needs and goals of particular patients, which may include a patient's resources, time, motivation, goals for training, cost of equipment or training, weather, and personal preference. Providing cross-training activities may decrease the chance of burn-out in regard to an exercise program [10–12].

Five primary components are included in the definition of physical fitness: [13] Adapted from Stephens, MB Exercise Prescription in Sports Medicine: Just the Facts.

1. Cardiorespiratory endurance, which is the ability of the cardiovascular and respiratory systems to take in and transport oxygen to metabolically active tissue
2. Muscular strength, which is the measure of maximal force generated by a muscular group against a fixed resistance
3. Muscular endurance, which represents the ability to repetitively move a muscle group against a set resistance before the onset of muscle fatigue
4. Body composition: The ratio of fat to lean tissue (muscle and bone) mass
5. Flexibility: The ability to move a particular joint through an entire range of motion

The basic components of a training session for a healthy person include a warm-up period (5–10 minutes), resistance/strength training (15–30 minutes), aerobic conditioning training (20–60 minutes), and a cool-down period (5–10 minutes) [11,12]. Warm-up exercises of low-intensity, low-impact exercise, and stretching allow for increased muscle temperature and blood flow, enhancing joint mobility [14]. The cool-down period allows redistribution of blood flow from working muscles, avoiding post-exercise weakness and syncope. Providing specific, written instructions may enhance compliance with recommendations. An example of an exercise prescription is found in Fig. 16.1.

The following exercise prescription is recommended specifically for you based on the exercise test you have just completed. During this test, we monitored your electrocardiogram as well as your blood pressure at various levels of activity.

 • Your training heart rate goal should be at least _____ but not above _____ during your exercise.
 • You should maintain your target heart rate for a minimum of 20 minutes of continuous activity, 3–5 times a week.
 • Flexibility and stretching exercises should always precede each exercise session. It is best to have a 5- to 10-minute warm-up session before exercise and a 5- to 10-minute cool-down session after exercise.

Chest pain of any type should lead to an immediate cessation of exercise. Please report any chest pain to my office. Feel free to call with questions and good luck!
_____M.D./D.O.

Fig. 16.1 Exercise prescription. (Adapted from Morrison and Norenberg [14] with permission from Elsevier.)

While the above example of a training session is to maximize health and exercise, many sedentary or obese patients may need a simpler approach, with lower exercise intensities. This simpler approach was espoused by the Surgeon General's Report that "Significant benefit can be obtained by including a moderate amount of physical activity. . .on most days of the week [9]."

Frequency and Duration of Training

The recommended frequency and duration of exercise for various stages of training vary depending on the health status of a patient, as well as their general level of fitness (whether they are beginning an exercise program or have advanced their initial training regimen). Initial guidelines may include low-intensity/low-duration exercise for myocardial infarction/coronary artery bypass grafting (MI/CABG) patients under direct supervision of a cardiac rehab program. This may involve a range of motion exercises, treadmill, or cycle versus relatively higher levels of activity and duration for healthy subjects involving walking, cycling, jogging, running, or swimming. Regardless of the patient's preexisting fitness, all exercise prescriptions should include the mnemonic FITT-PRO [15] which indicates the frequency, intensity, type, time, and progression of exercise. The frequency, intensity, and duration of exercise will increase as the relative fitness and needs of the patient allow. The ACSM on cardiorespiratory fitness for healthy adults recommends 20–60 minutes of continuous or intermittent aerobic exercise activity (with a minimum of 10-minute bouts throughout the day) 3–5 days a week for cardiorespiratory fitness in healthy adults [9,16]. The duration of the activity should correspond with the intensity of the exercise, whereby higher intensity exercise may be conducted for a shorter period of time (20 minutes or longer) and lower intensity exercise should be conducted for a longer period of time (30 minutes or longer).

Training of less than 2 days a week does not generally result in a meaningful increase in VO2 max(maximum oxygen uptake) [17–22]. However, in a study from the Cooper Clinic from Dallas, Texas, there was a decrease in all-cause mortality even among people with low to moderate fitness levels compared with the least fit group [23]. Additionally, cardiac patients who exercise regularly, even at lower than prescribed levels, show benefit. They achieve better control of angina and enhancement of physical working capacity. These effects are due to peripheral cardiovascular adaptations which increase the threshold at which they experience angina pectoris [7]. Improvement in VO2 max tends to plateau when frequency of training is increased to more than 3 days/week [18, 20, 22]. For cardiac patients, improvement in their overall VO2 max is particularly beneficial. These patients may subsequently feel more comfortable at any level of work, because the work may represent a lower percentage of their now higher maximal capacity.

Frequency and duration of training are influenced by the patient's demographics and medical conditions. Elderly patients may only be able to tolerate brief exercise sessions when beginning an exercise program. Therefore, multiple daily sessions of small relative duration may be more appropriate (1–3 times/day, 5–6 days/week) [11, 12]. The exercise should first focus on strength training and joint stability and then balance training should be considered [11, 15, 24]. For cardiac rehabilitation patients, the progression of exercise should be done in a controlled environment whereby a patient will progress through stages. These stages are set levels of defined exercise duration and intensity, related to the patient's underlying condition and function.

Intensity of Training

Quantity and Quality

The quantity and quality of exercise needed to obtain health benefits may differ from that which is needed for fitness benefits. Thus, an exercise prescription, which takes into account the specific goals and needs of the individual patient, is useful in generating recommendations. Significant health benefits are generated by exercising at even low levels, compared to a sedentary state. Exercise of a greater frequency and duration provides additional benefits [23, 25, 26].

Determining the intensity of an aerobic activity is done by measuring the energy required to perform that activity relative to its maximum metabolic cost. This measurement is the (VO2 max) [27]. To obtain a desired training intensity, this VO2 max or another equivalent index, such as the training heart rate, must be calculated.

Calculation of Training Heart Rate

Several methods exist for calculating the target heart rate (THR). General guidelines are available to the public via the American Heart Association (AHA) as well (Table 16.1). The target heart rate can be determined directly by using an age-related maximal heart rate formula, whereby the target heart rate max = 220 − age. Patients are then instructed to exercise at a range of 77–90% of this heart rate max based on their needs. It is important to note that this method of determining target heart rate is considered unreliable and is not recommended due to the variability of measured maximal heart rate, especially in older patients. For example, the standard deviation is 12 beats, so the range will be ±25 [9]. There is also a variability in the actual measured resting heart rate. One prior recommendation from Graves and Pollock et al. had suggested using 240 − age to determine heart rate (HR) max, especially over the age of 55 because of the variability in resting heart rates in this population to attempt to account for this variability [28].

The Karvonen method is another method of determining the target heart rate. In this method, the heart rate is determined by the following formula:

$$\text{THR} = \text{Maximum Heart Rate Reserve (Maximum HRR)} \times 0.7$$
$$+ \text{Resting Heart Rate (RHR)}$$

In this method, the maximal heart rate reserve (max HRR) is first calculated.

$$\text{Max HRR} = \text{Target Heart Rate Max} - (\text{resting heart rate})$$

The ACSM manual states that "until a multivariate regression equation is developed that accurately predicts maximal heart rate, obtaining the maximal heart rate through a maximal exercise test is preferred" [9]. Thus, for purposes of this discussion, THR max will be that determined by an exercise test, not the unreliable, age-based formula.

To achieve aerobic conditioning, a patient should attempt to maintain an exercise heart rate at 60–70% above this max HRR. An example of a 50-year-old man with a resting heart rate of 75 would have the following heart rate target:

Table 16.1 American Heart Association target heart rate ranges

Age (years)	Target HR(bpm)	Avg max. HR (bpm)
60	80–120	160
65	78–116	155
70	75–113	150
75	73–109	145

HR, heart rate; bpm, beats per minute
From McDermott and Mernitz [15], with permission.

$$\text{Target Heart Rate Max} = 175(\text{Measured directly by treadmill testing})$$
$$\text{Max HRR} = 175 - 75 = 100$$
$$\text{Target HR} = (60\text{--}80\%\text{of HRR}) + \text{resting HR} = (0.6 \times 100) + 75 = 135$$
$$= (0.8 \times 100) + 75 = 155$$

(Calculation of these two values allows for a training range for the individual: 135–155).

Another method for determining a training heart rate is based on a corresponding VO2 max, where

$$\text{Target VO2} = (\text{VO2 max} - \text{VO2 resting}) \times 0.7 + \text{VO2 resting}$$

A corresponding work rate may be calculated or a corresponding MET (metabolic equivalent) level can be obtained from published tables (Table 16.2). One MET is equivalent to the energy expended at rest. Because VO2 testing may not be available in all situations, THR and rating of perceived exertion are commonly used methods of determining intensity levels for exercise prescriptions aimed at improving cardiovascular fitness. The Linear 6-to-20 Borg Scale of Perceived Exertion is the most commonly used method to determine levels of perceived exertion [29].

Table 16.2 Approximate metabolic cost of activities

Metabolic cost	Occupational	Recreational
1–2 METS	Desk work	Standing, walking (1 MPH)
	Auto driving	Playing cards
2–3 METS	Auto repair	Walking (2 MPH)
	Manual typing	Golf (cart), playing piano
3–4 METS	Brick laying	Walking (3 MPH), cycling (6 MPH)
	Cleaning windows	Golf (pulling bag cart)
4–5 METS	Painting, masonry	Walking (3.5 MPH), cycling (8 MPH)
	Light carpentry	Golf (carrying clubs), raking leaves
5–6 METS	Digging garden	Walking (4 MPH), cycling (10 MPH)
	Light shoveling	Ice or roller skating
6–7 METS	Shoveling 10 minutes (10 lb)	Walking (5 MPH), cycling (11 MPH)
		Tennis (singles), lawnmowing (hand)
7–8 METS	Digging ditches	Jogging (5 MPH), cycling (12 MPH)
	Sawing hardwood	Basketball, ice hockey
8–9 METS	Shoveling 10/minute (14 lb)	Running (5.5 MPH), cycling (13 MPH)
		Basketball (vigorous)
10 plus METS	Shoveling 10/minute (16 lb)	Running: 6 MPH = 10 METS
		7 MPH = 11.5 METS
		8 MPH = 13.5 METS
		9 MPH = 15 METS
		10 MPH = 17 METS
		Squash, handball

Adapted from Morrison and Norenberg [14], with permission from Elsevier.

A Borg score of 11, or light exertion level, equates with approximately 30–49% of maximal oxygen uptake, while a Borg scale number of 15, or heavy exertion level, is approximately equivalent to 85% of maximal oxygen uptake. A simple method of measuring exercise intensity is the Talk Test, in which the patient is instructed to exercise at an intensity where they are able to talk in short sentences without undue shortness of breath [13].

Whichever method a clinician decides to use, one must become familiar with the specific details of the particular method and use the data produced from the exercise test. Once the THR has been established, it should be viewed as a general goal to achieve during exercise for a duration of 20 minutes, 3–5 times a week. Time, fatigue, motivation, goals for training, convenience, and boredom may all influence the adherence to an exercise regimen.

Generally, maintenance of aerobic conditioning should be prescribed as a range of 40–85% of heart rate reserve (HRR) or 13–15 Borg rating. Individual levels of fitness will also influence recommendations regarding intensity, as people with lower relative fitness can improve their fitness with relatively lower intensity training, while those with higher relative fitness levels require higher intensity activity to maintain or improve fitness.

Lower levels of exercise may be appropriate for elderly patients to prevent age-related declines in functional capacity; however more intense activity is required if the goal is to improve cardiovascular fitness. The influence of underlying medical conditions will be examined in a later section.

Duration and Frequency of Activity

Low-Intensity Activities Versus High-Intensity Activities

Duration has been discussed in some detail in discussion of the intensity of exercise because it is intrinsically linked to the intensity of exercise. Lower intensity activities need to be performed for longer than higher intensity activities to achieve similar training effects. Endurance training for long-distance running, biking, or swimming may require even longer duration of training to achieve endurance effects. The duration of exercise in relation to the exercise prescription and improvement in cardiovascular fitness has been discussed, with the general model of a warm-up phase, followed by a period of continuous activity for at least 20 minutes at the target heart rate, and completed with a cool-down phase. Flexibility sessions are included in both the warm-up and cool-down phases of physical activity. The ACSM recommends an accumulation of 30 minutes or more of moderate-intensity physical activity on most or preferably all days of the week [30]. Moderate physical activity is that which is within 3–6 metabolic equivalents (METS) of physical exertion, and is generally lower intensity physical activity, which may improve fitness for sedentary adults. Examples of physical activities in this range are listed in Table 16.2 and include fishing from the bank of a stream, walking 4 MPH on level ground, and light carpentry.

Physical activity beyond this low threshold will clearly lead to enhanced physical fitness, and exercise prescriptions should be tailored to meet the changing needs of a patient as they progress through various levels of cardiovascular fitness. The greatest improvement in VO2 max is felt to occur when large muscle groups are engaged in aerobic and rhythmic activities during prolonged bouts of exercise.

Not every patient requires an exercise prescription prior to embarking on a physical conditioning program. The recommendations for exercise testing are discussed in greater detail as part of a comprehensive evaluation of cardiovascular fitness in a preceding chapter. The exercise prescription should take into account the "individual's health status (including medications), risk factor profile, behavioral characteristics, personal goals, and exercise preferences" [9].

Importance of Frequency of Exercise

Moderate physical exercise should be performed on most or all days of the week. Cardiovascular fitness improvement requires exercising 3–5 days of the week at previously established levels of goal heart rate or physical exertion. Muscular resistance training is recommended for at least 2 days a week with at least 48 hours of rest in between sessions to promote recovery when involving the same muscle groups.

Specific Sample Exercise Prescriptions

Example 1

An overweight (BMI = 27) 55-year-old woman with no known cardiac risk factors desires a weight loss program. Her resting heart rate (HR) = 80; physical examination is essentially unremarkable; lab values including thyroid stimulating hormone (TSH), complete blood count (CBC), complete metabalic profile (CMP), and lipids are within normal limits. Twelve lead ECG is normal for age.

Exercise testing is indicated. Maximal heart rate is 165, and the ECG during exercise is unremarkable.

Prescription: Calculate THR by determining HR max (then determine a percentage of HR max as seen below or calculate using Karvonen formula)

HR max = 165

THR = 165 × 0.8 = 132

Karvonen formula calculation:

THR = (HR max − RHR) × 0.6 + RHR = (165 − 80) × 0.6 + 80 = 131

      (HR max − RHR) × 0.8 + RHR = (165 − 80) × 0.8 + 80 = 148

THR range: 131–148

Insert this THR into exercise Rx (Fig. 16.1) and counsel patient as to its meaning (theoretical goal).

The constant 0.6 or 0.8 used in the above equation is numbers commonly used in calculating THR; however this number ranges from 0.5 to 0.85 depending on a patient's particular level of fitness, whereby a lower number may be used with a more sedate patient and a higher number used in a fit patient [14].

Example 2

An asymptomatic 45-year-old type 2 diabetic nonsmoker presents with no family history of coronary artery disease. The patient is overweight (BMI = 26) and would like to start training for a local 5K race, but has never engaged in formal exercise on a regular basis. No end-organ damage from diabetes is seen, and diabetes is very well controlled on metformin only. Patient has no history of dyslipidemia, but is taking statin medication at the recommendation of his physician. CBC, CMP, and lipids are normal, recent hemoglobin A_{1C} (A1C) = 5.8%. Physical examination is unremarkable. Resting ECG is normal for age.

Exercise testing is indicated. ET results: HR max = 160 bpm; RHR = 70; ECG during exercise test (ET) is unremarkable.

Prescription: Calculate THR using Karvonen method

THR = (HR max – RHR) × (0.6 or 0.8) + RHR

THR = (160 – 70) × 0.6 + 70 THR = (160 – 70) × 0.8 + 70

THR range = 124–142

Insert this THR into exercise Rx (Fig. 16.1) and counsel patient as to its meaning (theoretical goal).

Example 3

A 70-year-old man presents with history of atrial fibrillation and subsequent electrical cardioversion 5 years ago. He has remained on coumadin, with no recurrent episodes of atrial fibrillation. His hypertension is well controlled on an angiotensin receptor blocker (ARB). He is not on a beta blocker due to resting heart rate of 70 and reported intolerance to side effects (fatigue, erectile dysfunction). He has plans to go on a hiking trip with Elderhostel Organization and would like to have cardiac fitness evaluation. Laboratory results are all normal, including CBC, CMP, and lipids. Physical examination is unremarkable.

Exercise testing is indicated.

ET results: HR max 150

RHR = 70 bpm

VO2 max = 8 METS

EKG = normal, no changes during testing

Prescription: Calculate exercise regimen on the basis of either HR max or perceived exertion and MET levels. (In this example, constant used is 0.7.)

(VO2 max – VO2 resting) × 0.7 + VO2 resting = Exercise MET level

(8 – 1) × 0.7 + 1 = 5.9 METS

5.9 METS can be converted to recommended exercise levels using metabolic chart (Table 16.2), converting this value into equivalent activity levels that include walking 4 MPH, cycling 10 MPH, canoeing 4 MPH, or stair-stepping 8″ @ 22 steps/minute.

Progression of Training

Stages of Change Model

The exercise prescription will include three stages of progression [9, 12]: starting, slow-to-moderate progression, and maintenance. Zimmerman et al. measured the likelihood of sustaining an active lifestyle via the stages-of-change model [31]. Patients in the *precontemplation* stage are unlikely to change their pattern of behavior as they have not seriously considered engaging in regular physical activity. These patients should be counseled about risk and encouraged to be more active. The *contemplation* stage involves patients who may be considering change, but often present barriers or excuses for not adopting a healthier lifestyle. These patients are ready for an exercise prescription, but need encouragement to overcome their barriers to change. Those in the *preparation/action* stage should have an individualized exercise prescription and be offered encouragement and follow-up to assess their progress. Individuals in the *maintenance* stage have incorporated exercise into their routine and need periodic updates of their exercise prescription so they do not become bored of their routine or drop out of it. Patients in this stage often pass through three phases of acclimation, improvement, and maintenance. Acclimation is a demanding phase with a high dropout rate as this phase often lasts several weeks and is psychologically demanding. Patients are encouraged to commit first to the frequency of the activity, then to duration, and finally to intensity. Improvement is the phase after patients have acclimated to their regular activity. Patients often achieve improvement in self-efficacy, fitness, and mood. Modifications of the exercise prescription in this phase are done to fit patient fitness goals. The final stage of maintenance involves additional changes besides the aforementioned psychological benefits. Physical characteristics of heart rate adaptations, improved fitness, and exercise tolerance are seen in these patients. The exercise prescription may be modified to account for changes in improved cardiovascular condition and enhanced muscular performance.

The starting phase of exercise introduces an individual to the exercise regimen with low-level exercise, allowing for time to adapt to the program, and avoiding muscle soreness and injuries which will prevent further progression. The duration of this stage is typically 2–6 weeks and will vary depending on the individual's ability to tolerate the program and their motivation to continue. Patients with medical conditions may have a prolonged stage, depending on the severity of their disease, the possibility of a hospital stay, and their prior exercise history. Cardiac rehabilitation patients may have 6 weeks in the starting phase, including their initial hospitalization, and subsequent follow-up care in the first 3–5 weeks following discharge [14].

In the second stage of progression, the duration and intensity of exercise are gradually and systematically increased. Most physicians agree that there is a greater risk of injury with increasing an activity level too rapidly. Activity level should not be increased by more than 10% per week. The ability of a patient to adapt to each level of training will determine the frequency and magnitude of progression. This second stage of progression generally lasts 6 months; however patients with low previous fitness levels including the elderly and those with cardiac disease may continue to progress for up to 2 years [14].

The maintenance stage of progression is attained when the individual has achieved a satisfactory level of fitness. A wider variety of activities may be provided to the patient at this stage to avoid burn-out, and enhance compliance with an ongoing exercise regimen. At this stage of training, further improvements in cardiovascular fitness are minimal.

Periodic exercise testing may be used to assess the effectiveness of a training program. The results of this testing are used to provide positive feedback to the individuals who have improved their fitness levels [32]. The frequency of re-evaluation is not well established and depends on the patient's clinical status. Cardiac patients may be re-evaluated 4–6 weeks after operation or intervention, and annually after that as part of their medical evaluation. For healthy patients, some authors recommend administering testing 12 weeks after entry into a dedicated exercise program if it is financially and logistically feasible [14, 33]. Many articles have examined the importance of patient–doctor communication, as well as the effect of a physician's recommendations on changing behavior [34–36]. It is essential that instructions are communicated in a concise and clear manner, with written direction whenever possible. Regular follow-up is needed to assess compliance with instructions and progress.

Exercise Prescription for Muscular Training

Muscular training may be preferred by some patients as the mode of exercise, and an exercise prescription should include recommendations in regard to muscular strength and endurance. Muscular exercises should be performed at least twice weekly [9]. Individuals should perform sets of exercises with three to five maximal strength repetitions using proper technique in order to develop strength training [37–41]. Muscle endurance training is achieved with several sets using lower resistance (8–20 repetitions) [38–41]. Muscle strength and endurance are achieved by the progressive overload principle. This principle involves increasing more than the normal resistance to movement or frequency and duration of usual activity [39–42]. Free weights or resistance machines are applicable types of muscular strength and endurance training modalities. In this type of exercise, the duration, or time of exercise, refers to the number of sets of a particular exercise that an individual performs. Two sets are typically performed for each muscle group. Type of activity may be leg presses; time is number of repetitions; intensity is the weight or resistance in that time and the frequency is $3\times$ per week.

The appropriate resistance training load may be determined by several methods. One method suggests that the patient start with the lightest weight on the stack [12, 43]. The patient is encouraged to perform 10–12 repetitions or exercises up to a Borg scale rating of no higher than 13 (somewhat hard). The patient then gradually progresses to the next higher weight using increments of 5–10 lb every 1–2 weeks until maximum benefit is achieved. Programs which last longer than 60 minutes per session tend to result in higher dropout rates [44].

Training intensities to produce strength gains rely on lower relative repetitions. Studies evaluating strength training involving only one maximal repetition of weight generally do not report any significant cardiovascular complications [45–47]; however this may result in higher percentage of muscle injuries, which is detrimental to sustaining and maintaining an exercise program. It is important to avoid the Valsalva maneuver when performing weight training. Large muscle groups should be worked before small ones, and an emphasis on good form with performance of the exercise slowly through the full range of motion will maximize potential benefits [48]. Rest periods between exercises should not exceed 1–2 minutes. Greater levels of resistance may result in additional strength gains but have inherently higher levels of injury from cardiac events or orthopedic injury [12, 49]. While greater frequencies of training [40, 50, 51] and additional sets and repetitions may elicit larger strength gains [40, 42, 52, 53], the difference in improvement is usually small.

The effect of strength training is specific to the particular muscle group being trained [40, 54, 55], as muscular training involving only the lower legs will obviously have little effect on promoting arm or shoulder strength gains. The need for a well-rounded strength training program which emphasizes all the major muscle groups of the body is thus established [16].

Low-risk individuals with a MET capacity of 10 or greater can be cleared to perform resistance training to fatigue [33]. Obviously, exercise in these individuals needs to take into account the possibility of muscle injury with maximum resistance training, and exercise should be ceased upon the event of dizziness, dysrhythmia, shortness of breath, chest pain, or other warning signals. Recommendations for healthy individuals are for a minimum of 8–10 exercises for both the upper and lower body 2–3 days a week [16]. Each exercise is performed once for 8–12 repetitions to fatigue. Cardiac patients may follow these guidelines as well; however the number of repetitions should be slightly higher (10–15 repetitions) and their rate of perceived exertion should be slightly lower (RPE < 15) [33]. Patients with type 2 diabetes are encouraged to perform resistance exercises 3 times a week, targeting all the major muscle groups, with a goal to progress to three sets of 8–10 repetitions at a weight that cannot be lifted more than 8–10 times [56]. Initial assessments and periodic re-evaluations are recommended to ensure exercises are done correctly and to maximize health benefits.

Exercise Prescription for Flexibility Training

Flexibility training should be performed at least 3 times a week and may be incorporated into the warm-up or cool-down phase of an exercise prescription. Flexibility training has multiple benefits including improving joint range of motion and function [57, 58] and enhancing muscular performance [59–61]. Debate exists in regard to the proven efficacy of stretching in injury prevention, but observational studies support stretching in these applications [62, 63]. It is important to stretch with warmed-up muscles, and not to do "cold stretching." Aging often results in limitation of range of motion and loss of tendon flexibility [58]. These changes result in reduced tensile strength and increased tendon rigidity [64]. Degenerative joint disease and osteophyte formation, as well as prior injuries, may lead to a loss of flexibility, which can decrease an individual's ability to accomplish activities of daily living or exercise.

A stretching program which exercises the major muscle/tendon groups (lower extremity anterior and posterior, upper extremity flexors and extensors, lower back, shoulder girdle, etc.) should be developed using static, or modified proprioceptive neuromuscular facilitation techniques (contract/relax, hold/relax, active/assisted) [14]. This program should include a 6-second contraction followed by a 10- to 30-second assisted stretch. At least four repetitions per muscle group should be completed for a minimum of 2–3 days/week [16].

General Considerations and Exercise in Special Populations

Older Patients

Starting an exercise program later in life can significantly reduce risk factors even if a person was sedentary when younger [15]. Regular physical activity helps prevent many common chronic medical conditions associated with aging including obesity, hypertension, diabetes, osteoporosis, stroke, depression, colorectal cancer, and premature death [65]. The fundamental concepts of the exercise prescription for older adults are the same as those for the general population. The goals of an exercise prescription for older adults may differ. Enhancement of physical fitness, improvement of overall health by reducing risk factors for chronic disease, increased functional capacity and independence, and promotion of safety during physical exercise are common goals of an exercise prescription in this population [66]. Prevention of musculoskeletal injury is a main goal of an individual exercise prescription in an older person. Proper warm-up and cool-down phases are important, and abrupt changes in frequency, duration, or intensity of activity should be avoided [66]. Recovery days should be provided in between exercise days as needed, and special attention to surfaces should be considered to prevent falls [66]. Emphasis on muscle power (how fast the muscle contracts) rather than strength alone may help patients retain the greatest physical capacity as they age [67,68]. Balance training methods including progressive resistance training may provide the greatest amount of functional capacity as older patients age [69,70]. Activities which may exacerbate an underlying condition should be avoided, such as weight-bearing exercise in a patient with advanced degenerative joint disease (DJD). Patients with arthritis/DJD should focus on pain-free range of motion exercises for flexibility training, incorporating their pain threshold as a guide in regard to exercise intensity [15]. Exercise should be avoided during arthritis flare-ups, and patients with rheumatoid arthritis may want to avoid morning exercise.

Nutrition is an important factor for optimal athletic performance regardless of age. Older patients require lower caloric intake to maintain their lean body mass, and with potentially fewer calories consumed, the nutritional quality of the calories consumed is of increased importance [66]. The potential of prescription drugs to affect caloric intake and food tolerance, as well as the effect on exercise tolerance, must be considered. Beta blockers may attenuate heart rate response and reduce exercise capacity, and other medications may impair thermoregulation, such as diuretics [15]. The elderly population is at greater potential risk for thermoregulation injuries relative to a younger population, so this issue should warrant special concern. Adequate fluid intake may be more challenging for the older population due to decreased sensitivity of the thirst mechanism and increased water output by the kidneys [66]. Recommendations to help avoid dehydration include consuming fluids on a regular schedule during activity and avoiding reliance on the thirst mechanism to trigger fluid intake. Approximately 4–6 oz of fluid should be consumed every 10–15 minutes of exercise, with a greater intake during hot or humid weather. Hydration status may be assessed by weighing before and after exercise. One pound of weight loss is equivalent to 16 oz (480 ml) of water [66].

Nutrient intake is another important factor in this population. Carbohydrates are the primary fuel for working muscles and should comprise at least 55% of total daily caloric intake [71]. Fat intake requirements do not change with aging and should comprise <30% of total daily caloric intake [71]. General guidelines suggest that protein intake should be 0.8 g/kg body weight, but older patients may require 1–1.25 g/kg to promote positive nitrogen balance, which helps maintain lean body mass [71]. A review of the micronutrients required for exercise in the elderly can be found in Table 16.3.

Diabetes

Patients with diabetes should aim to expend 1,000 kcal a week (the equivalent of walking 10 miles). If weight loss is a goal, then the goal should be 2,000 kcal per

Table 16.3 Micronutrient requirements for exercise in the elderly

Micronutrient	Recommended daily intake/comment
Riboflavin	1.5 mg/day
Vitamin B6	2.0 mg/day
Vitamin B12	2.8 μg/day
Folate	400 μg/day
Calcium	1,500 mg/day
	Deficiency of calcium or vitamin D may result in the loss of bone mass, increasing risk of stress fractures
Vitamin D	10–15 μg/day
Vitamins A, C, and E	May help reduce exercise-related tissue damage and promote repair
	Rare deficiencies if patients emphasize fruits and vegetables

Data from Anish [65], with permission from Hanley & Belfus.

week [15]. Before beginning an exercise program, patients should undergo a medical evaluation to assess cardiovascular, nervous, renal, and visual systems to rule out diabetic end-organ damage. At least 150 minutes/week of moderate-intensity aerobic physical activity (50–70% of max HR) and/or at least 90 minutes/week of vigorous aerobic exercise (>70% max HR) are recommended to improve glycemic control, assist with weight management, and reduce cardiovascular risk [56]. Physical activity should be distributed over 3 days a week, with no more than two consecutive days without physical activity [56]. Intense physical activity may cause an acute hypoglycemic effect, or post-exercise hypoglycemia, especially in patients taking insulin or oral hypoglycemic agents [72]. Because approximately 50% of the calories burned during exercise come from carbohydrate sources during moderate exercise (with most of the remainder coming from fat sources), a rough estimate for carbohydrate intake to avoid hypoglycemia can be calculated: for a 30-minute exercise session resulting in 10 kcal/minute above basal, the individual should ingest about 38 g of carbohydrate [73]:

$$(50\% \times 300\,\text{kcal} = 150\,\text{kcal, or } 37.5\,\text{g of carbohydrate})$$

It should be emphasized that this is a rough estimate and patients should consult their physicians and monitor their blood sugars carefully when instituting an exercise program to determine exact caloric/carbohydrate needs. Guidelines from the American Diabetes Association (ADA) exist to determine energy expenditure during common activities in order to more closely approximate the number of calories burned during specific types of physical activity [73]. High-quality data on the importance of exercise in diabetes and fitness in diabetes had been lacking until more recent studies examined these issues [74]. These recent studies examine with greater detail information which includes the physiology of exercise and prevention of diabetes [75, 76]. It is recommended that patients with diabetes only exercise when they are feeling well and blood sugars are under adequate control (serum glucose of 90–140). Type 1 patients should administer their insulin in the abdomen, away from exercising muscle groups which may increase absorption [13]. The pre-exercise glucose level could present a danger to exercise; at the least it may affect exercise tolerance.

Peripheral neuropathy may lead to changes in gait or balance and should be considered during weight-bearing activity in regard to foot care. Thermoregulation may be an issue in this population as well, due to the potential for polyuria and subsequent dehydration. Finally, the patient's heart rate and blood pressure response should be followed carefully in addition to the Borg scale of rate of perceived exertion (RPE), because autonomic neuropathy may limit the sensitivity of RPE [15].

The ACSM now recommends that resistance training be included in the exercise regimen for adults with type 2 diabetes. Resistance training can have a positive impact on the progressive declines in muscle mass, decreased functional capacity, decreased resting metabolic rate, increased adiposity, and increased insulin resistance seen with advancing age in this population [77].

Coronary Artery Disease

An individual exercise prescription is an important secondary prevention tool in patients with known coronary artery disease. All-cause mortality is reduced in patients suffering a myocardial infarction who participate in a program of cardiac rehabilitation [9]. The American Heart Association has information regarding the monitoring of cardiac rehabilitation patients with known cardiac disease which include staffing, supervision, and progression guidelines [32]. The individual needs, clinical status, vocational demands, and personal goals of each patient will affect the level of supervision needed with each individual patient.

Pregnancy

Physical activity has been determined safe for pregnant patients and should be encouraged. The American College of Obstetricians and Gynecologists has recommended 30 or more minutes of moderate exercise a day on most, if not all, days of the week in the absence of either medical or obstetrical complications [78]. As pregnancy progresses, the intensity of physical exercise may decrease and a woman should be counseled to avoid activities with a risk of falling. Any activity that consistently elevates core temperature such as saunas, hot tubs, or prolonged exercise should be avoided. Fluid intake should be regular and often to avoid dehydration and heat stress, and women should consult with their obstetrician prior to undertaking an exercise program to rule out any pregnancy-associated medical conditions which preclude exercise.

Obesity

Obese patients should focus on large muscle groups which increase total energy expenditure. The frequencies of exercise recommendations are unchanged from those given for healthy adults. Initial intensity of exercise should be 40–60% VO2 max with an emphasis on increased duration and frequency; progression to 50–75% VO2 max will help the patient burn calories faster; a more moderate activity such as walking would be preferred over a more vigorous physical activity if it will help promote compliance [15]. Aerobic intensity and duration may be maintained at or below the usual recommendations to promote compliance and lessen injury; non-weight-bearing activities may be required. However, for maintenance after weight loss, the current ACSM guidelines recommend up to 60 minutes a day, 6 days a week [9]. Equipment needs should be considered in regard to compliance with recommendations, as patients may be too large for standard treadmills, exercise bikes, or other equipment. As in many other populations, thermoregulation is a concern in the obese patient as well. Proper hydration and attire should be emphasized.

Pulmonary Disease

Patients with pulmonary conditions may need to focus on low-intensity exercise, with higher frequency, due to underlying restrictions in functional capacity. Those patients with impaired functional capacity will benefit most from daily exercise [15]. Patients should initially exercise 10–30 minutes per session until they progress to 20–30 minutes of continuous exercise [15]. An exercise subspecialist or pulmonologist may be required to assess a patient's response to exercise. Progression of exercise should be tailored to these recommendations. Walking or stationary bike is good form of exercise for this population, and emphasis on shoulder girdle and upper extremity muscles is important [15].

Hypertension

Patients should focus on aerobic activities that exercise large muscle groups. Special avoidance of Valsalva maneuver through proper breathing technique and breathing form should be encouraged. The effect of beta blockers and diuretics has been discussed previously in the section on elderly patients. The frequency and progression of exercise are otherwise similar to the healthy population.

Contraindications to an Exercise Program

A patient should not be enrolled in an exercise program if one of the medical conditions listed in Table 16.4 is present. These patients should be referred to the appropriate specialist for further recommendations in regard to their cardiovascular program.

Table 16.4 Contraindications to an exercise program

Poorly controlled angina
Severe dyspnea at low work loads
Moderate to severe uncontrolled hypertension at rest (diastolic BP >110)
Complex arrhythmias
Atrial fibrillation with a rapid ventricular response
Second- or third-degree heart block
Significant valvular or congenital heart disease
Significant orthopedic or pulmonary limitations
Chronic alcoholism
Recent physical or mental illness

Data from Vaitkevicius and Stewart [7].

Behavioral Issues Behind Developing and Maintaining an Exercise Program

Much progress has been made in the past decade in regard to research on physical activity and the methods and interventions to maintain behavioral change. A current initiative by the ACSM involves placing a greater prominence on physical activity by clinicians, including considering making level of physical activity level a standard vital sign. The components of this program are designed to create broad awareness that exercise is a form of medicine, provide tools/resources for physicians to more effectively refer patients for their physical activity needs, lead to policy changes in public and private sectors supporting physical activity referrals, and produce an expectation among the public and patients that their physician ask about and prescribe exercise, as well as be active themselves (www.exerciseismedicine.org/about.htm) [77].

Stronger effects of physical activity interventions are seen in those that use behavioral intervention, and this is best seen in the adoption phase of physical activity, although few studies have examined this effect on longer-term maintenance [79]. Multi-faceted approaches in health care settings that include behavioral strategies such as goal setting, problem solving, self-monitoring, and feedback, as well as supervised exercise and provision of equipment, have generally been more superior than advice only [79]. Worksite intervention is an area that requires more studies to determine comprehensive approaches to exercise maintenance as well as studies designed to test which intervention methods are most efficacious [79]. Media-based interventions seem to generate a recall of the focal message of the campaign, however, have shown mixed results in regard to attitude change, and have not impacted change in the targeted population for the most part [79]. More research is also needed to determine methods to combine both physical activity and healthy eating regimens.

Maintenance of physical activity level is another area requiring more research and study, as it appears that half or less of those who initiate the behavior will continue, irrespective of initial health status or type of program [79]. Many others who do not drop out of the program may adopt a sub-threshold intensity, frequency, or duration of exercise [79]. All of these issues again highlight the need for direct physician involvement in removing barriers to exercise, and encouraging adoption and maintenance of physical activity. Excellent materials for the education and counseling of patients are available from the National Institutes of Health [80], ACSM [9], and AHA [81]. Future efforts to promote physical activity will need to consider how people interact with their environment, as information has increased that environmental influences play a role even in the most motivated persons [82]. It is the duty of the physician to leverage their professional credibility to sell the idea of exercise as medicine to their patients so that many more patients will realize the benefits provided by a physically active lifestyle [82].

Summary

The development and maintenance of cardiovascular fitness, strength, muscular endurance, and flexibility are the goals of prescribing an exercise program and prescription. These goals are the same whether testing healthy subjects or those with disease. The individual prescription and recommendations must be tailored to fit the individual, taking into account coexisting conditions, patient resources/time constraints, and motivation. The basic components of an exercise program include frequency, intensity, duration, mode, and progression of training; however each of these factors must be individualized to fit the patient.

Exercise testing provides objective evidence which may be used in providing a concrete exercise program for a patient. This exercise program will be at a safe and effective level to achieve cardiovascular fitness or improvement. In order to achieve success with the progression of training, it is essential that the patients both understand the information being presented to them and be encouraged to be compliant with the given exercise program. The patient should be encouraged, even when their level of physical activity is lower than desired, and may need assistance in removing perceived or real barriers to progression of their exercise program. The primary care physician should emphasize the importance and effectiveness of cardiovascular fitness training in preventing cardiac disease, as well as improving general functioning and well-being of patients with known cardiac disease. Staying involved in a patient's care with regular follow-up and encouragement, and revisiting the rationale behind cardiovascular fitness, is essential to the long-term success of an exercise program.

References

1. US Public Health Service. The Surgeon General's Call to Action to Prevent and Decrease Overweight and Obesity. Rockville, MD, US Department of Health and Human Services, Public Health Service; Washington, DC, Office of the Surgeon General, 2001.
2. US Department of Health and Human Services. Healthy People 2010: Understanding and Improving Health. Washington, DC, UD Department of Health and Human Services, Government Printing Office, 2000.
3. Walsh JM, Swangard DM, Davis T, et al. Exercise counseling by primary care physicians in the era of managed care. Am J Prev Med 1999;16(4):307–313.
4. US Preventive Services Task Force. Behavioral counseling in primary care to promote physical activity: Recommendations and rationale. Guide to Clinical Preventive Services, 3rd ed. Rockville, MD, 2002.
5. Nawaz H, Adams ML, Katz DC. Weight loss counseling by health care providers. Am J Public Health 1999;89:764–767.
6. Wee C, McCarthy E, Davis R, et al. Physician counseling about exercise. JAMA 1999;282:1583.
7. Vaitkevicius PV, Stewart KJ. Postmyocardial infarction care, cardiac rehabilitation, and physical conditioning. In: Barker LR, Burton JR, Zieve PD (eds), Principles of Ambulatory Medicine. Williams & Wilkins, 1999, pp. 744–767.
8. American College of Sports Medicine. The recommended quantity and quality of exercise for developing and maintaining cardiorespiratory and muscle fitness in healthy adults. Med Sci Sports Exerc 1990;22:265–274.
9. Whaley MH, Brubaker PH, Otto RM, Armstrong LE, for The American College of Sports Medicine. ACSM's Guidelines for Exercise Testing and Prescription, 7th ed. Philadelphia, PA, Lippincott Williams & Wilkins, 2006.
10. Pollock ML, Schmidt DH (eds). Heart Disease and Rehabilitation, 2nd ed. Champaign, IL, Human Kinetics, 1995.

11. Pollock ML, Welsch MA, Graves JE. Exercise prescription for the rehabilitation of the cardiac patient. In: Pollock ML, Schimidt DH (eds), Heart Diease and Rehabilitation, 3rd ed. Champaign, IL, Human Kinetics, 1995.
12. Pollock ML, Wilmore JH. Exercise in Health and Disease: Evaluation and Prescription for Prevention and Rehabilitation, 2nd ed. Philadelphia, WB Saunders, 1990, pp. 485–620.
13. Stephens MB. Exercise prescription. In: O'Connor FG, Sallis RE, Wilder RP, St. Peirre P (eds), Sports Medicine: Just the Facts. New York, McGraw-Hill, 2005, pp. 91–94.
14. Morrison CA, Norenberg RG. Using the exercise test to create the exercise prescription. In: Evans CH (guest ed), Exercise Testing. Primary Care Clin Office Prac. Philadelphia, WB Saunders, 2001;28(1):137–158.
15. McDermott AY, Mernitz H. Exercise and older patients: Prescribing guidelines. Am Fam Phys 2006;74(3):437–444.
16. Pollock ML, et al. The recommended quantity and quality of exercise for developing and maintaining cardiorespiratory and muscular fitness, and flexibility in adults. Med Sci Sports Exerc 1998;30:975.
17. Davies CT, Knibbs AV. The training stimulus, the effects of intensity, duration and frequency of effort on maximum aerobic power output. Int Z Angew Physiol 1971;29:299–305.
18. Gettman LH, Pollock ML, et al. Physiological responses of men 1, 3, and 5 days, and 5 day per week training programs. Res Q Exerc Sports 1976;47:638–646.
19. Olree HD, Corbin B, Penrod J, et al. Methods of achieving and maintaining physical fitness for prolonged space flight. In: Final Progress Report to NASA. Grant No. NGR-04-002-004, 1969.
20. Pollock ML. The quantification of endurance training programs. In: Wilmore JH (ed), Exercise and Sports Sciences Reviews. New York, Academic Press, 1973, pp. 155–188.
21. Shephard RJ. Intensity, duration, and frequency of exercise as determinants of the response to a training regime. Int Z Angew Physiol 1969;26:272–278.
22. Wenger HA, Bell GJ. The interactions of intensity, frequency, and duration of exercise training in altering cardiorespiratory fitness. Sports Med 1986;3:346–356.
23. Blair SN, Kohn HW, Paffenberger RS Jr, et al. Physical fitness and all-cause mortality: A prospective study of healthy men and women. JAMA 1989;262:2395–2401.
24. Mazzeo RS, Cavanagh P, Evans WJ. Exercise and physical activity for older adults. Med Sci Sports Exerc 1998;30:1002.
25. Department of Health and Human Services. Physical Activity and Health: A Report of the Surgeon General. Atlanta, US Department of Health and Human Services, Centers for Disease Control and Prevention, National Center for Chronic Disease Prevention and Health Promotion, 1996.
26. Williams PT. Relationship of distance run per week to coronary heart disease risk factors in 8283 male runners: The national runner's health study. Ach Int Med 1997;3:346–356.
27. Graves JE, Pollock ML. Exercise testing in cardiac rehabilitation: Role in prescribing exercise. Cardiol Clin 1993;11:253–256.
28. Zimmerman GL, Olsen CG, Bosworth MF. A "stages of change" approach to helping patients change behavior. Am Fam Phys 2000;61:1409–1416.
29. Borg GA. Psychological basis of perceived exertion. Med Sci Sports Exerc 1982;14:337–381.
30. Pate RR, Pratt M, Blair SN, et al. Physical activity and public health: A recommendation from the Centers for Disease Control and Prevention and the American College of Sports Medicine. JAMA 1995;273:402–407.
31. Balady GJ, Ades PA, Comoss P, et al. Core components of cardiac rehabilitation/secondary prevention programs: A statement for healthcare professionals from the American Heart Association and the American Association of Cardiovascular and Pulmonary Rehabilitation Writing Group. Circulation 2000;102(9):1069–1073.
32. Welsh M, Pollack M. Using the exercise test to develop the exercise prescription in health and disease. In: Evans CH (ed), Primary Care. Philadelphia, WB Saunders, 1994; 21(3).

33. Hirvensalo M, Heikkmen E, Lintunen T, Rantenen T. The effect of advice by health care professionals on increasing physical activity of older people. Scand J Med Sci Sports 2003;13:231–236.
34. Epstein RM, Alper BS, Quill TE. Communicating evidence for preparticipatory decision making. JAMA 2004;291:2359–2366.
35. Teutch C. Patient-doctor communication. Med Clin North Am 2003;87:1115–1145.
36. Verrill D, Shroup E, McElveen G, et al. Resistive exercise training in cardiac patients. Sports Med 1992;13:171–193.
37. Berger RA. Effect of varied weight training programs of strength. Res Q Exer Sports 1962;33:168–181.
38. Edstrom L, Grimby L. Effect of exercise on the motor unit. Muscle Nerve 1986;9:104–126.
39. Fleck SJ, Kraemer WJ. Designing Human Resistance Training Programs, 2nd ed. Champaign, IL, Human Kinetics Publishers, 1997, pp. 15–29, 131–163, 230–317.
40. Sale DG. Influence of exercise and training on motor unit activation. In: Pandolf DB (ed), Exercise and Sports Sciences Review. New York, MacMillan, 1987, pp. 95–152.
41. Delorme TL. Restoration of muscle power by heavy resistance exercise. J Bone Joint Surg 1945;22:645–667.
42. American College of Sports Medicine. Guidelines for Graded Exercise Testing and Exercise Prescription, 4th ed. Philadelphia, PA, Lea and Febinger, 1991.
43. Pollock ML. Prescribing exercise for fitness and adherence. In: Dishman RK (ed), Exercise Adherence: Its Impact on Public Health. Champaign, IL, Human Kinetics Books, 1998.
44. Butler RM, Beierwaltes WH, Rodgers FJ. The cardiovascular response to circuit weight training in patients with cardiac diseases. J Cardiac Rehabil 1987;7:402–409.
45. Ghilarducci LE, Holly RG, Amsterdam EA. Effects of high resistance training in coronary artery disease. Am J Cardiol 1989;64:866–870.
46. Squires RW, Muri AJ, Anderson LJ, et al. Weight training during phase II (early outpatient) cardiac rehabilitation: Heart rate and blood pressure responses. J Cardiac Rehabil 1991;11:360–363.
47. Graves JE, Pollock ML, Jones AE, et al. Specificity of limited range of motion variable resistance training. Med Sci Sports Exerc 1989;21:84–89.
48. Crozier-Ghilarducci LE, Holly RG, Amsterdam EA. Effects of high-intensity resistance training on coronary artery disease. Am J Cardiol 1989;64:866–871.
49. Borms J, Vanroy P, Santens JP, et al. Optimal duration of static stretching exercises for improvement of coxofemoral stability. J Sports Sci 1987;5:39–47.
50. Gillam GM. Effects of frequency of muscle strength training on muscle strength enhancement. J Sports Med 1981;21:432–436.
51. Berger RA. Effect of varied weight training programs of strength. Res Q Exer Sports 1962;33:168–181.
52. Hettinger T. Physiology of Strength. Springfield, IL, Charles C. Thomas, 1961, pp. 18–40, 65–73.
53. Astrand PO, Rodahl K. Textbook of Work Physiology, 3rd ed. New York, McGraw-Hill, 1986, pp. 412–485.
54. Sale DG. Neural adaptation to resistance training. Med Sci Sports Exerc 1988;20: S131–S145.
55. Sigal RJ, Kenny GP, Wasserman DH, et al. Physical activity/exercise and type 2 diabetes: A consensus statement from the American Diabetes Association. Diabetes Care 2006;29: 1433–1438.
56. Hubley CL, Kozey JW, Stanish WD. The effect of static exercises and stationary cycling on range of motion at the hip joint. J Orthop Sports Physiol Ther 1984;6: 104–109.
57. Raab DM, Agre JC, McAdam M et al. Light resistance and stretching exercise in elderly women: Effect upon flexibility. Arch Physiol Med Rehabil 1988;69:268–272.
58. Bosco C, Tarkka I, Komi PV. Effect of elastic energy and myoelectrical potentiation of triceps surae during Stretch-shortening exercise. Int J Sports Med 1982;3:137–140.

59. Wilson GJ, Elliot BC, Wood GA. Stretch shorten cycle performance enhancement through flexibility training. Med Sci Sports Exerc 1992;24:116–123.
60. Worrell TW, Smith TL, Winegardner J. Effect of stretching on hamstring muscle performance. J Orthop Sports Phys Ther 1994;20:154–159.
61. Doucette SA, Goble EM. The Effect of exercise on patellar tracking in lateral patellar compression syndrome. Am J Sports Med 1992;20:434–440.
62. Hilyer JC, Brown KC, Sirles AT, et al. A flexibility intervention to reduce the incidence and severity of injuries among municipal firefighters. J Occup Med 1990;32:631–637.
63. O'Brien M. Functional anatomy and physiology of tendons. Clin Sports Med 1992;11: 505–520.
64. Stephens MB, O'Connor FC, Deuster PA. Exercise and Nutrition, Monograph, 283 ed., AAFP Home Study. Leawood KS, American Academy of Family Physicians, December 2002.
65. Anish EJ. The senior athlete. In: Mellion MB, Walsh WM, Madden C, et al. (eds), Team Physician's Handbook, 3rd ed. Philadelphia, Hanley & Belfus, 2002, pp. 95–108.
66. Foldvari M, Clark M, Laviolette LC, et al. Association of muscle power with functional status in community-dwelling elderly women. J Gerontol A Biol Sci Med Sci 2000;55: M192–M199.
67. Fielding RA, LeBrasseur NK, Cuoco A, et al. High-velocity resistance training increases skeletal muscle peak power in older women. J Am Geriatr Soc 2002;50:655–662.
68. Li F, Harmer P, Fisher KJ, et al. Tai chi and fall reductions in older adults: a randomized controlled trial. J Gerontol A Biol Sci Med Sci 2005;60:187–194.
69. Sherington C, Lord SR, Finch CF. Physical activity interventions to prevent falls among older people: update of the evidence. J Sci Med Sport 2004;(suppl 1): S43–S51.
70. Sacheck JM, Roubenoff R. Nutrition in the exercising elderly. Clin Sports Med 1999;18: 565–584.
71. MacDonald MJ. Post-exercise late-onset hypoglycemia in insulin-dependent diabetic patients. Diabetes Care 1987;10:584–588.
72. Devlin JT. Exercise therapy in diabetes. In: Leahy JL, Clark NG, Cefalu WT (eds), Medical Management of Diabetes Mellitus. New York, Marcel Dekker, 2000, pp. 255–266.
73. American Diabetes Association (ADA). Physicians Guide to Non-Insulin Dependent (Type 2) Diabetes (ADA Clinical Education Program), 2nd ed. ADA, 1998, pp. 36.
74. American Diabetes Association. Evidence-based nutrition principles and recommendations for the treatment and prevention of diabetes and related complications. Diabetes Care 2002;25:S50–S60.
75. Sigal RJ, Kenny GP, Wasserman DH, et al. Physical activity/exercise and type 2 diabetes. Diabetes Care 2006;29(6);1433–1438.
76. Sigal RJ, Wasserman DH, Casteneda-Sceppa C. Physical activity/exercise and type 2 diabetes. Diabetes Care 2004;27:2518–2539.
77. American College of Sports Medicine "Exercise is Medicine" Campaign. www. exerciseismedicine. org/about.htm
78. American College of Obstetricians and Gynecologists: Committee opinion. Exercise during pregnancy and the postpartum period. ACOG Tech Bull 2002;267.
79. Marcus BH, Williams DM, Dubbert PM, et al. Physical activity intervention studies: what we know and what we need to know. Circulation 2006;114:2739–2752.
80. US Department of Health and Human Services, National Institutes of Health, National Heart, Lung, and Blood Institute. Your guide to physical activity and your heart. NIH Publication No. 06-5714, 2006.
81. American Heart Association (www.americanheart.org). Accessed September 15, 2006. (click on Healthy Lifestyle, then Exercise and Fitness).
82. American College of Sports Medicine and the American Heart Association. Physical activity and public health: Updated recommendation for adults from the ACSM and the AHA. Circulation 2007;116;1081–1093.

Suggested Reading

1. ACC/AHA 2002 guideline update for exercise testing: summary article: a report of the American College of Cardiology/American Heart Association Task Force on Practice Guidelines (Committee to Update the 1997 Exercise Testing Guidelines). Circulation 2002;106(14):1883–1892.

2. Ades PA, Wasserman ML, Meyer WL. Skeletal muscle and cardiovascular adaptations to exercise conditioning in older patients. Circulation 1996;94:323–330.

3. Barry HC. Activity for older person and mature athletes. In: Safran MR, McKeag DB, Van Camp SP (eds), Manual of Sports Medicine. Philadelphia, Lippincott-Raven, 1998, pp. 184–189.

4. Beaver WL, Wasserman K, Whipp BJ. A new method for detecting the anaerobic threshold by gas exchange. J Appl Physiol 1986;60:2020–2027.

5. Belardinelli R, Georgiou D, Scocco V. Low intensity exercise training in patients with severe chronic heart failure. J Am Coll Cardiol 1995;26:975–982.

6. Buchfuhrer MJ, Hansen JE, Robinson TE. Optimizing the exercise protocol for cardiopulmonary assessment. J Appl Physiol 1983;55:1558–1564.

7. Carter JB, Banister EW, Blaber AP. Effect of endurance exercise on autonomic control of hear rate. Sports Med 2003;33:33–46.

8. Campbell AJ, et al. Randomized controlled trial of a general practice programme of home based exercise to prevent falls in elderly women. BMJ 1997;315:1065–1069.

9. Fiatrone MA, O'Neill EF, Ryan ND, et al. Exercise training and nutritional supplementation for physical frailty in very elderly people. N Engl J Med 1994;330:1769–1775.

10. Fletcher GF, Mills WC, Taylor WC. Update on exercise stress testing. Amer Fam Phys 2006;74(10)

11. Gulati M, McBride PE. Functional capacity and cardiovascular assessment: Submaximal exercise testing and hidden candidates for pharmacologic stress. Am J Cardiol 2005;96(8A)x

12. Hambrecht R, Fien E, Weigl C. Regular exercise corrects endothelial dysfunction and improves exercise capacity in patients with chronic heart failure. Circulation 1998;98:2709–2715.

13. Houts PS, et al. Using pictographs to enhance recall of spoken medical instructions. Patient Educ Couns 1998;35:83–88.

14. Kenney WL. Thermoregulation at rest and during exercise in healthy older adults. Exerc Sports Sci Rev 1997;25:41–76.

15. Kessels RP. Patients' memory for medical information. J R Soc Med 2003;96:219–222.

16. Kinderman W, Simon G, Keul J. The significance of the aerobic-anaerobic threshold transition for the determination of work load intensities during endurance training. Eur J Appl Physiol 1979;42:25–34.

17. Kraemer WJ, Adams K, Cafarelli E, et al. American College of Sports Medicine position stand. Progression models in resistance training for healthy adults. Med Sci Sports Exerc 2002;34:364–380.

18. Meyer T, et al. An alternative approach for exercise prescription and efficacy testing in patients with chronic heart failure: A randomized controlled training study. Am Heart J 2005;149(5):e1–e7.

19. Shrier I, Gossal K. Myths and truths of stretching: Individualized recommendations for healthy muscles. Phys sports Med 2000;28:57–63.

20. Sullivan MJ, Higginbotham MB, Cobb FR. Exercise training in patients with severe left ventricular dysfunction: Hemodynamic and metabolic effects. Circulation 1988;78:506–515.

21. Pate RR, Davis MG, Robinson TN, et al. Promoting physical activity in children and youth: A leadership role for schools. A scientific statement from the American Heart Association Council on Nutrition, Physical Activity, and Metabolism (Physical Activity Committee) in Collaboration with the Councils on Cardiovascular Disease in the Young and Cardiovascular Nursing. Circulation 2006;114:1214–1224.

Chapter 17
The Role of Gas Analysis and Cardiopulmonary Exercise Testing

Vibhuti N. Singh, Ajoy Kumar, and Joseph S. Janicki

Apart from the measurement of the vital signs, evaluation of exercise performance constitutes one of the most crucial parameters in the clinical assessment of a patient. Many different methods are currently employed by the health care providers in this regard, but most remain un-standardized and arbitrary. Generally, physicians depend on the clinical history and the information provided by the patients about their own ability to walk a certain distance or climb a certain number of steps. Physicians, then, assign the patients a "grade" by arbitrarily ascribing a New York Heart Association (NYHA) functional class, I–IV, to provide some semblance of objectivity to obtain a measure of their level of peak exercise ability. The information so obtained, however, still remains inherently subjective since it can be influenced by bias from both the patient and the physician. Furthermore, the exercise stress tests routinely performed for evaluation of chest pain do not adequately assess the exercise performance since the acquired parameters, such as "exercise duration" and "maximum heart rate achieved", do not necessarily show concordance with exercise capacity [1]. Medical literature, on the other hand, has consistently shown that the "accurate level" of exercise performance is highly predictive of and correlates strongly with the occurrence of future adverse cardiovascular events. The need, therefore, for evaluation of exercise performance with greater objectivity and precision cannot be overstated.

The use of gas analysis with stress testing, known as cardiopulmonary exercise (CPX) testing, is just such a test that can easily be performed in an outpatient setting by minor modifications to the regular stress testing assembly. CPX testing adequately provides the obviously much-needed precise and objective assessment of exercise performance. In addition to obtaining the electrocardiogram, heart rate, and blood pressure similar to a routine stress test, the CPX test also assesses breath-by-breath analysis of ventilation (VE), oxygen uptake (VO_2), and carbon dioxide production (VCO_2) and provides a much more comprehensive evaluation of the functional ability of a patient. Such information not only helps prognosticate future

V.N. Singh (✉)
Department of Medicine, Division of Cardiology, University of South Florida College of Medicine;
Clinical Research, Suncoast Cardiovascular Center, St. Petersburg, Florida, USA
e-mail: vsingh@health.usf.edu; vnsingh@post.harvard.edu

C.H. Evans, R.D. White (eds.), *Exercise Testing for Primary Care and Sports Medicine Physicians*, DOI 10.1007/978-0-387-76597-6_17

events but also assists in differentiating various etiologies of dyspnea involving the disorders of multiple distinct physiological systems, such as cardiac, vascular, pulmonary, and hematological system.

In this review, the underlying physiologic principles, various testing procedures, and the clinical applications of CPX testing are discussed along with descriptions of its utility not merely for diagnosis and prognosis, but also for formulating exercise training and monitoring the effectiveness of various exercise interventions.

History

Back in the eighteenth century, Laplace and Lavoisier described the physiology of muscles and stated that muscle contractions involve uptake of oxygen (O_2) and elimination of carbon dioxide (CO_2) by individual muscles. They also described the mechanisms underlying the ability of the musculoskeletal system to increase O_2 uptake and CO_2 elimination with increase in physical activity. Subsequently, in the early 1900s, Morgan and Murray published a four-quadrant diagram that depicted the interplay involved in O_2 uptake within the lungs, the transfer of O_2 into the bloodstream, and its final release to the individual muscles. More recently, the literature describing the physiology of muscular exercise has been enriched by many physiologists, including A.V. Hill, August Krogh, and Otto Meyerhof—all of whom have received Nobel prizes. Furthermore, with increasing use of mitochondrial enzyme assays, there has been expansion of knowledge regarding O_2 utilization at the tissue level [2]. One of the most enduring observations includes the description by A.V. Hill who stated that the maximal O_2 uptake (VO_2max) is primarily determined by the heart, and it is the limiting factor to exercise endurance [3].

Physiology of Gas Analysis

The ability to perform muscular activity is primarily determined by the quantity of O_2 that can be conveyed to the muscles by the cardiopulmonary unit and the ability of muscles to extract the oxygen. The so-called cardiopulmonary unit is made up of heart and lungs within the thoracic cavity. This unit ascertains O_2 delivery in accordance with and proportionate to the prevailing need, and it facilitates the elimination of CO_2 that is produced as the end product of tissue metabolism. O_2 delivery to the target tissues during rest or exercise is dictated by four main physiologic characteristics:

1. Central circulation (i.e., blood volume, O_2-carrying capacity, cardiac output, and baro-receptor activity)
2. Peripheral circulation (i.e., blood flow increment to exercising muscles and reduction to non-exercising tissues and higher O_2 extraction)

3. Respiratory activity (i.e., VE, ventilation–perfusion match, O_2 diffusion capacity, and O_2–hemoglobin affinity)
4. Muscular metabolism (i.e., slow-twitch versus fast-twitch fibers and untrained versus trained conditions) [4].

Oxygen Uptake at Rest Conditions

The cardiopulmonary unit is designed to constantly fulfill the oxygen requirements of the tissues on a beat-to-beat and breath-to-breath basis with extraordinary precision. Metabolic needs are continually assessed, and the cardiac output (CO) as well as ventilator activity (VE) is accordingly modified in an ongoing fashion. During the "rest" conditions, only a fourth (25%) of the total oxygen delivered to the tissues is absorbed and utilized [5]. For example, for a person weighing 80 kg, the amount of oxygen that is delivered to the tissues and muscles per minute in the "rest" conditions is usually in the range of 1085 ml/min (or 14 ml/kg/min) while the amount extracted by the tissues would be approximately 280 ml/kg/min (3.5 ml/kg/min).

Oxygen Uptake with Exercise and Maximal Oxygen Uptake (VO_2max) at Peak Exercise

Both O_2 delivery and tissue O_2 extraction increase proportionate to the elevation in O_2 utilization by tissues during exercise. The ventilation (VE) has the ability to increase almost 8- to 10-fold, and CO has the ability to rise about 4- to 5-fold along with increasing tissue O_2 extraction (>70%) as the demand for oxygen consumption escalates with exercise. VE generally does not limit the ability to perform aerobic work. Instead, the aerobic capacity is limited by the ability of CO to rise which depends on the cardiac reserve. Once this limit is reached, any further increase in work is not attended by a steep rise in O_2 utilization. A plateau is, thus, reached at that point, which is termed the "maximal oxygen uptake" *or* VO_2max [6]. Peak VO_2 achieved during sub-maximal stress is not the same as VO_2max; it is usually lower.

The VO_2max is a very important measure of cardiac reserve, and it is essentially a measure of functional capacity of the entire cardiovascular system [7]. It is the maximal amount of oxygen the tissues and muscles can assimilate and utilize during certain physical activity. For an average person weighing 70 kg, with a maximal attainable cardiac output of 20 l/min and arterio-venous O_2 difference of 120 ml/l, a VO_2max of 34 ml/kg/min should be achievable. Athletes tend to have a higher VO_2max because of a high level of muscular adaptation through consistent training effect. On the contrary, the patients with heart disease reside at the other end of the spectrum, where they are generally quite limited in their ability to increase the cardiac output when demanded by incremental exercise. In these conditions, their VO_2max tends to be lower, and such decrement is usually proportionate to the reduction in their cardiac reserve. Accordingly, the CPX-determined VO_2max can

Table 17.1 Classification of functional impairment in aerobic capacity and anaerobic threshold (cardiac/circulatory failure)

Class	Severity	VO_2max (ml/kg/min)	Anaerobic threshold (ml/kg/min)	Predicted cardiac index (l/sq-m/min)
A	Mild to none	> 20	> 14	> 8
B	Mild to moderate	16–20	11–14	6–8
C	Moderate to severe	10–16	8–11	4–6
D	Severe	6–10	5–8	< 4
E	Very severe	< 6	< 4	–

Modified from Weber et al. [13], with permission from Elsevier.

be used to not only ascertain the functional class of a cardiac patient but also predict the maximal cardiac output achievable at peak exercise when they are subjected to cardiopulmonary exercise testing [8] (Table 17.1).

Carbon Dioxide Generation at Rest Conditions

Tissue respiration and metabolism involve oxygen consumption and production of carbon dioxide (CO_2). The CO_2 is then transported via the venous system to the right atria and ventricles. Subsequently, it is delivered to the alveolar surfaces of the lungs via the pulmonary arteries and is transported to the atmosphere via the broncho-alveolar system through the expiratory process. Of the total O_2 assimilated through inspiration (VO_2), only about 75–80% of it is exchanged to CO_2 (VCO_2) under "rest" conditions. Thus, given the VO_2 of 280 ml/min (3.5 ml/kg/min) for an 80 kg person, the VCO_2 at "rest" conditions would be approximately 215 ml/min (2.7 ml/kg/min). The ratio of the carbon dioxide produced (VCO_2) and the oxygen delivered (VO_2) is called the *respiratory quotient* or *respiratory exchange ratio* or "R" (VCO_2/VO_2). Generally, the respiratory quotient at rest lies within the range of 0.75–0.80.

Carbon Dioxide Generation with Exercise and the Phenomenon of Anaerobic Threshold

During exercise, both VO_2 and VCO_2 tend to increase in parallel to each other until the heart becomes limited and unable to supply the O_2 at the requisite rate. Consequently, the working tissues begin to utilize the anaerobic metabolic pathways as a means of energy production. During these conditions, the cytosolic nicotinic adenine dinucleotide (NAD) is not oxidized fast enough by the mitochondrial proton (H^+) shuttle. Pyruvate, thus, becomes proton (H^+) receptor and is converted to lactate. The cytosolic NAD is re-oxidized allowing glycolysis to take place [9]. The lactate thus generated is, however, rapidly buffered by bicarbonate (HCO_3^-). It then produces excess CO_2 that serves as an added stimulant to increase the VE and to maintain the eucapnia. As the demand continues and the exercise accelerates,

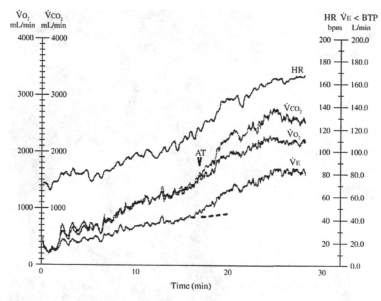

Fig. 17.1 Cardiopulmonary exercise (CPX) response. Shown are 2 min of rest, followed by incremental exercise. The responses include oxygen uptake (VO_2), carbon dioxide production (VCO_2), minute ventilation (VE), and heart rate (HR). Maximal O_2 uptake at the plateau in VO_2 occurred after the VCO_2 curve transected the O_2 curve at the anaerobic threshold (AT) associated with steeper rise in VE. (Adapted from Weber [5], with permission.)

the VE and VCO_2 begin to rise disproportionately relative to the VO_2—thereby resulting in an increased "R" value. The level of VO_2 at this point (about 60% of VO_2max) is referred to as the anaerobic threshold (AT). Any further exercise above the level of the AT causes a metabolic acidosis and an inability to achieve a steady state in the gas-exchange parameters. Figure 17.1 shows changes in VO_2, VCO_2, VE, and heart rate during incremental exercise in these conditions. In conclusion, the determination of AT along with VO_2max during CPX testing can be used in the differential diagnosis of disorders involving the organs which couple external respiration to cellular respiration, i.e., the main organ systems, such as the heart, lungs, peripheral vasculature, and the blood.

Available Gas-Exchange Systems for Gas-Exchange Testing and Gas Analysis

Appropriate "user-friendly" systems for respiratory gas-exchange monitoring (CPX testing) are now commercially available. Test results are obtainable in a digital manner during the test as well as printable at the test completion. SensorMedics Horizon System (SensorMedics Corporation, Anaheim, California, USA) is one of the newer systems that provides an online graphic display of VE, VO_2, and VCO_2. Subsequently, AT and VO_2max can then be calculated from these parameters using

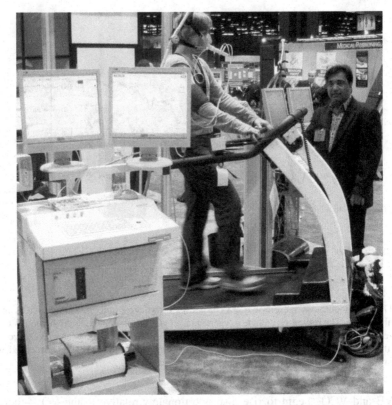

Fig. 17.2 Cardiopulmonary exercise (CPX) test. Patient wears a mask with mouthpiece tightly fitted and nose clamped for collection of oxygen and carbon dioxide while EKG and respiratory rate as well as minute ventilation are also monitored. The weight of the non-rebreathing valve is borne by the head by means of the headpiece. Oxygen consumption is determined during graded maximal exercise performance on a treadmill with continuous monitoring of 12 electrocardiogram leads and blood pressure

the built-in software and displayed in the form of a table or a graph. Some of the other systems currently available include Schiller System (Schiller America, Inc., Doral, Florida, USA; Fig. 17.2) and those from Warren E. Collins, Inc., Braintree, Massachusetts, USA; Datex Instrumentation, Helsinki, Finland; Hans Rudolph, Kansas City, Missouri, USA; and Validyne Engineering Corporation, Northridge, California, USA.

Methods of Exercise Testing and Gas Analysis in Medical Settings

Exercise testing along with gas analysis (i.e., CPX testing) has become a very important tool in evaluating the patients who present with dyspnea or fatigue. In such a patient population, the CPX testing allows an objective determination of the quality and severity of symptoms and helps differentiate the relative contributions of the cardiovascular or pulmonary dysfunction. Online dynamic measurements of VO_2, VCO_2, VE, respiratory rate, tidal volume, heart rate, and arterial pressure on a breath-to-breath basis are obtained by this method, and the data so gathered far surpass those obtained during static conditions, i.e., ejection fraction, lung volumes, vital signs at rest, as well as the ventilator capacity and airflows in sedentary conditions. Which type of exercise test is used for the purposes of dynamic testing and gas analysis depends on the nature and acuteness of the disease being evaluated, associated co-morbid conditions, and the availability of the hardware in the laboratory, such as a treadmill or a bicycle ergometer. While the parameters obtained during CPX testing are valuable in separating the abnormalities of the heart and lungs, and measuring the severity of dysfunction, they do not necessarily identify or diagnose the underlying pathologic defects or provide an etio-pathologic diagnosis. They merely provide the information regarding the extent of physiologic derangements. The physicians, then, have to consider the data so acquired, and add them to the information obtainable through other modalities, e.g., hemodynamic measurements, echocardiography, or pulmonary function testing, and in the end use their clinical judgment for making the final etiologic and pathologic diagnoses.

Noninvasive Treadmill Exercise Testing with Gas Analysis

Graded walking on a treadmill is the most commonly used form of exercise for the purpose of stress testing. The main hardware includes an electrically run treadmill which consists of a sturdy platform with a heavy-duty motor (2 or more horsepower). It essentially duplicates a person's daily walking routine. A number of exercise protocols can be programmed for different clinical use. Routine stress tests utilize the so-called Bruce protocol. The standard Bruce protocol, however, involves too steep an increment in speed and slope to be useful for a compromised patient. Therefore, a modified Naughton protocol, which involves much more gradual progression of exercise, is preferred by most clinicians for such patients (Table 17.2) [10]. The Naughton protocol generally involves several stages of exercise, each stage lasting for 2 min. The first two stages serve as a warm-up stage, and then the speed and grade begin to increase as we get into subsequent stages of exercise.

For the purposes of proper gas collection, the patient wears a tightly fitted mask equipped with a non-rebreathing valve and a mouthpiece that is designed to disallow any air leak. The nose is clamped in order to move all air through the mouth, and collect and measure respiratory rate, tidal volume, and the O_2 and CO_2 content of the expired air. Concomitant electrocardiogram (ECG) is also monitored and recorded along with the measurement of cuff blood pressure at each stage of exercise. The weight of the non-rebreathing valve is borne by the headpiece (Fig. 17.2). Continuous breath-by-breath analysis of VO_2, VCO_2, VE, and continuous telemetry with

Table 17.2 Modified Naughton treadmill exercise protocol and the level of everyday physical activities that are represented in each stage of work

Stage	Speed	Grade	Mets	Watts	Physical activities
1	1.0	0	1.5	10	Driving a car, sitting and writing or eating
2	1.5	0	–	–	Dressing, knitting, walking to bathroom
3	2.0	3.5	3.0	25	Shave self, wash entire body, food shopping
4	2.0	7.0	4.0	50	Sexual activity, raking leaves, plastering
5	2.0	10.5	5.0	75	Stacking firewood, mowing lawn (powered), walking downstairs
6	3.0	7.5	6.0	100	Scrubbing floors, gardening, walking upstairs
7	3.0	10.0	–	–	Lifting and carrying 65–80 lb, carpentry, climbing hills (no load)
8	3.0	12.5	–	–	Digging, snow shoveling, climbing (20 lb load)
9	3.0	15.0	8.5	150	Beyond this level workloads are compatible with very vigorous exercise (e.g., skiing, basketball)
10	3.4	14.0	10.0	175	
11	3.4	16.0	11.0	200	
12	3.4	18.0	–	–	
13	3.4	20.0	13.5	250	
14	3.4	22.0	–	–	

Adapted from Weber et al. [13], with permission from Elsevier.

heart rate monitoring is also acquired and displayed in real time on the computer screen. This information can be printed for later review and subsequent analysis.

The main parameter reflective of oxygen utilization is VO_2max. The VO_2max is defined as the value of VO_2 that generally varies way less than 1 ml/kg/min for at least 30 s duration or longer (plateau). It generally is identified by recording the VO_2 that finally stops rising and plateaus for at least two exercise stages despite a continuing increment in the workload. The VO_2max, by itself, generally reflects a value of oxygen consumption which is a little bit beyond the value that describes the point when AT is achieved. The AT usually occurs at about 60% of the aerobic capacity or the VO_2max.

The extent of exercise performed on a treadmill generally provides 10% higher aerobic capacity than that performed on a bicycle ergometer. This is because the former utilizes a group of larger muscles of the lower extremity [11]. The VO_2max is a very good objective measure of the functional impairment of a patient's functional capacity (Table 17.1). In general, a VO_2max of less than 20 ml/kg/min would indicate an abnormal decrease in the aerobic capacity of the subject [12].

Another parameter that is used to evaluate aerobic capacity is called the "anaerobic threshold" or the "AT" as mentioned above. The AT is derived in a number of ways by using multiple criteria [9]. These criteria define AT as the VO_2 at crossover point of the VCO_2 and VO_2 curves (Fig. 17.1), where "R", for the first time, is above 1.0. A concomitant disproportionate rise in the following parameters is also seen at that point:

(i) VCO_2, VE, R (VCO_2/VO_2),
(ii) Ventilatory equivalent for O_2 (VE/VO_2), and
(iii) End-tidal O_2 relative to end-tidal VCO_2.

It should be noted that the measurement of AT is reproducible in almost all patients with a wide range of cardiopulmonary dysfunction [10].

Respiratory parameters are also evaluated along with VO_2max and AT. The ventilatory response is one of those parameters. It mainly reflects an increase in the "minute ventilation" (VE) in response to the rise in tidal volume and respiratory rate with exercise.

In order to assess the ventilator reserve of a subject, one can calculate the ratio of the following two out of the several parameters obtained by routine pulmonary function testing. These parameters include "maximal ventilation" (VE_{max}) and "maximal voluntary ventilation" (MVV). Thus, the VE_{max}/MVV ratio would reflect the ventilator reserve. The VE_{max}/MVV ratio generally remains under 1.0 (unity) in patients who do not have significant pulmonary disease. The oxygen saturation in these patients generally does not drop below 90% (desaturation point). In contrast, patients with significant chronic obstructive pulmonary disease (COPD), restrictive lung disease, such as pulmonary fibrosis, pulmonary vascular disease, or pulmonary hypertension, and congenital cardiac disorders with right-to-left shunt tend to develop desaturation as well as VE_{max}/MVV ratio greater than 1.0 with progressive maximal exercise.

VE is an important parameter but it requires a reliable and accurate measurement of oxygen utilization before it can provide any meaningful prognosis. Therefore, the oxygen saturation should be not only measured with noninvasive pulse (or ear-lobe) oximeters but also re-checked by drawing an arterial blood sample and running acid–base gas (ABG) analysis. Generally, a maximal cardiopulmonary exercise test (CPX) that provides a measure of VO_2max is needed for meaningful inferences to be drawn for diagnostic purposes. A less than optimal CPX, nonetheless, still provides significant amount of information for differential diagnosis through estimation of such parameters as AT and VE, as well as the tendency and extent of desaturation.

Invasive Treadmill Exercise Testing with Gas Analysis

In most patients, the gas analysis and CPX testing, which is generally a noninvasive testing modality, can be complemented with invasive hemodynamic monitoring to better define the type and severity of an underlying cardiac or pulmonary dysfunction [13]. For this purpose, a flexible, balloon-tipped floatation pulmonary arterial catheter (similar to a Swan–Ganz catheter or a Berman catheter) inserted via a central vein (internal jugular or subclavian) can be used safely during the exercise. When used, the parameters obtained provide very valuable information. For example, a normal exercise response of the hemodynamic parameters would include a rise in the cardiac output (CO) due to an early rise in stroke volume and a progressive increase in the heart rate (CO = stroke volume × heart rate). As discussed below, the degree to which stroke volume increases in such circumstances is inversely proportional to the severity of heart failure. The patients classified as class A or class B show graded increment, while those classified as class D exhibit little or no increase in these parameters.

In the beginning, as an invasive cardiopulmonary exercise testing is performed, the right atrial (RA) pressure tends to remain invariant while pulmonary capillary wedge (PCW) pressure shows progressive increases with incremental exercise. However, as the exercise workload rises further, a point is reached where the stroke volume response begins to plateau, and thereafter, the RA and PCW pressures begin to show an increase by equal amounts for both. This latter response in filling pressures (i.e., PCW) has been attributed to the value and contributions of pericardial constraint [14].

At the time of the achievement of VO_2max, the tissue O_2 extraction approaches almost 70%. When the patient exercises around the AT, a rise in mixed venous lactate concentration occurs as the VO_2 begins to surpass 60% of the overall VO_2max. Radial or brachial artery catheterizations show a rise in systolic and mean arterial pressures during exercise while diastolic pressures remain unchanged or fall. Peripheral vasodilatation results in an approximately 50% decrement in systemic vascular resistance, frequently down to <600 dynes s/cm^5. The degree to which pulmonary systolic, diastolic, and mean pressures rise and pulmonary vascular resistance falls during exercise also depends on the severity of the underlying CAD and other cardiopulmonary disorders [15].

Bicycle Ergometer Exercise Testing with Gas Analysis

An alternative to walking on a treadmill is exercising on a bicycle ergometer. The bicycle ergometer is an equipment that consists of a mainframe, adjustable seat, handlebars, a flywheel, and a foot-crank assembly. As a patient exercises on a bicycle ergometer, the "resistance" is applied by tightening the "brake-pad"-type device to the wheel. The amount of workload experienced would be proportional to the amount of "resistance". The "workload" thus achieved along with pedaling frequency can be used to calculate the VO_2. Generally, pedaling frequency is kept constant (e.g., at 50 RPM). Therefore, the workload becomes directly proportional to and predictive of the VO_2. In addition, since the "workload" on the bicycle ergometer tends to be independent of a person's weight, VO_2 can be estimated even if O_2 uptake and CO_2

production are not measured. Some of the advantages of a bicycle ergometer over the treadmill include portability, less noisiness, small space requirement, and increased affordability. In addition, patients with hip joint and knee problems who are unable to use a treadmill can still be exercised on a bicycle ergometer by changing into an "arm" ergometer.

The bicycle exercise protocols usually start at the lowest workload setting, beginning with 15 or 25 W (90 or 150 kilopond-meter/min). Each subsequent stage of the protocol lasts for 2–3 min with the increment in workload of 15–25 W per stage. The relationship between work rate in watts (for ergometer) and mets (for treadmill) using modified Naughton protocol as an example is listed in Table 17.2 [10].

The VO_2max estimated through maximal exercise on a bicycle ergometer is generally quite reproducible; however, the value is approximately one-tenth lower than that estimated through maximal exercise on a treadmill. The VO_2max is similarly defined as the level of VO_2 that remains invariant by less than 0.75 ml/kg/min on increment in exercise at the plateau. The point of anaerobic threshold (or AT) is determined as described for the treadmill. Similar to the treadmill, the ventilator parameters estimated in response to gradually increasing workload on a bicycle ergometer are proportionate to the amount of resistance applied. Pulmonary artery catheter can be placed and invasive parameters can be determined during a bicycle ergometer exercise just as well as with the treadmill.

Clinical Applications of CPX Testing and Gas Analysis

Exercise testing with gas analysis is generally useful in the following clinical circumstances (Table 17.3).

Chronic Cardiac Failure

Generally, heart failure is described as a condition where the heart is unable to supply O_2 and substrate to the metabolizing tissues commensurate with their nutritional requirement. Louis N. Katz emphasized the need to differentiate the cardiac disorders that compromise O_2 uptake but spare the myocardium (e.g., valvular disease, constrictive pericarditis, or arrhythmias) from those that do (e.g., ischemic or dilated cardiomyopathy) [16]. Objectives for exercising the patients in the former category include

  (i) calculation of cardiac reserve using VO_2max and AT,
 (ii) determination of the severity of underlying disease,
(iii) objective assessment of the patient's functional capacity, which is generally not dependent on the left ventricular ejection fraction,
 (iv) monitoring of the progression of illness, and
  (v) assessment of the response to various therapeutic interventions.

Table 17.3 Clinical applications of exercise stress testing and gas analysis

1. Chronic cardiac failure
   a. Systolic dysfunction
   b. Diastolic dysfunction
   c. Chronotropic (heart rate-related) dysfunction
2. Non-myocardial circulatory disorders
   a. Valvular heart disease
   b. Pulmonary vascular disease
   c. Peripheral vascular disease
   d. Congenital heart disease
3. Chronic lung disorders
   a. Obstructive lung disease
   b. Restrictive lung disease
4. Differential diagnosis of exertional dyspnea
5. Miscellaneous clinical applications
   a. Heart transplantation
   b. Presurgical risk prediction
   c. Periodic follow-up assessments status-post-therapeutic
      interventions
   d. Post-myocardial infarction risk evaluation
   e. Hypertension and hypertrophic heart disease
   f. Pacemaker evaluation and bi-ventricular pacing
   g. Assessment of functional disability
   h. Exercise prescription
   i. Research applications

Systolic Cardiac Failure

Systolic cardiac dysfunction and heart failure usually result from ischemic or dilated cardiomyopathy. The extent of LV dysfunction is proportionate to the decrease in the VO_2max obtained on the cardiopulmonary exercise test. Therefore, if the VO_2max is known, the cardiac output (a measure of systolic LV function) can be easily predicted (see Table 17.1). Alternatively, VO_2max is the "noninvasive" marker or substitute for "cardiac output". Anaerobic threshold (AT) is another measure that can be used to calculate the cardiac output despite the fact that the AT is usually achieved at less than maximal exertion, the latter being the determinant of the VO_2max. This relationship between VO_2max, AT, and functional classes A, B, C, and D as well as invasively determined cardiac output (CO) is displayed in the four different examples shown in Fig. 17.3. Mixed venous concentrations of lactate were also determined via the invasive testing and added to the above parameters [8,17]. Whenever a patient is able to achieve over 70% of oxygen extraction, any reduction observed in VO_2max should be considered to be a result of dysfunction of the heart. Figure 17.4 shows the interdependence of the oxygen uptake and rise in cardiac output with incremental exercise. Invasive stress testing also provides an opportunity to measure the pulmonary capillary wedge pressure (PCW) which tends to rise as the cardiac reserve decreases with increasing workload. It usually remains

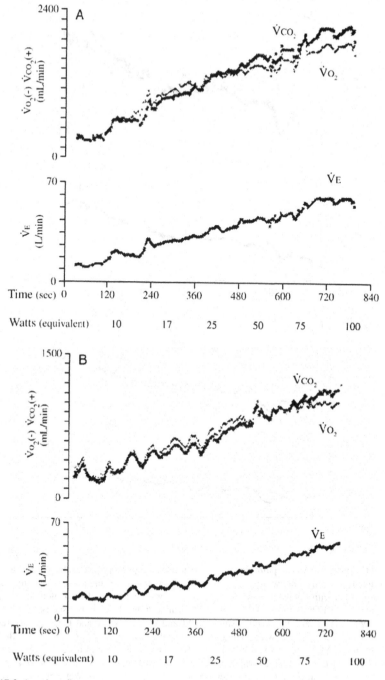

Fig. 17.3 (continued)

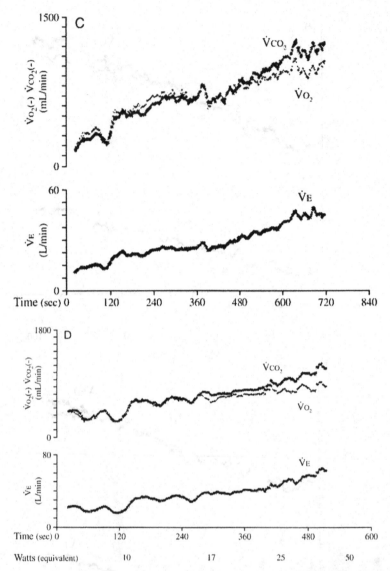

Fig. 17.3 (continued) Cardiopulmonary exercise testing (respiratory gas exchange during incremental exercise) in patients with varying degrees of chronic heart (myocardial) failure. (**A**) 61-year-old woman with idiopathic cardiomyopathy, who was functional class A, with an anaerobic threshold (AT) of 17 ml/kg/min, and VO₂max of 23 ml/kg/min, (**B**) class B response in a 58-year-old man with dilated cardiomyopathy exhibiting AT and VO₂max of 14 and 19 ml/kg/min, respectively, (**C**) a 45-year-old man with dilated cardiomyopathy who is class C on exercise with AT of 9 ml/kg/min and VO₂max of 13 ml/kg/min, and (**D**) class D response in a 42-year-old man with AT and VO₂max of 6 and 9, ml/kg/min, respectively. Class D patients are anaerobic during stage 1 or 2 of modified Naughton treadmill exercise protocol. (Modified from Weber and Janicki [10], with permission from Elsevier.)

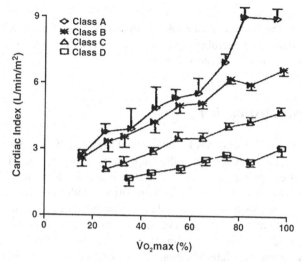

Fig. 17.4 Relationship between treadmill exercise cardiac index and normalized aerobic capacity (VO$_2$max) for patients with chronic heart failure of diverse origin and severity, subdivided according to each functional class. (From Weber and Janicki [8], with permission from Elsevier.)

below 18 mmHg in functional class A patients, rises above 25 mmHg in class B patients, and crosses over 30 mmHg with minimal workload in class C and class D patients. Clinically manifested pulmonary edema, however, does not correlate well with the extent of rise in the PCW (filling pressure). Instead, it is better predicted by the rise in "lactate threshold" and the "out of proportion" increment in ventilation (VE) [17]. The VCO$_2$ also augments in proportion to the VE in patients with decreased functional capacity, and their VEmax/MVV remains below 0.5. While functional class A and class B patients increase their VE by increasing their tidal volume, the VE increase in those in the functional classes C and D mainly occurs by increasingly rapid but shallower breathing rather than increment in the tidal volume.

Diastolic Cardiac Failure

Generally a third of all heart failure patients appear to have preserved systolic LV function. Their heart failure is usually a result of diastolic dysfunction. Certain clinical conditions affect the myocardial relaxation which causes diastolic dysfunction. Such conditions include hypertension, hypertrophic cardiomyopathy, myocardial ischemia, aging, heart transplant, and microvascular disease. Higginbotham et al. [18] and Kitzman et al. [19] have shown that in patients with hypertension, and in elderly individuals, the diastolic dysfunction leads to a decrease in cardiac output as determined by invasive monitoring. Proportionate decrease in the VO$_2$max estimated by the CPX testing is seen which correlates well with the extent of drop in the cardiac output with incremental exercise on the bicycle ergometer. In another study [20] among patients who had received cardiac transplants, stress testing with gas analysis revealed a decrease in aerobic capacity, abnormal heart rate response, as well as decreased stroke volume and cardiac output.

Chronotropic Dysfunction

Cardiac output is a product of stroke volume and heart rate ($CO = SV \times HR$). Since cardiac reserve is determined by cardiac output, the heart rate and rhythm tend to significantly affect the cardiac reserve. Atrial contraction importantly contributes to the cardiac output (atrial kick) especially in patients with somewhat compromised ventricular function, such as atrial fibrillation. Ventricular dys-synchrony also contributes to reduction in cardiac reserve in patients with conduction abnormalities and single ventricular pacemakers. Such ventricular dysfunction can be estimated through CPX testing and determination of AT and VO_2max [21]. In patients with pacemakers, fixed rate pacing has been shown to correlate with lower AT as compared with rate-responsive pacing.

Circulatory (Extra-Myocardial) Disorders

A variety of non-myocardial disorders can lead to cardio-circulatory failure, such as valvular disease, pulmonary vascular disease, peripheral arterial disease, congenital heart disease, pericardial disease, and anemia.

Valvular Heart Disease

Valvular abnormalities—both stenotic and regurgitant in nature—can lead to profound decrease in the ability of the heart to raise cardiac output during incremental exercise testing. Such abnormalities may lead to significant as well as symptomatic chronic circulatory failure [16].

In patients with mitral valve stenosis, significant decrease in the left ventricular filling occurs, and it subsequently results in reduction in the stroke volume during progressive exercise. These abnormalities are a consequence of rise in the heart rate and pulmonary vascular resistance, and the reduction in the diastolic filling period and the right ventricular output with incremental exertion. Donald and coworkers have described a method of determining the severity of mitral stenosis by measuring the cardiac output response to supine exercise and the amount of lactate production in the working limb [22].

Severity of mitral stenosis is generally estimated by calculation of the area of the mitral aperture through "pressure-half time calculation" noninvasively using the echocardiogram or invasively through the "Fick method" during right and left heart catheterization with serial oxygen concentration measurements. It should be noted that while these measurements of valve area are very important for determining the timing of valvular surgery, current methods of determining the area can be influenced by multiple confounding factors including vasomotor reactivity, vascular resistance, pulmonary vascular changes, and associated mitral regurgitation. CPX testing provides a measure of VO_2max and AT that can be used to better estimate the decrement in the functional capacity as affected by the severity of mitral stenosis.

Pre-operative evaluation of mitral stenosis should, thus, include not only determination of valve area but also measurement of cardiac reserve and patient's functional capacity though CPX testing that provides the missing information.

In patients with mitral regurgitation much less increment in atrial size and pulmonary pressure is seen. The incompetence of mitral and aortic valves generally creates a volume overload on the left ventricle (LV) which may not be apparent in the beginning stages. The progression of the LV dysfunction is often unpredictable. In the early stages, the dysfunction may only manifest itself on exertion, but eventually it progresses to more severe dysfunction. The resting cardiac output in patients with different degrees of LV dysfunction may be similar, and the extent of dysfunction may only be measurable with exercise challenge. This information is valuable, and it makes the CPX testing a valuable tool in the process of trying to accurately determine the extent of LV dysfunction in the patients with regurgitant valvular lesions. Furthermore, the decision regarding the timing of surgery in mitral and aortic regurgitation is a complex one that requires evaluation of the patient's cardiopulmonary status. Noninvasive CPX testing serves this purpose well. It also helps to monitor the change in functional status over time both prior to and following the surgery.

As valvular regurgitation progresses, it leads to increasing LV dysfunction causing the cardiac reserve to fall which can be assessed adequately by CPX testing. Subsequently, the patients can be classified into the four functional classes A–D [5] (Fig. 17.5). Marked elevation in filling pressures during invasive CPX testing can be seen in class C and class D patients, as well as in the class B patients with associated regurgitant valvular lesions. Dyspnea in these patients with "non-myocardial" failure tends to correlate well with lactate threshold similar to that seen in patients with myocardial failure. AT can be used as a substitute measure to VO_2max in those patients who are unable to exercise hard enough and fail to achieve the maximal aerobic capacity.

Pulmonary Vascular Disease

Pulmonary vascular disease, especially pulmonary hypertension, could develop as "primary" or "secondary" pulmonary hypertension. In this process, the medial wall of the pulmonary arteries develops hypertrophy of the smooth muscle cells along with the development of fibrosis in the interstitium. These changes result in the development of increased pulmonary vascular resistance and elevated pulmonary arterial pressures causing pulmonary arterial hypertension (PAH). As pulmonary pressure rises, it raises the outflow resistance for the right ventricle diminishing its

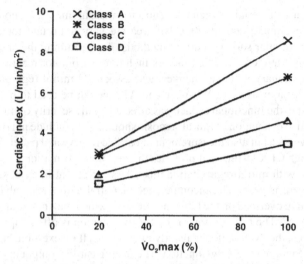

Fig. 17.5 The relationship between cardiac index and VO_2 attained during incremental treadmill exercise in patients with mitral or aortic valvular incompetence, or both, who are categorized according to their aerobic capacity. VO_2 uptake is normalized according to maximum O_2. (Modified from Weber and Janicki [10], with permission from Elsevier.)

cardiac output. Pulmonary venous hypertension, on the contrary, results from chronic left ventricular failure that raises passive resistance to the pulmonary venous return.

PAH leads to decline in cardiac output that can be ascertained and measured through the cardiopulmonary exercise testing where the reduced aerobic capacity would manifest as decreased VO_2max. Table 17.4 displays the hemodynamic responses to exercise during "invasive" CPX testing at both resting and peak exercise conditions. Maximal attainable cardiac output is not dissimilar to that in patients

Table 17.4 Resting and peak exercise hemodynamics for patients with nonhypoxic pulmonary vascular disease and pulmonary hypertension

	Resting	Exercise
PA (mmHg)	29 ± 9	47 ± 20
RVSP (mmHg)	52 ± 30	86 ± 37
RVDP (mmHg)	7 ± 4	16 ± 10
PCW (mmHg)	10 ± 3	22 ± 14
PVR (dynes s/cm^5)	412 ± 319	302 ± 331
CO (l/min/m^2)	2.8 ± 1.6	5.3 ± 2.2
MAP (mmHg)	106 ± 6	130 ± 8
Art O_2 sat (%)	97 ± 2	96 ± 2

PA, mean pulmonary artery pressure; RVSP and RVDP, right ventricular systolic and diastolic pressures, respectively; PCW, wedge pressure; PVR, pulmonary vascular resistance; CO, cardiac output; MAP, mean arterial pressure.

From Weber KT, Janicki JS. Pulmonary hypertension. *In* Weber KT, Janicki JS (eds.), *Cardiopulmonary Exercise Testing: Physiologic Principles and Clinical Application*. Philadelphia, Saunders, 1986, pp. 220–234, with permission from Elsevier.

with chronic congestive heart failure. Furthermore, the magnitude of decline in the cardiac output remains proportionate to the degree of elevation in the pulmonary arterial resistance. In fact, the patients in functional class D may exhibit pulmonary vascular resistance greater than 1,000 dynes s/cm^5. During incremental exercise, the patients with primarily PAH tend not to desaturate, always attain AT, and even attain VO_2max in most of the instances.

Furthermore, the CPX testing in the patients with hypoxic pulmonary vasoconstriction generally demonstrate elevations in the pulmonary arterial (PA) and right ventricular (RV) pressures. Pulmonary vascular resistance (PVR) tends to rise due to marked hypoxemia and desaturation. If supplemental O_2 is given, it can attenuate some of this response, and the rise in pulmonary arterial pressure becomes less steep.

Peripheral Arterial Disease

An objective assessment of functional limitation can be performed in the patients with occlusive peripheral arterial disease (PAD). Such patients usually stop exercising because of pain and claudication. Quantification of total exercise time and time to the onset of claudication can be used to develop an exercise prescription. Serial CPX testing can aid in monitoring the progress of such therapeutic interventions. Substantial increases in maximal calf blood flow have been documented following these exercise programs [23].

Congenital Heart Disease

Evaluation of functional capacity has been demonstrated to be useful in patients with many forms of congenital heart diseases in both determining the indication for surgical intervention and documenting the response to treatment. Furthermore, exercise testing can be of great value in confirming exertion-induced supra-ventricular or ventricular arrhythmias in patients with suggestive history. CPX testing has been shown to be particularly useful in a wide variety of congenital cardiac conditions, such as cyanotic defects, congenital complete atrioventricular heart block, dilated cardiomyopathy, syncope, suspected arrhythmias, aortic stenosis, pulmonic stenosis, repaired aortic coarctation, tetralogy of Fallot, Ebstein anomaly, and prior Fontan operation. CPX testing has also been shown to be beneficial in stratifying risk in those with adult congenital heart diseases. For example, an abnormal ventilator response to exercise (VE/VCO_2 slope) has been shown to be the strongest predictor of mortality in adult patients with non-cyanotic congenital cardiac defects [24].

Chronic Lung Disorders

In normal subjects and in patients with heart disease, VE and tidal volume do not exceed 50% of the MVV and vital capacity, respectively. Such persons have a ventilatory reserve that does not limit their exercise. Patients with obstructive or restrictive lung disease have reduced ventilatory reserve, along with altered lung mechanics, hypoxemia, pulmonary hypertension, and muscle fatigue causing impaired exercise performance [25, 26].

Chronic Obstructive Lung Disease

Ventilatory reserve diminishes primarily as a result of "wasted" ventilation of the "under-perfused" areas of the lungs in the patients with chronic obstructive lung disease (COLD). Their VE (ventilation) tends to be disproportionately greater for the degree of exertion. Furthermore, the VO_2 in such patients is usually higher at baseline (rest) and continues to stay higher for any workload as exercise progresses. These patients fail to achieve their VO_2max. When the COLD is severe, patients fail to even achieve their AT but with one distinct difference—they do not exhibit desaturation. Rather, oxygen saturation may rise due to added ventilation of previously underventilated areas with low ventilation/perfusion ratio. On the contrary, in patients with emphysema who have diminished gas-exchange surface area, desaturation develops early.

Restrictive/Interstitial Lung Disease

Patients with interstitial pulmonary disorders commonly present with exercise-induced dyspnea. They tend to be tachypneic, with shallower breathing (lower tidal volume) and low maximal ventilator volume (MVV). They develop desaturation with exertion quickly. The CPX appears to be more sensitive than pulmonary function tests (PFT) in such patients. For example, the ventilator reserve can be noted to decrease on CPX test long before the development of identifiable abnormalities on the PFT.

Exertional Dyspnea and Fatigue: Role of CPX with Gas Analysis

When breathing is perceived to be inappropriately difficult relative to the level of physical activity, it is called "shortness of breath" or "dyspnea" [10]. It may be caused by a number of possible conditions, such as cardiac, circulatory, pulmonary vascular, interstitial, airway, and chest wall disorders. Dyspnea occurs when ventilation (VE) is too high for the level of VO_2. Evaluation of dyspnea must include thorough analysis of historical, physical, and routine laboratory data. However, CPX is of immense value for assessing its severity in an objective and reliable manner. Inclusion of airflow and arterial O_2 saturation helps in estimating MVV by multiplying FEV_1 by 35. An encroachment by VE on more than 70% of MVV cannot be sustained for more than a few minutes before reaching VO_2max in patients with lung disease. Generally, in patients with co-existent cardiac and pulmonary diseases, it is difficult to establish the predominant cause. In such circumstances, the CPX test,

Table 17.5 An approach to assess exercise dyspnea in patients with cardiac and pulmonary diseases

Measurements

- Resting pulmonary function
- Breath-by-breath gas exchange and airflow; ear oximetry at rest and exercise
- Progressive exercise to exhaustion to determine maximum O_2 uptake (VO_2 max) and anaerobic threshold (AT)

Steps

- If AT and VO_2max are attained without O_2 desaturation, myocardial or circulatory failure is responsible
- If O_2 desaturation occurs during exercise, this suggests lung disease, pulmonary vascular disease, or a right-to-left intracardiac shunt
- If VO_2max and AT are not attained due to dyspnea, then an impairment in ventilation is suggested
- If more than 50% of vital capacity or maximum voluntary ventilation (MVV) is used by maximum exercise tidal volume and minute ventilation, respectively, then lung disease is dominant. Heart disease patients use less than 50% of MVV. A malingerer has an erratic respiratory response to exercise, evident at low levels of work and disappearing at higher levels when the chemical drive to respiration dominates

Modified from Weber KT, Janicki JS, Likoff MJ. Exercise testing in the evaluation of cardiopulmonary disease. *Clin Chest Med*, 5:173–180, 1984, with permission from Elsevier.

along with measurement of airflow and O_2 saturation by ear oximetry, can be used to differentiate disorders of ventilation from circulation (Table 17.5) [17]. The patients with pulmonary vascular or interstitial pulmonary disease may be unable to sustain alveolar ventilation at a level commensurate with appropriate arterial O_2 saturation and develop dyspnea. In patients with chronic airway disease, the need to move air through partial obstructed airway augments the respiratory muscle workload. The airflow in these patients is already compromised at rest, and with exertion it will increase approaching peak expiratory flows even before attaining the end-points of AT or VO_2max.

Miscellaneous Applications of Gas Analysis and CPX Testing

Cardiopulmonary exercise testing with gas analysis is invaluable in the objective assessment of the functional reserve of the heart and lungs. Such assessment has been found to be quite helpful in predicting the peri-operative risk in patients undergoing cardiac allograft transplantation and many non-cardiac surgeries [27]. Furthermore, the CPX testing has an important role in determining "functional disability", providing "exercise prescription", and stratifying the risk for patients following acute myocardial infarction.

Certain examples of such conditions and value of CPX testing are outlined below:

Heart Transplantation

CPX testing can provide an objective and reproducible assessment of the degree of myocardial dysfunction through determination of VO_2max and AT which together represent cardiac reserve. It has become most valuable in patients with systolic dysfunction from ischemic or dilated cardiomyopathy. Such patients are potential candidates for allograft heart transplantation. Static physiologic parameters, such as ejection fraction (EF), resting cardiac output, or pulmonary wedge (PCW) pressure, fail to adequately predict the severity of heart failure or patient's functional capacity, and are not used as the main parameters in decision-making process prior to heart transplantation. Determination of another clinical parameter, the New Heart Association (NYHA) functional class, which is usually obtained as part of patient history, suffers from lack of reliability due to unavoidable subjective bias from the patient or the physician.

In these situations, the CPX testing with determination of VO_2max and AT has proven to be an indispensable tool that addresses both cardiac reserve and functional capacity, and predicts survival [28, 29]. The cardiac transplantation task force in its 1993 report recommends transplantation based on clinical criteria and functional assessment data from CPX test results [30]. According to this criteria, the class A patients with preserved cardiac reserve and class B patients with only minimal reduction in LV function would not meet the criteria for heart transplant. Serial CPX testing can be performed in these patients to assess recovery or deterioration and timing of the heart transplantation surgery if they were to deteriorate. Class C patients ($VO_2max < 16\,ml/kg/min$) with moderate decrease in cardiac reserve are probable candidates for transplantation, while those in functional class D ($VO_2max < 10\,mg/kg/min$) are candidates for urgent transplant since they have a poor 1- to 2-year survival. Therefore, the CPX testing with gas analysis becomes critical in risk stratification, and identification of candidate with various degrees of cardiac dysfunction, and helps triage them for the urgency or non-urgency of allograft transplantation.

Furthermore, CPX testing, especially serial CPX testing, is quite useful in patients after the transplant for assessing the gain in cardiac and ventilatory reserves. Some of the poor prognostic findings include blunted heart rate response (due to denervation) and findings suggestive of diastolic dysfunction. These findings would indicate continuing limitations in their exercise performance.

Presurgical Risk Prediction

Cardiopulmonary exercise testing with gas analysis has been shown to much more precisely predict the peri-surgical cardiovascular risk prior to major operations. Surgical stress appears to mimic the stress of exercise including the requirements for higher oxygen consumption and increased ventilation as well as augmentation in cardiac output—the parameters that depend on the cardiac and pulmonary reserves. These parameters can be predicted by estimating the VO_2max and AT through CPX testing [27]. In the literature, there appears to be ample evidence to suggest that functional class A and B patients tend to have better prognosis than those in classes C and D.

Follow-Up Evaluations Subsequent to Therapeutic Interventions

Some of the commonly used therapeutic interventions in patients with heart failure include use of vasodilating and/or ionotropic drugs. If these drugs are successful, they show favorable alterations in multiple parameters, such as the resting and exercise cardiac output, O_2 uptake, O_2 delivery to exercising muscles, and the work of breathing—both during rest and exercise conditions. Studies involving the use of hydralazine and minoxidil showed improvement in resting cardiac output without significant improvement in the exercise capacity. On the other hand, nitrates have been shown to enhance aerobic capacity. An alpha-1 receptor antagonist, trimazosin, exhibited mixed results. Captopril, an angiotensin-converting enzyme inhibitor, brought about a significant increase in treadmill exercise duration in a multicenter randomized study within 2 weeks of therapy that was sustained beyond 16 weeks of treatment. Serial improvement in functional capacity has been documented by gas analysis testing with the intermittent use of intravenous ionotropic infusions of dobutamine as well as of amrinone (a phospho-diesterase inhibitor) used as inpatient or home infusion therapy.

Post-myocardial Infarction Risk Assessment

The risk of repeat cardiovascular events in the survivors of acute myocardial infarction is generally predictable by evaluation of the presence of inducible ischemia and the extent of left ventricular (LV) dysfunction. LV function, however, is just a static measurement. Instead, a dynamic assessment of exercise capacity by CPX testing provides a better objective measure of cardiac output during increasing levels of exercise, and subsequently, a better prediction of future cardiac outcomes. In a follow-up study, the patients who completed at least 6 min or two stages of the standard Bruce protocol (peak $VO_2 > 14$ ml/kg/min; $\geq$ class B) showed almost a 99% 1-year survival. In another study, those subjects who completed 72 W on the bicycle ergometer (peak $VO_2 > 17$ ml/kg/min) exhibited a 9-year survival of over 88%.

Hypertension and Hypertrophic Heart Disease

Patients with hypertension and left ventricular hypertrophy (LVH) frequently develop diastolic dysfunction and a decrement in exertional capacity. LVH has been shown to be an independent predictor of future outcomes. Some studies have demonstrated decreased exercise capacity and decline in VO_2max as well as exercise cardiac output as measured by CPX testing and gas analysis.

Pacemaker Function Evaluation and Role in Bi-ventricular Pacing

Assessment of exercise performance in patients with single-chamber and dual-chamber pacemakers, especially in patients with some degree of left ventricular dysfunction, has gained increasing importance in recent years. In patients with LV dysfunction and left bundle branch block who received bi-ventricular pacing as part of cardiac resynchronization therapy (CRT), a significant improvement in peak VO_2 was demonstrated by performance of gas analysis through CPX. The improvement in oxygen uptake correlated with an increment in LV ejection fraction, a decrement in the extent of mitral regurgitation, and an improvement in the patient's clinical symptoms. Several studies have demonstrated improvement in distance walked in 6 min as well as peak VO_2 after CRT due to decreased mitral regurgitation, improved autonomic nervous system function, and increased left ventricular efficiency [31, 32].

Assessment of Functional Disability

CPX testing provides an objective assessment of disability that is usually not available from merely obtaining the functional history. Generally the disability would be assessed by the relative difficulty to sustain physical activity above AT and the ability to attain a VO_2max and to continue even for very short duration.

Pediatric Populations

The role of CPX testing in the pediatric population has been evolving rapidly. Exercise testing is commonly used in children to assess the signs and symptoms that are induced or aggravated by exercise to diagnose arrhythmias and to evaluate the need for medical and surgical treatments. Exercise testing can also be helpful in this population before certain athletic, vocational, or recreational activities as well as to obtain baseline data and perform serial follow-ups after particular interventions. In children with congenital cardiac defects, CPX testing can be used to evaluate prognosis [33].

Exercise Prescription

Metabolic energy requirements have already been documented for a wide range of daily activities in which people generally engage. It becomes easier to write an appropriate exercise prescription once the degree of disability has been determined by CPX testing. Accurate measurement of VO_2max is essential instead of just predicting the exercise capacity by looking at the exercise stage or duration [34]. Since most cardiac patients would have an abnormally lower VO_2 for any level of workload, the CPX testing helps avoid over-prescription of exercise.

Research Applications

In addition to its contributions in the evaluation and management of patients with cardiovascular disorders, the assessment of aerobic capacity with CPX testing can be used as an important research tool. Serial assessments of exercise capacity following the baseline assessment are frequently used to evaluate the benefits of particular pharmacologic and device interventions. It can also be used to perform objective assessment of functional capacity in asymptomatic population since low levels of habitual physical activity are associated with increased risk of future cardiovascular events. Impaired functional capacity predicts increased risk to a greater degree than demographics and presence of standard risk factors in both men and women [35].

Pitfalls in CPX and Gas Analysis Interpretation

The data obtained from CPX testing are generally reliable and reproducible, but occasionally there may be pitfalls in the collection and interpretation of metabolic data obtained during exercise [36]. The role of a skilled technician performing the test cannot be overemphasized. The technician has to go over the minute details regarding the "breathing through the tight-fitted mask", need for putting the best effort in, and devise ways for the patient to communicate with them in some form of sign language. In addition to giving adequate instructions to the patient prior to testing, continuous encouragement throughout the test may be needed. System leaks, i.e., breathing around the mouthpiece, nasal breathing, or sampling line breaks can affect the data acquisition and must be checked frequently by a good technician.

Conclusions

Evaluation of exercise performance is an integral part of every medical history, but it is currently accomplished by simply asking patients to describe their functional ability and assigning a NYHA functional class. The routine exercise test adds very little information beyond recording heart rate and arterial pressure. The addition of gas analysis to exercise testing, called CPX testing, provides the crucial, but hitherto missing, objective data with breath-by-breath analysis of utilization of O_2, production of CO_2 and ventilation to determine aerobic capacity (VO_2max) and anaerobic threshold (AT) along with airflow and oximetry measurements [37]. Primary cardio-circulatory causes of dyspnea can be differentiated from primary ventilatory causes reliably by CPX testing. Patients with cardiac or circulatory causes of dyspnea who are able to achieve their VO_2max use less than 50% of MVV at maximum exercise VE and do not develop arterial desaturation with exercise. Those with ventilatory causes of dyspnea fail to cross AT and achieve VO_2max, utilize >70% of MVV at maximum exercise VE, and develop arterial desaturation with exercise [5].

CPX testing can be useful for physicians in many areas of medicine. For the cardiologist and pulmonologist, it helps to differentiate disorders of the heart from lungs that cause dyspnea, determine the timing of valve or transplant surgery, assist with prognosis, and monitor the responses to therapy. Physicians in occupational or industrial medicine use CPX to determine work capacity or disability. It is also applicable for personalized exercise prescriptions for people interested in rehabilitation. The physicians in sports medicine can use CPX to obtain objective information central to monitoring the progress of exercise training program [10]. Pre-operative CPX predicts postoperative morbidity and mortality in elderly and in patients with cardiopulmonary diseases [27]. In the current cost-conscious healthcare system, CPX proves to be a cost-effective test because it is objective and more directly targeted to the issues than conventional assessment tests.

References

1. Clark, AL, Poole-Wilson, PA, Coats, AJS. Effects of motivation of the patient on indices of exercise capacity in chronic heart failure. *Br Heart J*, 71:162–165, 1994.
2. Holloszy, JO, Booth, FW. Biochemical adaptation to endurance exercise in muscle. *Annu Rev Physiol*, 38:273–291, 1976.
3. Mitchell, JH, Bloomquist, CG. Maximal oxygen uptake. *N Engl J Med*, 284:1018–1022, 1971.
4. Saltin, B, Rowell, LB. Functional adaptation to physical activity and inactivity. *Fed Proc*, 39:1506–1513, 1980.
5. Weber, KT. Principles and applications of cardiopulmonary exercise testing. *In* Fishman, AP (ed.), *Pulmonary Diseases and Disorders*, 3rd ed. New York, McGraw Hill, 1998, pp. 575–588.
6. Taylor, HL, Buskirk, E, Henschel, A. Maximal O_2 uptake as an objective measure of cardiorespiratory performance. *J Applied Physiol*, 8:73–80, 1955.
7. Mitchell, JH, Sproule, BJ, Chapman, CB. The physiological meaning of the maximal O_2 intake test. *J Clin Investigation*, 37:538–547, 1958.
8. Weber, KT, Janicki, JS. Cardiopulmonary exercise testing for evaluation of chronic cardiac failure. *Am J Cardiol*, 55(Suppl A):22A–31A, 1985.
9. Wasserman, K (ed.). *Exercise Gas Exchange in Heart Disease*. Armonk, NY, Futura, 1996.
10. Weber, KT, Janicki, JS (eds.). *Cardiopulmonary Exercise Testing: Physiologic Principles and Clinical Applications*. Philadelphia, Saunders, 1986.
11. Page, E, Cohen-Solal, A, Jondeau, G et al. Comparison of treadmill and bicycle exercise in patients with chronic heart failure. *Chest*, 106:1002–1006, 1994.
12. Pollock, ML, Wilmore, JH, Fox, SM. *Health and Fitness Through Physical Activity*. New York, Wiley, 1978.
13. Weber, KT, Janicki, JS, McElroy, PA. Cardiopulmonary exercise (CPX) testing. *In* Weber KT, Janicki JS (eds.), *Cardiopulmonary Exercise Testing: Physiologic Principles and Clinical Applications*. Philadelphia, Saunders, 1986, pp. 151–167.
14. Janicki, JS. Influence of the pericardium and ventricular interdependence on left ventricular diastolic and systolic function in patients with heart failure. *Circulation*, 81:III-1500–III-20, 1990.
15. Janicki, JS, Weber, KT, Likoff, MJ, Fishman, AP. The pressure-flow response of the pulmonary circulation in patients with heart failure and pulmonary vascular disease. *Circulation*, 72:1270–1278, 1965.
16. Katz, LN, Feinberg, H, Shaffer, AB. Hemodynamic aspects of congestive heart failure. *Circulation*, 21:95–111, 1960.

17. Weber, KT, Janicki, JS. Lactate production during maximal and submaximal exercise in patients with chronic heart failure. *J Am Coll Cardiol*, 6:717–724, 1985.

18. Higginbotham, MB. Diastolic dysfunction and exercise gas exchange, *In* Wasserman, K (ed.), *Exercise Gas Exchange in Heart Disease*. Armonk, NY, Futura, 1996, pp. 39–54.

19. Kitzman, DW, Sheikh, KH, Beere, PA, et al. Age-related alterations of Doppler left ventricular filling indexes in normal subjects are independent of left ventricular mass, heart rate, contractility and loading conditions. *J Am Coll Cardiol*, 18:1243–1250, 1991.

20. Kao, AC, Van Trigt, P III, Shaeffer-McCall, GS, et al. Central and peripheral limitations to upright exercise in untrained cardiac transplant recipients. *Circulation*, 89:2605–2615, 1994.

21. Treese, N. Exercise gas exchange to evaluate cardiac pacemaker function. *In* Wasserman, K. (ed.), *Exercise Gas Exchange in Heart Disease*. Armonk, NY, Futura, 1996, pp. 257–270.

22. Donald, KW, Gloster, J, Harris, EA, et al. The production of lactic acid during exercise in normal subjects and in patients with rheumatic heart disease. *A Heart J*, 62:494–510, 1961.

23. Gardner, AW, Montgomery, PS, Flinn, WR, Katzel, LI. The effect of exercise intensity on the response to exercise rehabilitation in patients with intermittent claudication. *J Vasc Surg*, 42:702–709, 2005.

24. Dimopoulos, K, Okonko, DO, Diller, GP, et al. Abnormal ventilator response to exercise in adults with congenital heart disease relates to cyanosis and predicts survival. *Circulation*, 113:2796–2802, 2006.

25. Gallagher, CG. Exercise limitation and clinical exercise stress testing in chronic obstructive pulmonary disease. *Clin Chest Med*, 15:305–326, 1994.

26. Marciniuk, DD, Gallagher, CG. Clinical exercise testing in interstitial lung disease. *Clin Chest Med*, 15:287–303, 1994.

27. Older, P, Smith, R, Courtney, P, et al. Preoperative evaluation of cardiac failure and ischemia in elderly patients by cardiopulmonary exercise testing. *Chest*, 104:701–704, 1993.

28. Mancini, DM, Eisen, H, Kussmaul, W, et al. Value of peak exercise oxygen consumption for optimal timing of cardiac transplantation in ambulatory patients with heart failure. *Circulation*, 83:778–786, 1991.

29. Stevenson, LW. Role of exercise testing in the evaluation of candidates for cardiac transplantation. *In* Wasserman, K (ed.), *Exercise Gas Exchange in Heart Disease*. Armonk, NY, Futura, 1996, pp. 271–286.

30. Mudge, GH, Goldstein, S, Addonizio, LJ, et al. 24th Bethesda conference: Cardiac transplantation. Task Force 3: Recipient guidelines/prioritization. *J Am Coll Cardiol*, 22:21–31, 1993.

31. Karvounis, HI, Dalamaga, EG, Papadopoulos, CE, et al. Improved papillary muscle function attenuates functional mitral regurgitation in patients with dilated cardiomyopathy after cardiac resynchronization. *J Am Soc Echocardiogr*, 19:1150–1157, 2006.

32. Abraham, WT, Fisher, WG, Smith, AL, et al. Multicenter InSync Randomized Clinical Evaluation (MIRACLE). Cardiac resynchronization in chronic heart failure. *N Engl J Med*, 346:1845–1853, 2002.

33. Paridon, SM, Alpert, BS, Boas, SR, et al. Clinical stress testing in the pediatric age group: A statement from the American Heart Association Council on Cardiovascular Disease in the Young, Committee on Atherosclerosis, Hypertension, and Obesity in Youth. *Circulation*, 113:1905–1920, 2006.

34. Ekelund, LG, Haskell, WL, Johnson, JL, et al. Physical fitness as a predictor of cardiovascular mortality in asymptomatic North American men: The Lipid Research Clinics Mortality Follow-up Study. *N Engl J Med*, 319:1379–1384, 1988.

35. Fleg, JL, Pina, IL, Balady, GJ, et al. Assessment of functional capacity in clinical and research applications: An advisory from the Committee on Exercise, Rehabilitation and Prevention, Council on Clinical Cardiology, American Heart Association. *Circulation*, 102:1591–1597, 2000.

36. Milani, RV, Lavie, CJ, Mehra, MR. Cardiopulmonary exercise testing, how do we differentiate the cause of dyspnea. *Circulation*, 110:e27–e31, 2004.

37. Singh, VN. The role of gas analysis with exercise testing. *Primary Care* 28:159–179, 2001.

Chapter 18
Testing Athletic Populations

David E. Price, Eric T. Warren, and Russell D. White

Exercise is important in promoting a low-risk lifestyle and research continues to show its beneficial effects on cardiovascular health [1]. Athletes are known for their cardiopulmonary fitness and low incidence of cardiovascular disease. However, athletes may still develop coronary artery disease (CAD), arrhythmias, or other cardiac problems that may remain silent until a life-threatening event occurs. These tragic events, although rare, often prompt questions in the public and media about the most effective screening methods to detect diseases responsible for sudden death in athletes.

Current cardiovascular screening strategies, using the American Heart Association (AHA) expert consensus panel recommendations, are lacking across the entire spectrum of sporting, from high school to professional levels [2–4]. In addition, the AHA recommends symptom-limited, maximal electrocardiographic (ECG) exercise testing (ET) for athletes with a moderate to high risk of cardiovascular disease. This applies to men over 40 years or women over 50 years or postmenopausal with one or more independent coronary risk factors [5, 6] (Table 18.1). ET use in asymptomatic or low-risk individuals to screen for CAD is controversial and probably should not be done, given the low pretest probability of identifying cardiovascular disease. Master athletes (age >60) also frequently manifest false-positive findings on ET, furthering the controversy on how to apply the ET to this special population [7]. This chapter will examine the use of ET in identifying ischemia in these at-risk asymptomatic or symptomatic athletes, as well as its use as a training tool for determining functional capacity, fitness level, and the effectiveness of a training program.

D.E. Price (✉)
Department of Family Medicine, Carolinas Medical Center – Eastland, Charlotte, NC 28212, USA
e-mail: david.price@carolinas.org

C.H. Evans, R.D. White (eds.), *Exercise Testing for Primary Care and Sports Medicine Physicians*, DOI 10.1007/978-0-387-76597-6_18
© Springer Science+Business Media, LLC 2009

Table 18.1 Coronary artery risk factors used for risk stratification

Positive factors

Family history
1. Myocardial infarction or
2. Coronary revascularization or
3. Sudden death
   (history of above occurring in male first-degree relative before age 55 years; history of above occurring before age 65 in female first-degree relative)

Cigarette smoking
1. Current smoker or
2. Those who quit smoking in previous 6 months

Hypertension
1. Currently on antihypertensive medication or
2. Systolic blood pressure $\geq$ 140 mmHg or
3. Diastolic blood pressure $\leq$ 90 mm Hg
   (confirmed on two separate occasions)

Hypercholesterolemia
1. Total serum cholesterol >200 mg/dl or
2. High-density lipoprotein cholesterol <40 mg/dl or
3. Low-density lipoprotein cholesterol >100 mg/dl if CHD[a]
   or CHD risk equivalent
   $\geq$130 mg/dl if $\geq$2 risk factors
   $\geq$160 mg/dl if 0–1 risk factors

Impaired fasting glucose   Fasting blood glucose $\geq$110 mg/dl

Obesity
1. Waist girth >102 cm (men) or >88 cm (women)

Sedentary lifestyle
1. Persons not participating in regular exercise program or
2. Not meeting the minimal physical activity recommendations from the U.S. Surgeon General's report

Negative factors

High serum high-density
lipoprotein cholesterol   >60 mg/dl

[a] CHD, coronary heart disease

Adapted from [6], with permission from the American Medical Association.

Indications

General indications for exercise testing include diagnosis of ischemia, prognosis of a cardiac event, and exercise prescription. Guidelines for these indications were originally applied to adult men with intermittent pretest probabilities of coronary artery disease (CAD) to produce results with the greatest sensitivity and specificity [8]. These indications apply to athletes as well, but they are a special population, in that they usually have few risk factors for cardiovascular disease and lead a low-risk lifestyle. However, some athletes may still be at risk for cardiovascular disease and therefore still need to be screened appropriately. Their stress test must be interpreted in light of unique resting electrocardiograms (ECG) and cardiac responses to stress testing. They also may require special protocols to obtain the most accurate results. Athletes generally are divided into two categories to screen for cardiovascular disease: symptomatic and asymptomatic. Only asymptomatic patients should be tested for exercise prescription.

Symptomatic Athlete

An athlete is considered symptomatic if he or she has any positive findings based on the AHA recommendations on history and physical examination [2]. Symptomatic athletes are divided into two further categories based on age. Those athletes less than 35 years of age are most at risk for congenital morphologic abnormalities of the heart, with hypertrophic cardiomyopathy (HCM) and congenital coronary artery anomalies being the most common potentially fatal cardiac conditions in the United States [9, 10]. Arrhythmogenic right ventricular cardiomyopathy (ARVC) is the most common in Europe [11]. ECG and echocardiography are the initial tests of choice in these younger athletes as most of the silent but lethal conditions such as HCM can be detected by these means [2, 12]. Once HCM or other morphologic abnormality is ruled out, an ET may be performed to rule out ischemia, the proposed means by which sudden death occurs from coronary artery anomalies [9].

Symptomatic athletes older than 35 years are most at risk for CAD, which accounts for over 75% of sudden deaths in this age group [10]. The risk of sudden death in older athletes versus young athletes is much higher and epidemiological data estimate a risk of about 1/15,000–1/18,000 as compared to 1/100,000–1/300,000 in the younger athlete [13]. Accordingly, a physician should not take an athlete's symptoms lightly and assume he or she could not have CAD.

The two main mechanisms thought responsible for exercise-related sudden death in older athletes are coronary spasm and plaque rupture [10]. Exercise dilates normal coronary arteries but may induce coronary spasm in areas of atherosclerotic plaque. Contraction of these non-compliant plaques in the face of higher systolic blood pressure, and shear from increased velocity of blood flow during strenuous physical activity, may induce plaque rupture. Even in areas of non-occlusive disease, strenuous activity may induce ischemia and subsequent ventricular fibrillation leading to sudden death [10].

For symptomatic athletes over age 35, ET has good sensitivity (50–70%) and specificity (80–90%) and should be used when appropriate in the workup of any older athlete with possible ischemia. The AHA recommends symptom-limited, maximal ET for adult subjects with an intermediate pretest probability of CAD based on gender, age, and symptoms [14] (Table 18.2). While other clinical findings such as multiple coronary artery disease risk factors, dyspnea on exertion, or resting ECG abnormalities may suggest the possibility of CAD, the most predictive clinical

Table 18.2 Pretest probability of coronary artery disease by age, gender, and symptoms*

Age (years)	Gender	Typical/definite angina pectoris	Atypical/probable angina pectoris	Non-anginal chest pain	Asymptomatic
30–39	Male	Intermediate	Intermediate	Low	Very low
	Female	Intermediate	Very low	Very low	Very low
40–49	Male	High	Intermediate	Intermediate	Low
	Female	Intermediate	Low	Very low	Very Low
50–59	Male	High	Intermediate	Intermediate	Low
	Female	Intermediate	Intermediate	Low	Very Low
60–69	Male	High	Intermediate	Intermediate	Low
	Female	High	Intermediate	Intermediate	Low

*No data exist for patients less than age 30 or older than age 69, but presumably the prevalence of CAD increases with age. In a few cases, patients with ages at the extremes of the decades listed may have probabilities slightly outside the given ranges.
High, >90%; intermediate, 10–90%; low, <10%; and very low, <5%.
Adapted from [14], with permission.

finding is a history of chest pain or discomfort [14]. In fact, diabetes has only a modest impact, and smoking and hyperlipidemia have only a minimal impact on pretest probability [14].

While athletes over the age of 35 may still have morphologic cardiac abnormalities like HCM, they are not usually a major cause of sudden death in this age group. Usually if the abnormalities are serious enough, the patient will have had onset of symptoms or even sudden death at an earlier age. That is not to say that these older athletes cannot have sudden death from abnormalities such as HCM, but usually they develop congestive heart failure (CHF) or ischemic heart disease (IHD) from the obstruction, and therefore present earlier with symptoms related to these conditions [15]. Further explanation regarding the evaluation and management of the symptomatic athlete is described more in depth in Chapter 20.

Asymptomatic Athlete

Asymptomatic athletes are considered those without positive findings based on the AHA recommendations on history and physical examination [2]. ET is not recommended as a routine screening tool for the detection of early CAD in asymptomatic athletes because of the low predictive value and high rate of false-positive and false-negative results. However, in athletes with a moderate to high risk of CAD, the AHA recommends symptom-limited, maximal ET. This applies to men over 40 years or women over 50 years or postmenopausal with one or more independent coronary risk factors [5, 6] (Table 18.1).

Asymptomatic athletes may choose to use ET for training purposes to measure certain physiologic variables and then conduct interventions to determine if enhancement of each or all of these variables impacts their performance. Performance in endurance sports (e.g., distance running, cycling) has been shown to be dictated by three basic physiologic variables: maximal aerobic power ($VO_{2\,max}$), lactate threshold, and economy [16]. Elite athletes continuously strive for the competitive edge in their respective events, and performance-related testing has thrived in response. State-of-the-art sports medicine centers around the country now offer sophisticated testing for physiologic data crucial to enhancing athletes' performance ranging from youth sports participants to Olympic competitors.

An athlete's performance and ability to affect change on these physiologic variables is mostly a function of his genetics and training history, as well as the sport he has chosen. Exercise testing can evaluate a key variable such as an athlete's $VO_{2\,max}$ and provide information about the genetically determined range on that performance characteristic. However, looking at a single time point is not an accurate way of determining how an athlete will be able to improve that variable because it will vary with training. Most testing then is performed over time, during the athlete's training period prior to an event, so that changes to the training regimen can be made to enhance performance. $VO_{2\,max}$ rarely improves more than 20–25% with training and adaptations to training vary markedly between individual athletes, such that accurate prediction of a potential "best" determination of a physiologic variable becomes difficult [16]. Still, with repeated exercise testing, most athletes are able to improve their performance by making modifications to their training that cause increases in their $VO_{2\,max}$, lactate threshold, and economy. Eventually, maximal benefit is achieved, at which point there is very little additional improvement seen in these parameters [16].

Specific training techniques can affect each of the above physiologic variables in a different manner and exercise testing can record these objective measurements. For example, to improve maximal oxygen uptake ($VO_{2\,max}$), high-intensity, short-interval training is necessary, whereas longer duration intervals (e.g., Fartlek training in running) or sustained high-intensity exercise is necessary to improve lactate threshold [16].

Much research has been done to attempt to predict how well an athlete will perform in his sport. There is a strong relationship between treadmill velocity at the onset of plasma lactate accumulation and running performance at all distances [17]. Thus, many athletes determine their heart rate at 75% $VO_{2\,max}$ as this has been found to correlate very precisely with lactate threshold in highly trained distance runners [18].

Protocols

Proper protocol selection for testing athletes depends on the indication for the exercise test. In symptomatic athletes, the goal is to discover the cause of their symptoms, usually by trying to diagnose underlying ischemia or an arrhythmia, rather than testing exercise capacity or other physiologic parameters, the usual goal in asymptomatic athletes. The Bruce protocol has had the most published data and is typically the most widely used. Its use in athletes, regardless of whether they are symptomatic or not, is debatable. As Buchfuhrer and Myers have shown, the optimal protocol selected should allow the athlete to reach his expected maximum metabolic equivalent (MET) at 10 min of exercise [19, 20]. This time frame may be difficult to adhere to in well-trained athletes who frequently go much further on the standardized Bruce protocol. The Bruce protocol also has shown poor correlation between estimated oxygen uptake and measured uptake [20].

The ramped Bruce protocol, a newer protocol, may be more appropriate for both the symptomatic and asymptomatic athletes. The ramped Bruce protocol is similar to other ramped protocols that employ continuous steady increases in workload without abrupt changes as in the Bruce and other conventional stage protocols (Balke and Ware, Astrand, Costill) [21–23] (see Fig. 2.1). Although there is hemodynamic comparability among these ramp and stage protocols [19, 20, 24, 25], there are marked variations in VO_{2max} and METS achieved in conventional protocols compared with ramp protocols. Myers et al. showed that the measured and predicted VO_{2max} and METS were significantly more accurate for ramp protocols that employ smaller increments in work over the test period than conventional protocols [20]. Using smaller increments in work also produces a higher VO_{2max} than large increments [19]. Finally, studies have shown that the ramp protocols may be better than the Bruce protocol for achieving a level of stress adequate for CAD detection in the symptomatic patient [19, 26, 27].

Ramp protocols may be individualized or standardized, and there exist proponents for both [20, 26]. Individualization allows the physician to determine the maximum workload, speed, and time of the test, with the computer adjusting the grade every few seconds to arrive at the maximum. This protocol however does not allow serial comparison for the same patient or between patients as in a standardized protocol.

Many athletes prefer a specific training speed or pace, and protocols like the Astrand [22] and Costill [23] employ a constant speed with a staged increase in grade. Athletes do not become frustrated with a very slow pace and still finish in a reasonable amount of time. Both ramp and stage protocol specifics and selection are discussed more in depth in Chapter 3.

Most athletes attain higher VO_{2max} values on a treadmill compared to other ergometers [28]. However, numerous studies have shown that elite athletes in their specific sports (e.g., cycling, rowing) are able to attain higher VO_{2max} values than when tested on a treadmill [29–31]. The importance then of sport-specificity in fitness testing cannot be overemphasized.

The Athletic Heart Syndrome

The athletic heart syndrome is the term given to the constellation of specific morphologic and electrophysiologic alterations of the heart in response to vigorous athletic training [32]. There exists a continuum of adaptations depending on the type of exercise the athlete is engaged in. Endurance athletes who engage in dynamic exercise such as running or cycling develop a volume-overloaded state. The heart adapts to the increased plasma volume by increasing left ventricular end-diastolic diameter and left ventricular wall thickness, a process known as eccentric hypertrophy. This results in a higher stroke volume and cardiac output. Vagal tone is enhanced and sympathetic tone is diminished with dynamic exercise, resulting in low resting heart rates. Normally, with increasing exercise intensity, systolic blood pressure (BP) will increase and diastolic BP will remain about the same or decrease slightly. In well-trained athletes however, diastolic BP may decrease dramatically as peripheral and pulmonary resistance falls to accommodate increasing capillary volume.

Athletes who perform static exercises such as weightlifting develop a pressure-overloaded state with little change in parasympathetic tone. The heart adapts to this state with an increased absolute and relative wall thickness without significant changes in end-diastolic diameter, a process known as concentric hypertrophy. Pacemaker function, heart rate, and conduction, however, remain relatively unaffected [33].

There are many physical exam and ECG findings of athletic heart syndrome that would be considered pathologic in a sedentary individual but are considered normal in an athlete. Palpation may reveal a slowed pulse, with increased amplitude secondary to the increased stroke volume. Auscultation may expose third and fourth heart sounds as well as systolic ejection murmurs. The systolic murmurs are usually grade 1 or 2 and have the clinical characteristics of benign flow murmurs. They may be found in up to half of athletes engaged in dynamic activities [32]. A multitude of ECG findings may be seen in athletes including alterations in rate, rhythm, conduction, repolarization, and precordial voltage. Most of these effects are derived

Table 18.3 The athletic heart syndrome*

Benign findings	Pathologic findings
Physical exam	Physical exam
Grades 1 and 2 systolic ejection murmurs Split S_2 S_3 or S_4	Systolic murmurs at the lower sternal border augmented by Valsalva and decreased with squatting Diastolic murmurs
ECG changes Sinus arrhythmia Sinus bradycardia First-degree heart block	ECG changes Downsloping ST-segment depression ST elevation with broad T waves Significant Q waves (anterior or inferior pattern)
Second-degree heart block (Mobitz 1) Junctional escape beats Voltage criteria for hypertrophy Early repolarization Incomplete right bundle branch block P wave increases in amplitude and duration Tall, peaked T waves T-wave flattening or inversion that normalizes with exercise Prominent U waves	Delta waves (Wolff–Parkinson–White) Second-degree heart block (Mobitz 2) Third-degree heart block Prolonged QT interval LVH with ST-T wave strain pattern

*These findings assume an asymptomatic athlete. If an athlete is symptomatic or a possible pathologic finding is found, further workup is indicated.
Adapted from Marolf et al. [15], with permission from Elsevier.

from an increase in parasympathetic tone and decreased sympathetic drive. Common findings include sinus bradycardia, sinus arrhythmia, first degree AV block, and voltage criteria for hypertrophy. ST-segments may show early repolarization and T waves may be inverted at rest but normalize with exercise. Table 18.3 summarizes the various physical exam and ECG findings that are associated with athletic heart syndrome along with findings that should generally be considered pathologic [32]. Interestingly, a study by Pelliccia et al. examining the clinical significance of abnormal ECG patterns in trained athletes showed that even athletes with striking ECG abnormalities suggesting cardiovascular disease were almost always innocent consequences of long-term intense athletic training. Thus, although further workup is often indicated for these grossly abnormal ECGs, it is reassuring that most of these athletes will not have a cardiovascular abnormality [34].

Interpretation

Interpretation of the EST in athletes requires special attention because highly trained athletes' ECG and cardiovascular responses differ from untrained individuals as discussed above. Familiarity with athletic heart syndrome and its associated findings on physical exam and ECG is required for accurate interpretation. The criteria for a positive EST are no different from that of the general population: 1.0 mm or more of horizontal or downsloping ST-segment depression during exercise, recovery, or both [35]. Upsloping ST-segment depression of 1.5 mm or greater at 80 ms beyond the J point is also considered positive. These cutoffs, however, may lead to more false-positive tests in athletes, a finding noted by Spirito et al. [36]. The majority of those athletes with false-positive tests were found to have left ventricular masses above the 95th percentile of the control population. Left ventricular hypertrophy on resting ECG more frequently correlates with benign ST-segment depression. But when significant ST-segment depression occurs during exercise, remains depressed for several minutes during recovery, and has a downsloping pattern, true ischemia is more likely [37]. ST-segment depression usually occurs maximally after the ventilatory threshold is reached, though its depth is usually greater in non-athletes compared with athletes [38].

If it remains uncertain whether a finding on EST is significant or a manifestation of athletic heart syndrome, discontinuation of training may help distinguish between benign and pathologic findings. A detraining period of 8 weeks should produce a rapid and progressive decrement in morphology, and repeat ECG and echo findings should normalize. Any abnormalities on repeat EST at this time should be considered pathologic and further workup with stress imaging should be considered [37, 39].

Summary

Healthy-appearing asymptomatic athletes may have underlying cardiovascular disease with the potential to cause life-threatening events. Other athletes may present symptomatically with a number of signs and symptoms suggestive of cardiovascular disease. Exercise testing may be a valuable diagnostic test in the management of both of these athletes. Given the media hype surrounding the deaths of several high-level athletes over the years, new standards and precedents now exist because of the potential legal implications [40]. It is important for physicians to be aware of guidelines that exist based on these precedents to avoid potential pitfalls and clarify the standard of care in the evaluation of competitive athletes. Physicians should strictly adhere to the recommendations from the American Heart Association in testing both symptomatic and asymptomatic athletes. Athletes may alternatively wish to use ET as a training tool to evaluate and improve performance. In either case, it is imperative to choose a proper protocol in which to test the athlete, as well as be familiar with the normal variants exhibited by well-trained athletes, to properly interpret their test.

References

1. ACSM. Resource manual for guidelines for exercise testing and prescription, 4th ed. Baltimore, Williams and Wilkins, 2001.
2. Maron BJ, Thompson PD, Ackerman MJ, et al. Recommendations and considerations related to preparticipation screening for cardiovascular abnormalities in competitive athletes: 2007 update. A scientific statement from the American Heart Association Council on nutrition, physical activity, and metabolism, American Heart Association. Circulation 2007; 115: 1643–55.
3. Pfister GC, Puffer JC, Maron BJ. Preparticipation cardiovascular screening for US collegiate student-athletes. JAMA 2000; 283:1597–99.
4. Glover DW, Maron BJ. Profile of preparticipation cardiovascular screening for high school athletes. JAMA 1998; 279:1817–19.
5. Maron BJ, Araújo CG, Thompson PD, Fletcher GF, de Luna AB, Fleg JL, et al. Recommendations for preparticipation screening and the assessment of cardiovascular disease in masters athletes: an advisory for healthcare professionals from the working groups of the World Heart Federation, the International Federation of Sports Medicine, and the American Heart Association Committee on Exercise, Cardiac Rehabilitation, and Prevention. Circulation 2001; 103:327–34.
6. Expert Panel, on Detection, Evaluation, and Treatment of High Blood Cholesterol in adults. Summary of the third report of the National Cholesterol Education Program (NCP) expert panel on detection, evaluation, and treatment of high blood cholesterol in adults (Adult Treatment Panel III). JAMA 2001; 285:2486–97.
7. Hood S, Northcote RJ. Cardiac assessment of veteran endurance athletes: a 12 year follow-up study. Br J Sports Med 1999; 33:239–43.
8. Bryant BA, Limacher MC. Exercise testing in selected patient groups, elderly, and the asymptomatic. In Evans CH (ed.), Exercise Testing: Current Patient Management. Primary Care 1994; 21:517–34.
9. Virmani R, Burke AP, Farb A. The pathology of sudden cardiac death in athletes. In Williams RA (ed.), The Athlete and Heart Disease: Diagnosis, Evaluation, and Management. Philadelphia, Lippincott, Williams and Wilkins, 1999.
10. Basilico FC. Cardiovascular disease in athletes. Am J Sports Med 1999; 27:108–121.
11. Corrado D, Basso C, Thiene G. Sudden Death in young athletes. Lancet 2005; 366(suppl 1):S47–S48.

12. Corrado D, Basso C, Schiavon M, et al. Screening for hypertrophic cardiomyopathy in young athletes. N Engl J Med. 1998; 339:364–69.
13. Lee IM, Hsieeh CC, Paffembarger RS Jr. Exercise intensity and longevity in men: the Harvard Alumni Health Study. JAMA 1995; 273:1179–84.
14. ACC/AHA Guidelines for Exercise Testing: a report of the American College of Cardiology/American heart Association Task Force on Practice Guidelines (Committee on Exercise Testing). JACC 1997; 30(3):268.
15. Marolf GA, Kuhn A, White RD. Exercise testing in special populations: athletes, women, and the elderly. Primary Care 2001; 28:58.
16. Pate RR, Durstine JL. Exercise Physiology and its role in clinical sports medicine. So Med J 2004; 97:881–85.
17. Farrell PA, Wilmore JH, Coyle EF, et al. Plasma lactate accumulation and distance running performance. Med Sci Sports Exerc 1979; 11:338–44.
18. Tananka K, Matsuura Y. Marathon performance, anaerobic threshold, and onset of blood lactate accumulation. J Appl Physiol 1984; 57:640–43.
19. Buchfuhrer MJ, Hansen JE, Robinson TE, Sue DY, Wasserman K, Whipp BJ. Optimizing the exercise protocol for cardiopulmonary assessment. J Appl Physiol 1983; 55:1558–64.
20. Myers J, Buchanan N, Walsh D, Kraemer M, McAuley P, Hamilton-Wessler M. Comparison of the ramp versus standard exercise protocols. J Am Coll Cardiol 1991; 17:1334–42.
21. Balke B, Ware R. An experimental study of physical fitness of air force personnel. US Armed Forces Med J 1959; 10:675–80.
22. Astrand PO, Rodahl K. Textbook of Work Physiology. New York, McGraw-Hill, 1986, pp. 331–65.
23. Costill DL, Fox EL. Energetics of marathon running. Med Sci Sports Exerc 1969; 1:81–86.
24. Froehlicher VF, Brammell H, Davis G, Noguera I, Steward A, Lancaster MC. A comparison of the reproducibility and physiologic response to three maximal treadmill exercise protocols. Chest 1974; 68:331–36.
25. Pollock ML, Bohannon RL, Cooper KH. A comparative analysis of four protocols for maximal treadmill stress testing. Am Heart J 1976; 92:39–46.
26. Webster MWJ, Sharpe DN. Exercise testing in angina pectoris: the importance of protocol design in clinical trials. Am Heart J 1989; 117:505–08.
27. Will PM, Walter JD. Exercise testing: improving performance with a ramped Bruce protocol. Amer Heart J 1999; 138:1033–37.
28. Harrison MH, Brown GA, Cochrane LA. Maximal oxygen uptake: its measurement, application, and limitations. Aviat Space Environ Med 1980; 51:1123–27.
29. Basset FA, Boulay MR. Specificity of treadmill and cycle ergometer tests in triathletes, runners and cyclists. Eur J Appl Physiol 2000; 81:214–21.
30. Bouckaert J, Pannier JL, Vrijens J. Cardiorespiratory response to bicycle and rowing ergometer exercise in oarsmen. Eur J Appl Physiol 1983; 51:51–59.
31. Aziz AR, Chia MY, Teh KC. Measured maximal oxygen uptake in a multi-stage shuttle test and treadmill-run test in trained athletes. J Sports Med Phys Fitness 2005; 45:306–14.
32. Huston TP, Puffer JC, Rodney WM. The athletic heart syndrome. N Engl J Med 1985; 313:24–32.
33. Holly RG, Shaffrath JD, Amsterdam EA. Electrocardiographic alterations associated with the hearts of athletes. Sports Med 1998; 25:139–48.
34. Pelliccia A, Maron BJ, Culasso F, et al. Clinical significance of abnormal electrocardiographic patterns in trained athletes. Circulation 2000; 102:278–84.
35. Grumet J, Hizon J, Froelicher V. Special considerations in exercise testing: protocols, equipment, and testing athletes. In Evans CH (ed.), Exercise Testing: Current Applications for Patient Management. Primary Care 1994; 21:459–74.
36. Spirito P, Maron BJ, Bonow RO, et al. Prevalence and significance of an abnormal St-segment response to exercise in a young athletic population. Am J Cardiol 1983; 51:1663–66.
37. Ellestad MH. Stress Testing: Principles and Practice, 4th ed. Philadelphia, FA, Davis, 1996.

38. Kitagawa T, Mizushima Y, Sato H, et al. ECG-ST level, maximal oxygen uptake, and ventilatory threshold during treadmill exercise test in athletes and non-athletes. Vivo 1996; 10: 307–11.
39. Futterman LG, Myerburg R. Sudden death in athletes: an update. Sports Med 1998; 26: 335–50.
40. Paterick TE, Paterick TJ, Fletcher GF, et al. Medical and legal Issues in the cardiovascular evaluation of competitive athletes. JAMA 2005; 294:3011–18.

Chapter 19
Exercise Testing for the Symptomatic Athlete

Karl B. Fields

Many physicians consider exercise tolerance testing for athletes to be counterintuitive in that these individuals routinely perform high-level activity that would stress the cardiovascular system. However, numerous case reports of high-level athletes experiencing cardiac death have underscored the importance of identifying the athlete with symptoms that warrant evaluation. An additional challenge of deciding who merits testing is the labeling of individuals as athletes and the differentiation between symptoms of physiologic stress and pathophysiology.

Who is an athlete? If one considers that the American College of Sports Medicine (ACSM) definition for vigorous exercise requires the exertion of only a six metabolic equivalent (MET) workload [1], most of our younger and middle-aged patients routinely exceed this level. The current ACSM recommendations for physical activity qualify as moderate activity and easily can exceed the level defined as vigorous. Thus, a physician who strongly believes in the value of exercise tolerance testing (ETT) screening for athletes finds that most men above age 45 and smaller numbers of women above age 55 fall into the level of risk that merits testing (based on performance of work loads of moderate level for individuals with two or more risk factors or vigorous level with or without risk factors). For the athlete with symptoms, the nature of the symptoms outweighs any considerations of age or cardiac risk factors in the decision to perform testing.

Identifying the symptomatic athlete also poses unique challenges, as strenuous aerobic activity always stresses the cardiopulmonary system. The description of the complaint must seem different or out of proportion to what an athlete experiences with exhaustive effort. In pediatric age groups and young adults, chest pain usually arises from a non-cardiac origin. Above age 30, chest pain in adults requires the subjective interpretation of the individual physician as to whether the complaint represents typical, atypical or non-anginal pain. Fortunately, guidelines help direct testing of both men and women with this complaint based on the pretest probability

K.B. Fields (✉)
Moses Cone Health System, Greensboro, NC; Department of Family Medicine,
University of North Carolina at Chapel Hill, Greensboro, NC, USA
e-mail: bert.fields@mosescone.com

C.H. Evans, R.D. White (eds.), *Exercise Testing for Primary Care and Sports Medicine Physicians*, DOI 10.1007/978-0-387-76597-6_19

353

of coronary artery disease. See Table 2.1 for data summarizing probability based on age, gender and type of pain.

The American College of Cardiology/American Heart Association (ACC/AHA) guidelines of 2002 [3] underscore that virtually all adult men and many women with chest pain whether defined as athletes or not would be reasonable candidates for testing. The summary recommendations are as follows:

- Patients with pretest probability of 10–90% adjusted for age, gender and symptoms
- Patient must have stable chest pain if symptomatic
- Patients with electrokardiogram (EKG) such as right bundle branch block (RBBB) or <1 mm of ST-segment depression can be tested

These three points are considered Class I recommendations.

While chest pain guidelines direct physician decision making for ordering an ETT, less information is available to weigh the seriousness of other symptoms. The complexity of other symptoms relates to the type and level of activity done. Dyspnea, for example, while a key symptom in the cardiac patient, occurs routinely with maximum effort in sport. Thus the clinician must decide whether the dyspnea was out of proportion to the effort exerted, atypical in the time of onset, of prolonged duration or associated with other troubling symptoms. Similarly, palpitations often occur with arrhythmias. Since intense effort requires maximal heart rate (HR), individuals may describe their heart rate as "racing" after a particularly vigorous effort. Tachycardia or very irregular rhythms early in exercise would always suggest the possibility of pathology, as would arrhythmias associated with collapse during exercise. However, for tachycardia at maximal exercise or at the completion of exercise, relying on history to distinguish symptoms related to effort from those associated with cardiac disease is often not possible.

Excessive fatigue in an adult athlete also raises the question of cardiac dysfunction. Athletes routinely push themselves to the point of fatigue and sometimes experience fatigue for several days after a prolonged effort. For example, marathoners may require a few weeks to recover from a hard race. Triathlon training often requires working at multiple sports, sometimes on the same day. The total time and intensity of workouts can determine the degree of fatigue experienced afterwards. However, when well-trained individuals begin noticing fatigue early in workouts or on efforts that are usually considered light training days, this becomes an important observation. In men above 40 and women above 50, this type of complaint should trigger consideration of cardiac screening. Syncope represents a serious symptom in most medical patients. However, post-exercise collapse and even brief syncope are relatively common after road races, cross country events and marathons. These episodes carry a less serious prognosis. They typically arise from decreased blood volume and hypotension once muscle activity ends and venous return to the heart drops off. For this reason, race directors have learned to keep runners walking at the end of events until they recover somewhat. Collapse or syncope during the performance of exercise, though, always increases the likelihood that cardiac causes underlie the symptoms. Whether secondary to arrhythmia or ischemic change, ETT may reveal the cause and is part of the standard evaluation.

The following cases demonstrate the use of ETT to evaluate symptoms in athletes. These cases all have diagnostic findings on ETT. Follow-up in these cases ranges from 5 to 15 years and offers further evidence to support the conclusions derived from ETT. The quality of some of the tracings is due to their age. Many cases do not have a clear diagnosis even after ETT, and in those situations the full range of cardiac testing may be necessary. The symptoms experienced in these patients are not specific but seemed significant enough to the author to initiate further testing. As in all clinical medicine, judgment rather than specific evidence-based medicine (EBM) determines diagnostic assessment of individual patients. However, when possible, the author has offered clinical studies that help influence the ultimate interpretation of these test findings.

Case Studies

Case 1A: Chest Pain in a 50-Year-Old Athlete

JB is a 50-year-old computer instructor who has remained thin and active his entire life. Currently, he exercises by running approximately 3 miles, 5 times weekly and routinely does physical work, such as gardening and cutting trees. Recently he began having sharp, somewhat tight feeling, mid-chest pain, almost always occurring about 9 minutes into his runs. He would slow down for about 2 minutes and then be able to complete the remainder of the run without symptoms. His breathing would feel constricted when this occurred, but he never experienced radiation of chest pain, nausea, extreme fatigue or any other symptoms. He has a history of allergic rhinitis and wonders if his symptoms are coming from exercise-induced asthma (EIA). He comes to the office requesting a trial of albuterol to see if this will resolve his chest pain and tightness. Risk factors include a positive family history of coronary artery disease and a low high density lipoprotein (HDL) of 30. We recommend an ETT before considering the diagnosis of EIA (Fig. 19.1A).

At 9 minutes into the test, the patient experiences very mild chest tightness—not severe enough that he feels he should stop exercising. Continuous monitoring reveals ST depression beginning in inferior leads and gradually increasing in II, III, AVF and in V_5 and V_6. EKG tracing at 9 minutes and 13 seconds shows significant changes. EKG findings of ST-segment depression persist, as shown on 3-minute recovery tracing. Note the patient is asymptomatic at this point and all symptoms resolved within 30 seconds of exercise cessation. Fit athletes often demonstrate rapid heart rate recovery as we note in Fig. 19.1C, even though the ST-segment depression persists and appears downsloping in V_5 and V_6.

Based on results of this test, this patient was sent for catheterization and found to have a 90% occlusion of the mid-right coronary artery. Other vessels were free of disease and his ejection fraction was normal. He underwent successful angioplasty and returned to his normal running routine within 3 months.

A

B

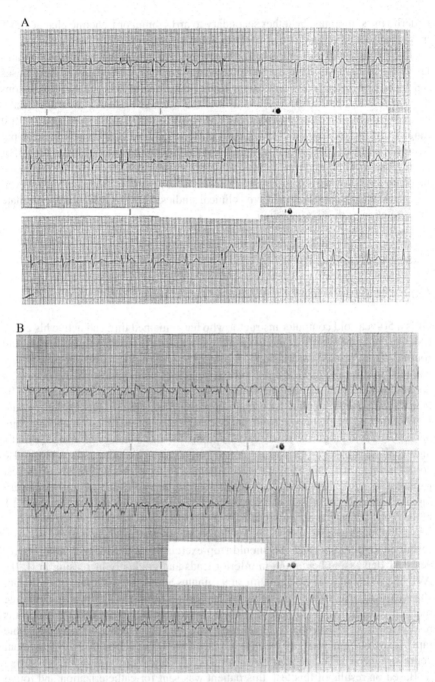

Fig. 19.1 (**A**) Resting tracing appears normal in this active 50-year-old patient. (**B**) EKG tracing at 9 minutes and 13 seconds shows significant changes. (**C**) The patient demonstrated rapid heart rate recovery, even though the ST-segment depression persists and appears downsloping in V_5 and V_6

C

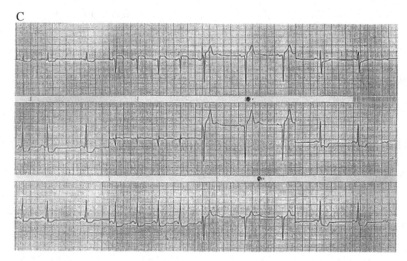

Fig. 19.1 (continued)

Teaching points from this case include the importance of evaluation of chest pain in any adult athlete. In a 50-year-old man, whether you feel the chest pain history represents non-anginal pain or atypical angina, the patient would still fall into a pretest probability that ranges from 20 to 65%. These statistics clearly make this individual a good candidate for ETT (Class I ACC). Even assuming that the patient described symptoms that the doctor believes represents EIA, recommending an ETT in an individual pursuing vigorous exercise who also has two major risk factors and age as variables would be the correct choice of action (Class II ACC) [3].

Case 1B: 57-Year-Old White Man with Sharp Chest Pains

This same patient remained active and had uneventful yearly follow-ups until returning 7 years after angioplasty in 2001. He complains of decreased energy on his 3-mile runs and occasional sharp chest pains that resolve after 20–30 seconds of walking. We perform an ETT the next day.

This EKG looks almost identical to the one performed 7 years earlier (Fig. 19.2). One difference is that on this ETT all ST-segment depression has returned to normal by the 1-minute recovery tracing. While this patient quickly normalizes his EKG changes and chest pain and can perform almost 10 metabolic equivalents (METs) of activity before developing these symptoms, his history suggests that he has been exceeding his anginal threshold with vigorous activity. Considering that the patient has known cardiac disease and is status post-angioplasty, we refer him for invasive testing. Catheterization shows triple vessel disease and the patient undergoes successful bypass surgery. He has returned to full activity since surgery and remains asymptomatic to date.

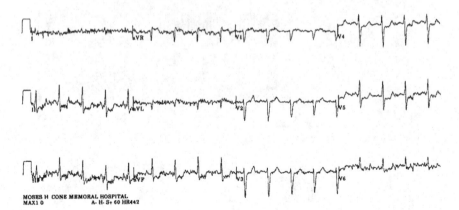

MOSES H CONE MEMORAL HOSPITAL
MAX1 0   A- H- S+ 60 HR442

Fig. 19.2 The same patient shown in Fig. 19.1 is seen 7 years later. His EKG looks almost identical to the one performed 7 years earlier. One difference is that ST-segment depression has returned to normal by the 1-minute recovery tracing

Teaching points of this follow-up testing include that once a patient has known heart disease, any suggestive symptoms, even when very mild, warrant ETT investigation (Class I ACC) [3]. Following angioplasty, stress imaging may provide more information than standard ETT. However, in this case we could schedule the ETT quickly and chose to go ahead. Even though epidemiologic studies of stress testing show that individuals having had a prior myocardial infarction (MI) and achieving 10.7 MET workloads have only average risk of death for their age group [4], this patient could not be considered at average risk. Since he had already demonstrated that he was symptomatic with his current activities, he would have to be considered at higher risk.

Case 2: 48-Year-Old Marathon Runner with Shortness of Breath

RD has run for 20 years, completing numerous marathons and averaging 40 miles of training per week. In preparation for a marathon, he notes that he becomes short of breath if he eats too soon before running. He has a history of reflux, but has not noticed any chest pain or "heartburn" symptoms. He also notes that on the previous week's 18-mile run he felt extremely fatigued at 14 miles, even though he was able to complete the full distance. He has a blood pressure (BP) of 115/70 mmHg, pulse of 52, total cholesterol of 150 and no other classic risk factors. He does admit to extreme marital stress.

Resting tracing shows increased voltage but a vertically oriented heart (Fig. 19.3A). He also has nonspecific ST and T wave changes. At 13 minutes the

A Resting

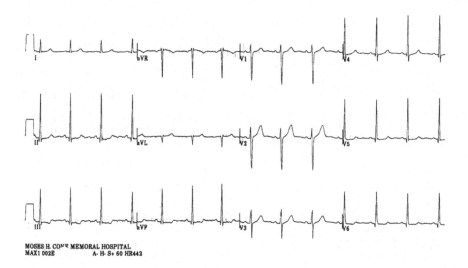

MOSES H. CO^R MEMORAL HOSPITAL
MAXI 002E   A- H- S+ 60 HR442

B   **13 Minutes**

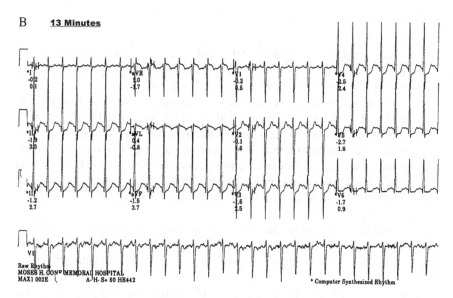

Raw Rhythm
MOSES H. CON^R MEMORAI HOSPITAL
MAXI 002E (A-JH- S+ 60 HR442   * Computer Synthesized Rhythm

Fig. 19.3 (**A**) Resting tracing shows increased voltage but a vertically oriented heart. (**B**) At 13 minutes the patient has some upsloping ST-segment depression in several leads and more planar appearing ST-segment depression of 1.7 mm in lead V_6. (**C**) At 3 minutes of recovery the patient demonstrates downsloping ST-segment changes with T wave inversion

C   **Recovery - 3 Minutes**

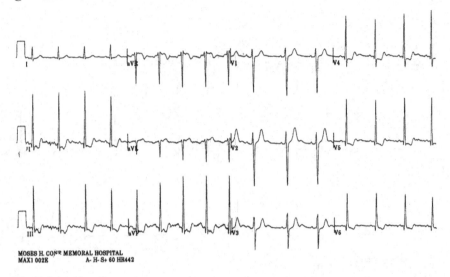

MOSES H. CONE MEMORAL HOSPITAL
MAX1 002E   A- H- S+ 60 HR442

Fig. 19.3 (continued)

patient has some upsloping ST-segment depression in several leads, and more planar appearing ST-segment depression of 1.7 mm in lead V_6 (Fig. 19.3B). At 13 minutes and 43 seconds he reaches his maximum exercise tolerance.

At 1 minute of recovery the patient has a somewhat limited heart rate recovery of about 15 beats – much less than expected for a well-conditioned distance runner. Many runners will recover 30 beats per minute so that they return to a HR of <100 in 3 minutes. This is a heart rate recovery approach often used in distance training to determine when the runner can do a repeat interval training run. This recovery rate would be in the poor category for 1 minute in a distance runner who has been training consistently. Note also that by 3 minutes he does have a HR recovery to a rate of less than 100.

At 3 minutes of recovery the patient demonstrates downsloping ST-segment changes with T wave inversion (Fig. 19.3C). The ST changes increase until beginning to resolve at 9 minutes post-exercise. He remains asymptomatic throughout this monitoring.

RD is sent for catheterization that reveals a 95% right coronary artery occlusion and smaller lesion in the distal left anterior descending coronary artery and one diagonal. These are successfully stented and the patient returns to marathon running within 18 months.

On a visit for an orthopedic running injury, 27 months post-stenting, RD admits to having some chest pain which he feels is a worsening of his reflux symptoms. He is sent for catheterization after counseling and found to have triple vessel disease. He undergoes successful bypass surgery and has resumed marathon running at present.

Several teaching points emerge from Case 2. Shortness of breath in a runner that is out of proportion to effort represents a cardiac equivalent symptom until proven otherwise. Many individuals with reflux, or, as in Case 1, with a history of possible asthma symptoms, tend to deny the significance of symptoms that may represent cardiac disease. Fatigue experienced at 14 miles of a standard long run would also have to be considered atypical and a possible cardiac symptom. While 14 miles of running is extreme for most individuals, this athlete was used to that degree of exertion and typically completed these runs with less effort. This patient had no major risk factors identified prior to diagnosis. He also followed medical management faithfully after his angioplasty but, nevertheless, had rapidly progressive coronary artery disease.

Poor heart rate recovery has been documented in some studies to be a predictor of coronary artery disease. In one analysis [5], at completion of a Bruce protocol, individuals were asked to continue walking at 1.5 MPH on a 2.5% grade. Those who had heart rate recovery of 12 beats or less at 1 minute had high risk of coronary artery disease. Similarly, other studies have looked at 2 minutes recovery ranges and found that individuals with recovery of less than 22 beats per minute at 2 minutes post-test were at greater risk [6, 7]. Well-conditioned distance runners usually drop 30 beats or more in 1 minute. This patient's decline of only 15 beats may have been an indirect marker of his coronary artery disease (Class 2, LOE B).

Case 3: 48-Year-Old Man with Fatigue

GB is a male construction worker, who comes in for a medical check because he wants to begin playing softball again. He notes he has been more fatigued at work and feels that getting back into sports will give him more energy. Since he has been sedentary and wants to begin an exercise program we recommend an ETT (Class II ACC).

The resting tracing reveals poor R wave progression in anterior leads and non-specific ST and T waves changes (Fig. 19.4A). At only 5 minutes, GB reaches a maximum predicted HR and also shows marked ST-segment depression in inferior and lateral leads (Fig. 19.4B). This represents an exercise tolerance level of less than 6 METS. GB was referred for catheterization and had triple vessel coronary artery disease. He underwent successful bypass surgery.

Multiple teaching points arise from this case: The first is the subjective nature of fatigue as a complaint. Some clinicians would consider that this ETT was done for a symptomatic patient with fatigue representing a potential cardiac symptom. Others would not interpret such general symptoms as being specific to exercise and therefore as not specific enough to warrant testing. In this scenario, screening based on sedentary lifestyle and desire to begin an exercise program is suggested (Class II) but not a Class I recommendation [3]. This type of patient represents a dilemma in interpretation of ETT guidelines, and the clinician's judgment determines the course of action.

A

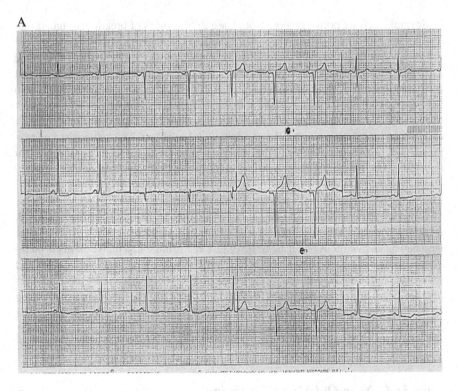

B

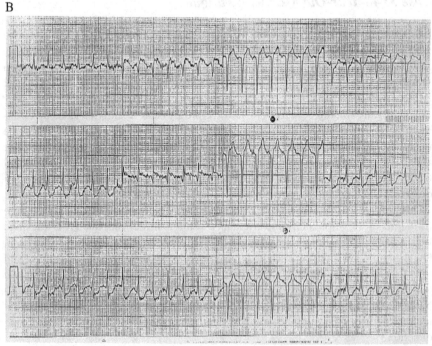

Fig. 19.4 (**A**) The resting tracing reveals poor R wave progression in anterior leads and nonspecific ST and T waves changes. (**B**)At only 5 minutes, GB reaches a maximum predicted HR and also shows marked ST-segment depression in inferior and lateral leads

A second teaching point is the significance of poor fitness level. This patient achieved less than 6 METS of a work load. This type of poor performance is associated with left main coronary artery disease, triple vessel disease and marked deconditioning. Along with the significant ST-segment depression, this poor exercise tolerance made referral for invasive testing an easy decision in this case. However, had this individual not shown ST-segment depression, he probably still would have merited invasive or at least additional testing to try to explain the low exercise tolerance. Age-adjusted relative risks of death for patients with an exercise tolerance of less than 6 METs range from 4.0 to 4.5 times normal whether they have known cardiovascular (CV) disease or not [4]. (Class I, LOE A)

A final point is that occupation and appearances both can deceive the clinician in making judgments about a patient's cardiac fitness. This patient was not excessively obese and appeared no worse than the average man his age. His work consisted of heavy construction involving lifting and shoveling. He had never had chest pain with work activities. In spite of this, the patient's ETT suggests that he would be symptomatic with much of the standard work involved in construction. This again raises the question of whether his complaints of fatigue were actually a cardiac equivalent symptom.

Case 4: 46-Year-Old Marathoner with Syncope

GR, an experienced marathoner, traveled to Minneapolis to run the Twin Cities marathon. He awakened at 4 AM to go to the bathroom and "blacked out," hitting his head against the door. He thinks he was briefly unconscious, but in any regard, aroused quickly and felt fine. He ate breakfast and went to the race, finishing the marathon uneventfully.

Two weeks later he came into the office for assessment. His wife has insisted he get some evaluation for his blackout spell, as he had another near syncopal episode in his kitchen when he had difficulty swallowing a bagel. He notes that several times he has had dizzy episodes while eating difficult to swallow foods.

His physical exam is entirely normal, with the exception that his resting heart rate averages 42. His BP is consistently 110/70 mmHg without significant orthostatic change. As part of his overall workup, cardiac, pulmonary and neurological tests are scheduled to assess his syncope. Cardiac tests demonstrate some interesting findings, as noted on ETT and Holter. His echocardiogram (ECHO) is normal with an excellent ejection fraction.

Holter monitor showed the following changes (Fig. 19.5A–C): This 6 beat run of ventricular tachycardia was entirely without symptoms. These two strips show isolated periods of complete heart block. In the second strip the patient has a pause of approximately 3.8 seconds. Both of these episodes occur entirely without symptoms.

The author discussed the worrisome Holter results with a consulting electrophysiologist and based on the excellent ejection fraction and absence of symptoms during the ventricular arrhythmia and during the brief episodes of complete heart block, we decided to proceed with the ETT.

Resting tracing for ETT reveals bradycardia and prominent voltage with a normal axis (Fig. 19.5D). Maximum HR was reached only after the completion of seven stages of the Bruce protocol and a total of 21 minutes on the treadmill. There is no sign of arrhythmia or of heart block. No ST-segment depression or T wave change occurs (Fig. 19.5E).

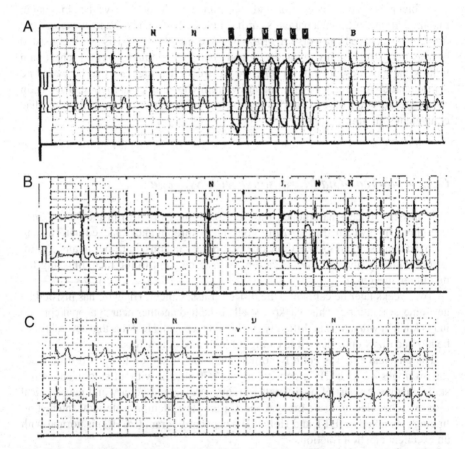

Fig. 19.5 (**A–C**) Holter monitor showed the following changes. This six beat run of ventricular tachycardia was entirely without symptoms. These two strips show isolated periods of complete heart block. (**B**) In the second strip the patient has a pause of approximately 3.8 seconds. Both of these episodes occur entirely without symptoms. (**D**) Resting tracing for ETT reveals bradycardia and prominent voltage with a normal axis. (**E**) Maximum HR was reached only after the completion of seven stages of the Bruce protocol and a total of 21 minutes on the treadmill. There is no sign of arrhythmia or of heart block. No ST-segment depression or T wave changes occur

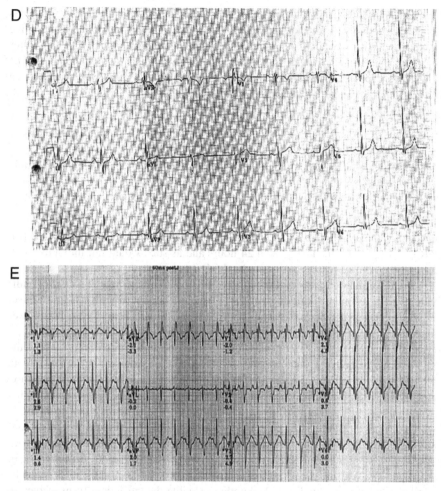

Fig. 19.5 (continued)

This level of performance ranks above 99th percentile expected for any age athlete. How does the clinician determine what course of action to follow in a case of this complexity?

Several teaching points underscore the approach we followed with this case after considerable discussion with multiple cardiology experts. EKG changes with clearly associated symptoms carry far more significance than those which seem unrelated. The Holter shows two distinctly concerning rhythm disturbances – ventricular tachycardia and complete heart block. When these abnormalities were noted, the patient was keeping an event diary and felt no symptoms and clearly did not have any of the pre-syncopal feelings that he had experienced before.

Studies of elite marathoners demonstrate that high-grade ventricular arrhythmias in athletes actually occur commonly. One study looked at a group of 355 competitive athletes with runs of three or more preventricular contractions (PVCs) on Holter monitor. The authors divided the athletes into three groups, based on the number of PVCs recorded in 24 hours, and noted the number in each group who were proven on workup to have cardiac problems.

- Group A > 2,000 PVCs per 24 hours – 21 of 71 athletes had cardiac abnormalities
- Group B > 100 but < 2,000 PVCs per 24 hours – 5 of 153 had cardiac abnormalities
- Group C < 100 PVCs in 24 hours – 0 of 131 had cardiac abnormalities

Only one athlete from Group A of the 355 total ultimately had a cardiac event [8]. GR had a total of only 15 PVCs in 24 hours and as such would fall into a low-risk group based on the results of this study *(LOE B)*.

Less information exists about benign forms of complete heart block. For individuals with second or third degree heart block and known structural heart disease, or who experience syncopal episodes correlated with their heart block, pacemaker insertion is clearly indicated. Athletic hearts lead to a variety of rhythm changes. Excessive vagotonia in athletes may lead to syncope and marked bradycardia during valsalva maneuvers, such as straining to urinate or swallowing. In this athlete we had a history of two provocative factors in his syncope evaluation – urination and swallowing. By history, the only activity that had repetitively produced his symptoms was difficulty swallowing. Were the complete heart block pathologic, we would have trouble explaining the excellent ECHO results and the exceptionally high performance on stress testing. These recurrent episodes associated with swallowing suggest that a likely diagnosis is carotid sinus hypersensitivity [9]. In these patients, carotid sinus massage may induce asystole for up to 3 seconds, similar to what was noted in GR. Another possible diagnosis is a form of benign congenital complete heart block, which occurs with an incidence of 1 in 15,000 to 1 in 20,000 live births [10]. Other acquired forms of heart block can follow viral infections.

Based on our assumption that this individual had athletic vagotonia and probably carotid sinus hypersensitivity, our instructions were to avoid swallowing foods that were difficult, particularly bagels, pizza crust or large pieces of meat. Following this dietary change he has not had any presyncopal events. He has returned for yearly stress tests for 10 years and has had two repeat Holter monitors. Subsequent Holters have been normal and his ETT results still reveal extremely high fitness levels. The patient continues to race in competitive cycling events at age 57 – several in excess of 100 miles. He has not exhibited any further signs of complete heart block by EKG or of ventricular tachycardia and has required no cardiac intervention.

Case 5: 39-Year-Old Male Former Runner Who Wants to Start Training Again

RB enters the office saying he wants an ETT as he knows he has risk factors. He is not clear whether he has any symptoms but may occasionally feel an irregular beat when stressed. He has a family history of heart disease, has been sedentary for 5 years and has a cholesterol of 214.

During the stress test he reaches a maximum heart rate in about 9 minutes and 30 seconds of the Bruce protocol (Fig. 19.6A). The patient has reached approximately 10 METs of a work load which is average for his age. He has no significant ST or T wave change. However, a rhythm change appeared near maximal exercise (Fig. 19.6B). No further PVCs occur during recovery and the patient was asymptomatic with this 3 beat run. How dose one advise him regarding risk?

At maximal exercise, athletes tend to become anaerobic and can experience ventricular irritability. This patient is more concerning, as he has not maintained good conditioning. However, his benign recovery phase is reassuring, based on the following study of multiple ETT results. This prospective study related the timing of PVCs to clinical outcomes over 5 years, and underscores the fact that while PVCs frequently occur in ETTs, special attention should be paid to those individuals who demonstrate these in recovery.

- Prospective study of 29,000 patients of whom 70% were men with a mean age of 56
- Clinically indicated tests terminated by symptoms

A

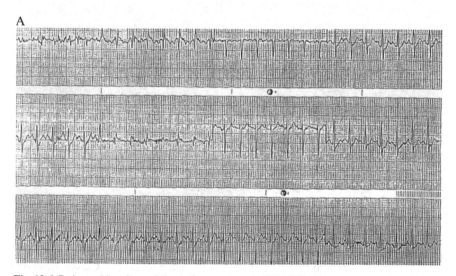

Fig. 19.6 Patient achieved a work load of approximately 10 METS, which was average for his age. At higher heart rates after 9.5 minutes of testing he shows some ventricular irritability, and has a run of 3 PVCs. He had an unremarkable recovery tracing and no symptoms with the arrhythmia

B

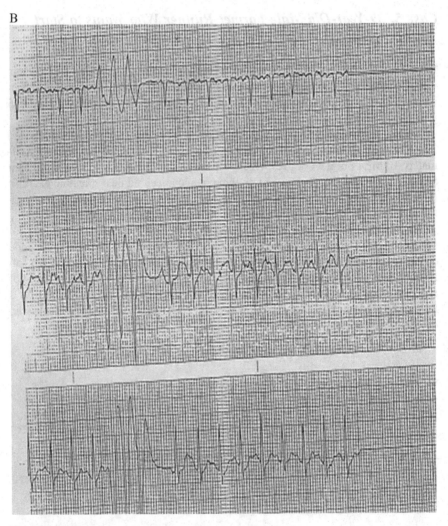

Fig. 19.6 (continued)

- 3% had PVCs only during exercise
- 2% had PVCs only during recovery
- 2% had PVCs during both

After controlling variables, PVCs during recovery but not during exercise were associated with increased risk of death within the next 5 years [11] (Class I, LOE A).

RB began his running program and within 1 year had lost 20 pounds. He also dropped his cholesterol by 30 points and his systolic blood pressure by 15 mmHg. On repeat testing 15 months after his initial test he exceeded 12 MET work load (good for age) and had no PVCs.

Case 6: 51-Year-Old Female Water Aerobics Instructor with Palpitations

SJ, an active swimmer, began noticing palpitations, at times following teaching a water aerobics class and other times after a stressful event. She never had chest pain, but would feel some dizziness as if her head were spinning with these events. They occurred infrequently and her examination and laboratory tests proved unremarkable, so we chose to do an ETT (Fig. 19.7A).

Maximal exercise occurred at about 9 minutes into the testing, which was good for the patient's age and represented a workload of 9.5 METs. She had no symptoms and an unremarkable EKG tracing with a maximum HR of ~160. During recovery she developed her classic palpitation symptoms after about 5 minutes. On the tracing shown in Fig. 19.7B, her HR is approximately 185 with a classic pattern of supraventricular tachycardia (SVT) and she shows significant ST-segment depression, probably related to her rate being well above 100% of her maximum predicted HR.

SJ responded well to medical management and reported no significant bouts of palpitations at the 5-year follow-up after this ETT. Teaching points in this case include that the recovery period is an integral part of the complete ETT assessment. For most cases of SVT, the ETT is not likely to yield the diagnosis. However, since SJ's symptoms warranted the testing, we were able to quickly establish a diagnosis and prescribe an effective treatment. The ETT could also be used in follow-up to assess the effectiveness of medication in controlling a rhythm disorder.

Summary and Discussion

This chapter offers six cases to illustrate key symptoms that may herald cardiac disease. Chest pain, shortness of breath, fatigue, syncope and palpitations all can be serious signs of heart dysfunction or have completely benign explanations. The ETT becomes one key tool in risk stratification to decide how to proceed with clinical management.

Chest pain is among the most common symptoms seen in emergency departments and many offices. Good analysis of pretest probability helps guide the use of ETT. Certainly the ETT offers a number of advantages in that the exercise tolerance independent of EKG helps predict risk category. In addition, ETT costs much less than most other cardiac tests. ETT can identify the workload that provokes anginal symptoms in certain patients, which may determine whether it is safe to return to work or recreational activities without invasive intervention. ETT is generally indicated in most men with nonanginal chest pain, atypical angina or typical angina. In women, the test is more useful in those with atypical or typical angina. Exceptions would be those men and women with extremely low risk (<10%) of coronary artery disease or exceptionally high risk (> 85–90%).

The seriousness of shortness of breath with exercise becomes a subjective decision on the part of the physician. In cases with very confusing histories, cardiopul-

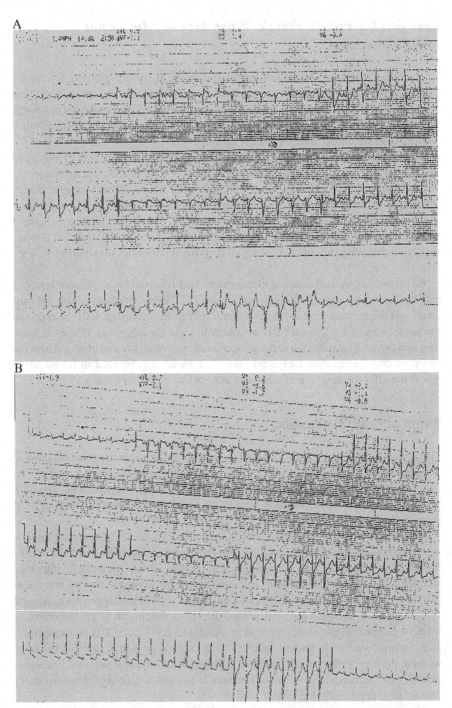

Fig. 19.7 (**A**) Maximal exercise occurred at about 9 minutes into the testing, which was good for the patient's age and represented a workload of 9.5 METs. She had no symptoms and an unremarkable EKG tracing with a maximum HR of approximately 160. During recovery she developed her classic palpitation symptoms after about 5 minutes. (**B**) The patient's HR is approximately 185 mmHg with a classic pattern of supraventricular tachycardia (SVT) and she shows significant ST-segment depression, probably related to her rate being well above 100% of her maximum predicted HR

monary testing adds the ability to measure gas exchange and to see if pulmonary dysfunction causes the patient's symptoms. When the physician has a strong suspicion that EIA may be causing the shortness of breath or chest tightness (such as that of RD in Case 1), peak flow measures can also be checked before, during and after the performance of the ETT. In patients with an intermediate risk of coronary artery disease, this complaint should be considered a cardiac equivalent symptom until coronary artery disease has been excluded as a diagnosis.

Fatigue that correlates with poor fitness has a serious prognosis. Meyers correlated poor fitness with cardiac outcomes in two large groups of 6,213 men referred for ETT [4]. Results showed that 3,679 of these individuals had significant cardiac or pulmonary disease, and 2,534 had no known serious medical problems. Mortality of these two groups was compared based on their fitness levels. When compared to all the standard cardiac risk factors in both the group with and without cardiac or pulmonary disease, fitness was the best predictor of mortality [4]. Meyers also noted that those who could perform greater than an 8 MET workload on ETT had low risk even if they had any of the following negative risk factors: hypertension, chronic obstructive pulmonary disease, diabetes, smoking, body mass index >30 or cholesterol >220 mg/dl.

In fact, for each MET of fitness gained (usually about 1 additional minute on most ETT protocols), patients had a 12% improvement in survival. Thus the 48-year-old man in Case 3 who reached a maximum heart rate in only 5 minutes (< 6 METs) had a poor prognosis based on his exercise tolerance regardless of his EKG changes or any preexisting risk factors.

Syncope has many potential etiologies. However, syncope noted during the performance of exercise always requires the exclusion of cardiac disease. In Case 4, GR had several concerning episodes but none of these involved exercise. His exercise tolerance actually fell into the top 1% of any age group. Cardiovascular syncope carries a poor prognosis and represents the spectrum from severe coronary artery disease to ventricular arrhythmias to obstructive valvular or subvalvular structural anomalies.

These diagnoses would be incompatible with GR's ability to perform an ETT at this level and also may have shown changes on his ECHO. One important factor to consider in testing athletes is that athletic individuals commonly demonstrate rhythm disturbances. Before determining that the arrhythmia represents pathology and not the physiologic response of an athletic heart, every effort should be made to establish if symptoms occur with the observed EKG changes. Even though we demonstrated two potentially serious rhythm changes in this patient, we could not correlate these with any symptoms.

Finally, palpitations often represent the patient's awareness of a rhythm disturbance. While in Case 6 we identified SVT in the recovery phase, a negative ETT would not have excluded significant arrhythmia. In fact, a 24-hour Holter or a longer term event monitor frequently is required to make a specific diagnosis. Recently, reports suggest that certain supraventricular rhythm problems such as atrial fibrillation may actually be more common in endurance athletes even though they are associated with low cardiovascular mortality [12]. Fitness may not protect against all cardiovascular problems; as such, palpitations require the same intensity of diagnostic search in the athletic as in the nonathletic individual.

In this group of six athletic patients, three ultimately required stenting, coronary artery bypass graft or both. Two of the individuals were allowed to continue vigorous exercise in spite of identification of ventricular rhythm abnormalities and, in one case, transient complete heart block. These two individuals required no medical treatment. SJ was able to resume her aerobic teaching after using medications to control SVT. In each case, the ETT led to the ultimate decision of what clinical path to follow. With follow-up ranging from 5 to 15 years, each of these patients remains active in athletic pursuits, which ultimately may be the greatest benefit to their health.

Acknowledgments The author would like to thank Teresa Rasco for her editing and help with the preparation of this manuscript.

References

1. American College of Sports Medicine. Guidelines for Exercise Testing and Prescription, 6th ed. Lea and Febiger, eds. Philadelphia: Lippincott, Williams & Wilkins, 2000.
2. Garber AM, Hlatky MA. Stress testing for the diagnosis of coronary heart disease. In: UpToDate Version 15.1, 2007.
3. Gibbons RJ, Balady GJ, Bricker JT, et al. ACC/AHA 2002 guideline update for exercise testing: summary article. A report of the American College of Cardiology/American Heart Association Task Force on Practice Guidelines (Committee to Update the 1997 Exercise Testing Guidelines). Circulation 2002;106:1883.
4. Myers J, Prakash M, Froelicher V, Do D, Partington S, Atwood JE. Exercise capacity and mortality among men referred for exercise testing. NEJM 2002;346:793–801.
5. Nishime EO, Cole CR, Blackstone EH, Pashkow FJ, Lauer MS. Heart rate recovery and treadmill exercise score as predictors of mortality in patients referred for exercise ECG. JAMA 2000;284(11):1392–1398.
6. Shetler K, Marcus R, Froelicher VF, Vora S, Kalisetti D, Prakash M, Dat D, Myers J. Heart rate recovery: validation and methodologic issues. J Am Coll Cardiol 2001;38(7):1980–1987.
7. Mora S, Redberg RF, Sharrett AR, Blumenthal RS. Enhanced risk assessment in asymptomatic individuals with exercise testing and Framingham risk scores. Circulation 2005;112(11): 1566–1572.
8. Biffi A, Pelliccia A, Verdile L, Fernando F, Spataro A, Caselli S, Santini M, Maron BJ. Long-term clinical significance of frequent and complex ventricular tachyarrhythmias in trained athletes. J Am Coll Cardiol 2002;40(3):446–452.
9. Olshansky B. Neurocardiogenic (vasovagal) syncope and carotid sinus hypersensitivity. In: Rose BD, ed. UpToDate. Waltham, MA: Version 15.1, 2007.
10. Arnsdorf MF. Congenital third degree (complete) atrioventricular block. In: Rose BD, ed. UpToDate. Waltham, MA: Version 15.1, 2007.
11. Frolkis JP, Pothier CE, Blackstone EH, Lauer MS. Frequent ventricular ectopy after exercise as a predictor of death [erratum appears in N Engl J Med 2003;348(15):1508]. N Engl J Med 2003;348(9):781–790.
12. Karjalainen J, Kujala UM, Kaprio J, Sarna S, Viitasalo M. Lone atrial fibrillation in vigorously exercising middle aged men: case-control study. BMJ 1998;316:1784–1785.

Part IV
Case Studies

Chapter 20
Case Studies: Lessons Learned from Interesting Cases

Corey H. Evans, H. Jack Pyhel and Russell D. White

In this chapter we illustrate many of the concepts discussed in earlier chapters with cases accumulated over years of experience performing exercise testing. It is hoped the cases will illustrate concepts through both electrocardiogram tracings and discussion. Jack Pyhel, a cardiologist with over 30 years' experience doing exercise testing, also has encountered many interesting treadmill cases shared in this chapter. All of these cases, other than being interesting, have taught valuable lessons. We hope the lessons we have learned can be passed on to the reader. Some of these cases occurred more than 20 years previously and the records were not available for illustration, plus some of the tracing are older so please bear with the tracing quality. The name at the end of each case indicate the contributor.

Case 1: Where's the Defibrillator?

A very healthy appearing 42-year-old gentleman was sent by his family practice doctor for a treadmill exam with a history of atypical chest pain. He had no family history of premature heart disease, hypertension, diabetes, dyslipidemia, or recent tobacco use.

Using a Bruce protocol he exercised into the tenth minute of exercise, Stage IV of the Bruce protocol, 4.2 miles per hour at 16% grade. His heart rate was 162 beats per minute and he was starting to tire. He had no chest pain or ST-segment change. There was no arrhythmia up to that point. Suddenly, without warning, one of the most malignant appearing episodes of ventricular tachycardia that I have ever encountered occurred. I jammed on the stop button of the treadmill as he was becoming extremely lightheaded and presyncopal. Fortunately the episode subsided spontaneously and no further treatment was necessary. He never had any chest pain and after his 6 minute recovery while I was explaining exactly what had happened he innocently asked if using cocaine could have something to do with this arrhythmia.

C.H. Evans (✉)
St. Anthony's Hospital, St. Petersburg, FL; Private Practice Family Physician, Florida Institute of Family Medicine, St. Petersburg, FL, USA
e-mail: email@coreyevansmd.com

C.H. Evans, R.D. White (eds.), *Exercise Testing for Primary Care and Sports Medicine Physicians*, DOI 10.1007/978-0-387-76597-6_20
© Springer Science+Business Media, LLC 2009

Not even 1 minute later the door to the treadmill room opened and a technician came walking in, whistling, carrying the defibrillator and told me she borrowed it from the treadmill room to use in another room in the hospital.

Lesson Learned

In 30 years I have never had to cardiovert or resuscitate anyone undergoing a treadmill examination. The one time I may have needed a defibrillator it was not there. To this day when I do a treadmill I walk in the room and look for the defibrillator. Do not let this happen to you.
H. Jack Pyhel

Case 2: Severe Ischemia Presenting as Dyspnea

A 77-year-old woman presented with 6 months of dyspnea on exertion and one episode of chest pain. Two prior physicians attributed the dyspnea to her age, without exercise testing. On exercise testing, ST-segment depression developed at 2:30 minutes on the Bruce protocol, and the test was stopped at 4:20 minutes due to severe ischemia (Fig. 20.1A). The heart rate and blood pressure were normal. Downsloping ischemia developed in recovery and lasted for 12 minutes (Fig. 20.1B). The following indications of severe ischemia were seen: ST-segment depression beginning before 5 METS of exercise, downsloping ST-segment depression, ST-segment depression in more than five leads, and ST-segment depression lasting more than 8 minutes into recovery. At cardiac catheterization she had a 98% left main lesion. She underwent two vessel by-pass and did well, living for more than 13 additional years.

Lesson Learned

Dyspnea can be due to myocardial ischemia and we need to exercise patients to find the cardiac etiology. Look for signs of severe ischemia and ensure these patients are fully evaluated as revascularization can prolong life expectancy.
Corey H. Evans

Case 3: Nitroglycerin—Friend or Foe?

A 74-year-old woman was referred for a treadmill after episodic chest pain. By history the pain was quite typical of angina pectoris, occurred with exertion, and was relieved shortly after resting. Her doctor had not prescribed any medication and she had never used nitroglycerin previously. Her past history was significant for dyslipidemia and a family history of heart disease but she was a nonsmoker and did not have hypertension or diabetes.

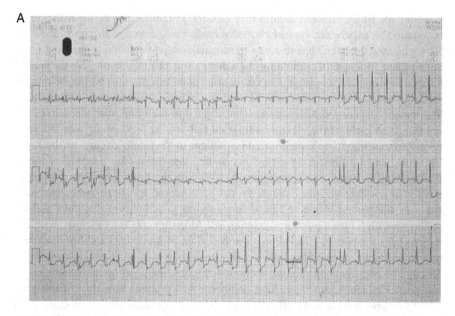

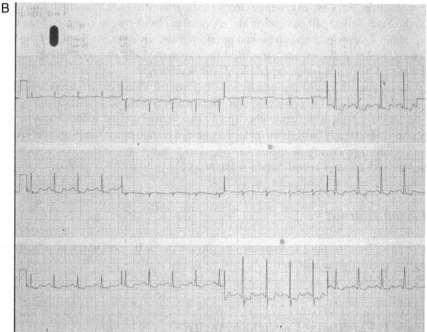

Fig. 20.1 (**A**) Electrocardiogram at peak exercise showing 2–4 mm of upsloping and horizontal ST-segment depression. Test was terminated due to these changes. (**B**) Downsloping ST-segment depression developed in recovery and lasted for 12 minutes

Using the Bruce protocol she did very well for 5 minutes. During the fifth minute she started to experience typical chest discomfort associated with rather dramatic ST-segment depression. The test was terminated just a few seconds later and I had her sit down. Because of continuing chest discomfort I had the nurse give the patient a single sublingual nitroglycerin as I have done hundreds of times before. Within 40 seconds the heart rate dramatically slowed and exhibited a long period of asystole. The patient lost consciousness and as she slipped to the floor, with the help of the nurse, all 12 leads of the electrocardiogram fell off. At this point I was left with no electrocardiographic recording and a patient in "asystole", lying on the floor. The nurse and I immediately picked her up and laid her on the treadmill. I raised the treadmill to a grade of approximately 10% with the head down. We worked as quickly as possible to replace the electrodes on the chest. By the time the electrodes were on, the patient was noted to be in profound sinus bradycardia, pale, and di-aphoretic with a blood pressure less than 70. Although still unconscious, within a minute later the patient's blood pressure had risen to around 90 and her heart rate had come back into the 60s. Lying on the treadmill with her head down and her feet up she regained consciousness about 4 minutes later, sat up and immediately lost consciousness again for at least another 3 or 4 minutes. Finally, I suspect the effect of nitroglycerin wore off; she regained consciousness and could carry on a conversation. Her post-experience electrocardiogram was back to normal. She went on the have cardiac catheterization and eventual coronary by-pass surgery. I ran into her about 7 years later and she asked me if I remembered her. At the time I did not remember her, and then she mentioned the experience she had with nitroglycerin. Let me tell you, this is one experience I will never forget.

As coronary care director of a major city hospital, I have experienced two other similar cases in the intensive care unit when patients were administered nitroglyc-erin for very typical ischemic chest pain. This nitroglycerine induced severe hy-potension and bradycardia is an under-recognized complication of nitroglycerin use. It is believed secondary to intense vasovagal response probably due to venous pool-ing and reduction of venous return to the heart [1–4].

Lesson Learned

Use nitroglycerin under appropriate circumstances but be alert to the possibility of a significant adverse reaction.
H. Jack Pyhel

Case 4: Exertional Cervical Arthritis

EC was a 58-year-old Caucasian man who presented with left shoulder and neck pain. He had been previously diagnosed with cervical spine disease by an orthopedic surgeon and prescribed sulindac (Clinoril). He presented for a refill of his medica-tion and requested a different medication since sulindac was no longer effective.

He described increasingly more frequent episodes of the described "arthritis pain" when he mowed his yard with a push mower and performed other activities. The "arthritis pain" was related to activity and had not occurred with rest. Because of the relationship of the symptoms to activity an exercise test was recommended. His only other risk factor for coronary artery disease was treated hypertension. His baseline electrocardiogram was within normal limits. At 6 minutes and 42 seconds into the Bruce protocol he complained of neck and right shoulder discomfort (Fig. 20.2A). The test was terminated at 7 minutes and 38 seconds (Fig. 20.2B). In recovery he developed progressive horizontal and downsloping ST-segment depression. At 7 minutes and 30 seconds into recovery he was given nitroglycerin (Fig. 20.2C).

Summary

1. He achieved 100% of his maximum predicted heart rate and 9.5 METS of work with exercise stress testing. His ST-segment changes persisted past 8 minutes into recovery with exercise stress testing.

A

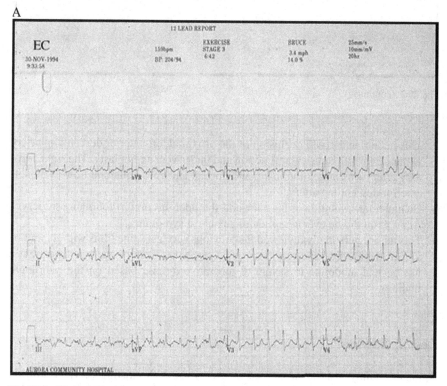

Fig. 20.2 (**A**) At 6:42 minutes patient had onset of "neck pain" and abnormal upsloping to horizontal ST-segment depression. (**B**) Maximal electrocardiogram showing 3 mm horizontal ST-segment depression in V$_4$. (**C**) Downsloping ST-segment depression in recovery

B

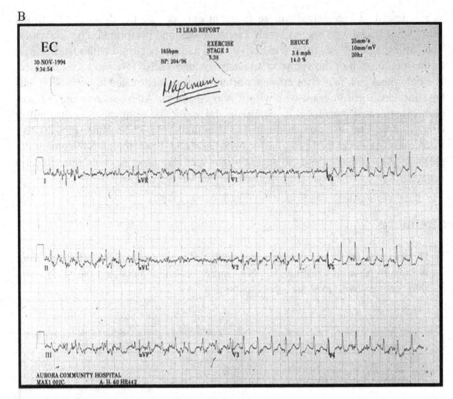

Fig. 20.2 (continued)

2. This patient had 100% occlusion of the proximal left anterior descending artery with normal left ventricular function and underwent angioplasty. The right coronary artery was large, dominant, and normal and gave collateral flow to the left anterior descending artery.
3. He had total resolution of his neck and shoulder discomfort following surgery.
4. At no point did he ever complain of any chest symptoms.
5. This author personally reviewed his previous cervical spine films with the radiological department and two orthopedic surgeons. Each of them independently felt he had moderate to severe degenerative disease based on the radiologic findings.

Lesson Learned

Angina certainly can be interpreted as exacerbation of existing cervical arthritis made worse by exertion. The stress test usually reveals that the "arthritis pain" is angina.

Russell D. White

C

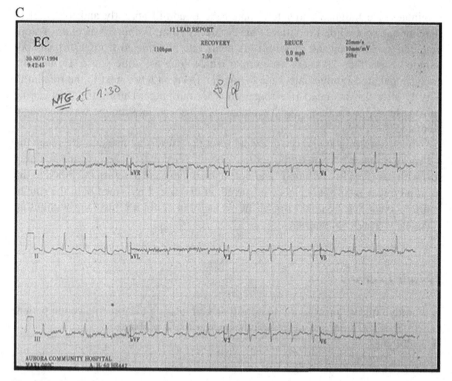

Fig. 20.2 (continued)

Case 5: The Athlete with Syncope

A 35-year-old man, a very good runner, came for a treadmill exam having experienced a syncopal spell several weeks previously. The patient's coach told me that the gentleman had been running 1 mile repeats in exactly five minutes and 25 seconds and had finished three of the repeats. He walked over to a water fountain, bent down to get a drink, and fell down unconscious on the ground. He was quite diaphoretic, extremely pale, had a thready to impalpable pulse, and awakened about 1 minute after falling. Fortunately, he was not hurt and was alert and responsive on awakening. He had never experienced a similar spell but had on occasion after running hard been somewhat lightheaded during his recovery periods.

Because this runner was superbly trained I elected to put him on the "Olympic protocol" established in 1984 prior to the Olympics and administered to the marathon runners. The protocol is in 2 minute stages starting at 3.5 miles an hour, quickly rising to 10 miles an hour with no elevation. The protocol continues at 10 miles an hour raising the grade 2% each 2 minutes until fatigue. This athlete reached 6% elevation and had been running at a 6 minute per mile pace for at least

8 minutes. He fatigued and I terminated the treadmill abruptly and told him to stand in one spot while I monitored his cardiac rhythm. Within 30 seconds of stopping and standing on the treadmill his heart rate plummeted from 170 beats per minute to less than 20 beats per minute with a long asystolic pause. He became presyncopal, and I immediately made him lie down on a bed next to the treadmill. Shortly after this his heart rate rose into a normal range. During the bradycardic episode he did not exhibit any hypotension. I suspect his syncope was vasovagal mediated.

While exercising at a very strenuous level the exercising muscles are receiving a disproportionate portion of the cardiac output. Terminating exercise and standing still with his "legs full of blood" and no exercising muscle to return the blood to the heart a typical vasovagal episode occurred, in his case. I informed both the runner and the coach that he could run all he wanted but could not just stop without an adequate warm-down period.

Lesson Learned

A thorough history prior to the treadmill and simulating the experience the patient experiences will frequently give you the answer to the problem.
H. Jack Pyhel

Case 6: Severe Ischemia Manifesting as Gastroesophageal Reflux

GR was a 48-year-old Caucasian man who presented for a refill of his cimetidine (Tagamet) prescribed for the treatment of his gastroesophageal reflux disease. He remarked that the Tagament was no longer working and requested a different medication. GR described typical symptoms of indigestion but the symptoms were more severe with activity and exertion. Because of this association he was scheduled for an exercise test. His risk factors for coronary artery disease included cigarette smoking, elevated cholesterol (253 mg/dl), and a positive family history. His mother had suffered an acute myocardial infarction at age 51.

His resting electrocardiogram was within normal limits (Fig. 20.3A). At 1 minute and 9 seconds into the Bruce protocol he experienced epigastric pain (Fig. 20.3B). Note the peaked T waves, an early sign of myocardial ischemia. The test was continued and at 2 minutes and 50 seconds he suddenly developed ST-segment elevation. The test was terminated. I thought he had suffered an acute myocardial infarction (Fig. 20.3C). In recovery the ST-segment elevation persisted although the epigastric pain resolved (Fig. 20.3D). The patient was transferred to the Emergency Department, an intravenous line was placed and lab was drawn for biomarkers along with serial electrocardiogram tracings. He was stabilized and there was no evidence of an acute myocardial infarction. He was then transferred to the cardiology service where he underwent angiography.

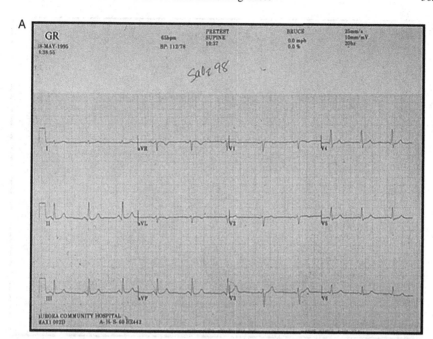

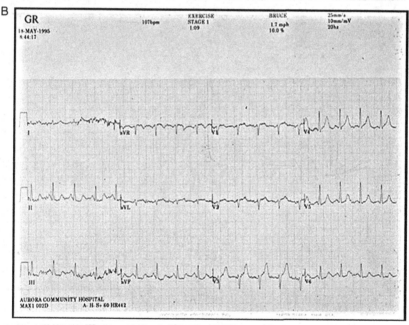

Fig. 20.3 (**A**) Normal resting electrocardiogram. (**B**) Electrocardiogram at 1 minute and 9 seconds into the Bruce protocol, the patient experienced epigastric pain. Note the peaked T waves, an early sign of myocardial ischemia. (**C**) Marked J point and ST-segment elevation with exercise causing termination of the test. (**D**) In recovery, the ST-segment elevation slowly resolved

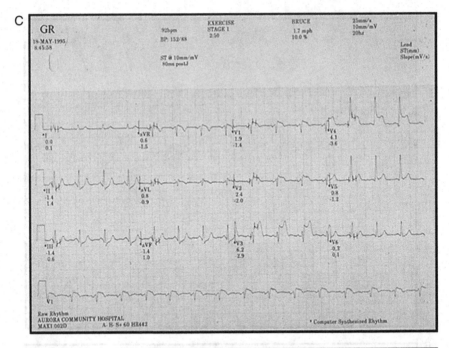

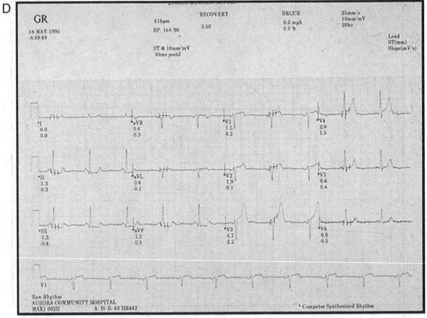

Fig. 20.3 (continued)

Summary

1. His chief complaint was epigastric pain and there was a remote history of peptic ulcer disease. He did not complain of chest pain.
2. At 1 minute 9 seconds into Stage I of the exercise test (Bruce protocol) he complained of epigastric pain. His electrocardiogram revealed ST-segment elevation in V_1, V_2, and V_3 with peaking of T waves in V_3, V_4. In addition early ST-segment depression was noted in leads II, III, and aVF.
3. At 2 minutes 50 seconds into exercise stress testing his electrocardiogram showed sudden ST-segment elevations in $V_1 - V_4$ and the test was terminated.
4. Angiography revealed severe two-vessel disease involving the left anterior descending artery (95% obstruction) and the right coronary artery (90% obstruction). Left ventricular function was normal.
5. He underwent two-vessel coronary by-pass surgery and his epigastric pain resolved.

Lesson Learned

As discussed in Case 3, angina can present in atypical ways. ST elevation is a sign of severe ischemia and when seen, necessitates termination of the test and further workup.
Russell D. White

Case 7: The Athlete with Paroxysmal Atrial Fibrillation

A 63-year-old male triathlete who engaged in at least one and sometimes as many as all three sports on an almost daily training regimen was referred to me when he was found to be in atrial fibrillation by his family doctor. When I initially saw him in my office he was in sinus rhythm but being an extremely type A personality had been recording his heart rate before and after exercise for almost 5 years. On occasion he would notice very fast, irregular rhythms after completing vigorous workouts which would last several hours and in retrospect were representative of paroxysmal atrial fibrillation. There was no history of hypertension, diabetes, or previous cardiovascular problems. An echocardiogram revealed good left ventricular function, very mild mitral insufficiency, and no left atrial enlargement. Because he had experienced some chest discomfort on several occasions I elected to proceed with a treadmill exam.

Using the Bruce protocol he exercised into Stage V at which point he was running 5 miles an hour at an 18% grade. His heart rate "maxed out" and he became fatigued. I stopped the treadmill at a heart rate of 168 beats per minute and no ST-segment change. Within 30 seconds into recovery he went into atrial fibrillation with a heart rate of almost 200 beats per minute (Fig. 20.4). There was some ST-segment

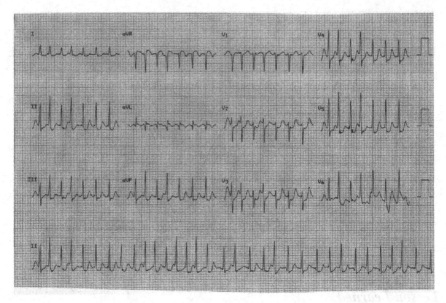

Fig. 20.4 Thirty second recovery electrocardiogram showing rapid atrial fibrillation with some lateral ST-segment depression suggesting ischemia

depression which persisted for the next 7 or 8 minutes in the absence of any chest pain. Fortunately he did have an isotopic test, the isotope having been given 1 minute prior to termination of the exercise. His perfusion study was entirely normal despite having the ST-segment change. He was still in atrial fibrillation after 20 minutes in the treadmill lab and went home with prescriptions for digoxin and atenolol, for rate control. He has subsequently been seen by an electrophysiologist and is scheduled for ablation.

Lesson Learned

With extreme sympathetic stimulation, at peak exercise, atrial fibrillation can present with an extremely rapid rate. If indeed the patient also had associated significant coronary obstructive disease the rapid rate may well precipitate subendocardial ischemia or non-transmural myocardial infarction.
H. Jack Pyhel

Case 8: Severe Ischemia

CA was a 62-year-old Caucasian man who was followed for hypertension and type 2 diabetes mellitus for 6 years. He had lost 48 pounds following his diagnosis of diabetes and his initial prescription for metformin was discontinued. His most recent

A1C was 6.1%. He denied any chest pain or shortness of breath but did complain of occasional dizziness when standing up after lying down for any length of time. He ran 3 miles on the treadmill 4–5 days per week with no symptoms. Orthostatic blood pressures in the office were normal. An exercise test was recommended due to his symptoms. His resting electrocardiogram was within normal limits.

At 11 minutes and 50 seconds into the Bruce protocol he developed ST-segment depression in leads II, III, aVF, V_5 and V_6. ST-segment elevation was noted in leads aVR, aVL, and V_1. The test was terminated (Fig. 20.5A). At 1 minute into recovery he developed downsloping ST-segment changes in leads I, aVL, and V_2 with ST-segment elevation in leads III and aVF (Fig. 20.5B). At 3 minutes into recovery he developed peaked T waves in leads II, III, and aVF with marked T wave inversion in leads aVL and V_2. There was downsloping ST-segment depression in lead I and horizontal ST-segment depression in V_5 (Fig. 20.5C). At 6 minutes into recovery he developed horizontal ST-segment depression in leads II and aVF with downsloping ST-segment depression in leads V_4, V_5, and V_6 (Fig. 20.5D). At 7 minutes into recovery he developed downsloping ST-segment depression in leads I, II, aVF, V_5, and V_6 with inverted T waves in lead V_2 (Fig. 20.5E). The patient was left in the hospital stress laboratory with electrocardiogram leads attached and two nurses in attendance. A cardiologist was summoned and the patient was scheduled for immediate angiography.

Summary

1. The patient had a normal resting electrocardiogram with dramatic changes in the post-exercise period.
2. At angiography the patient had diffuse and severe coronary artery disease.
3. He underwent quintuple coronary by-pass surgery and has done well since.
4. He later admitted his "running on the treadmill" was a slow walk.
5. In summary, he had severe heart disease with a paucity of symptoms.

Lesson Learned

Many of our patients, especially those with diabetes, have severe myocardial disease with a minimum of symptoms. We need to have a low threshold to evaluate these patients with an exercise test.
Russell D. White

Case 9: Adenosine Stress Test in the Patient with Atrial Fibrillation

An 82-year-old woman with bad spinal stenosis and inability to walk on the treadmill presented for an adenosine *stress test*. She had a history of atrial fibrillation for a number of years with a well-controlled ventricular response. There was also a history of hypertension and type 2 diabetes along with a metabolic-like form of

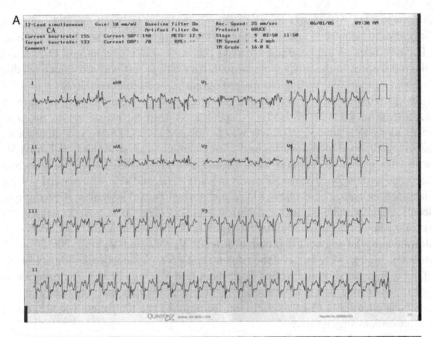

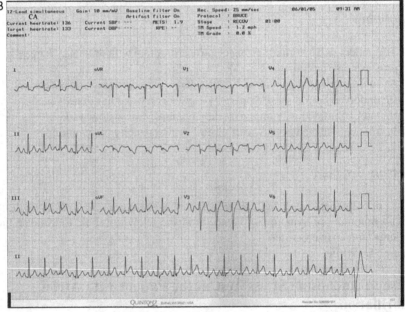

Fig. 20.5 (**A**) ST-segment depression in leads II, III, aVF, V$_5$, and V$_6$. ST-segment elevation was noted in lead aVR. The test was terminated. (**B**) 1 minute recovery electrocardiogram showing downsloping ST-segment changes in leads I, aVL, and V$_2$ with ST-segment elevation in leads III and aVF. (**C**) Three minute recovery electrocardiogram showing both peaked T waves and T wave inversion. (**D**) Significant inferior and lateral downsloping ST-segment depression is seen at 6 minutes in recovery. (**E**) Continued inferior and lateral downsloping ST-segment depression

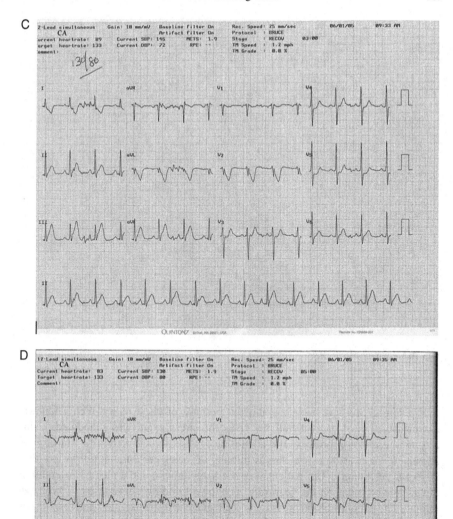

Fig. 20.5 (continued)

E

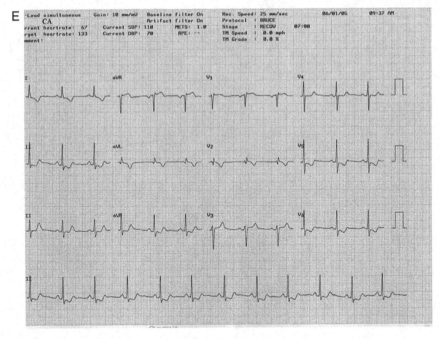

Fig. 20.5 (continued)

dyslipidemia. She had been hospitalized because of chest pain which I felt was somewhat atypical but with all her risks the stress exam was scheduled. Using a 6 minute infusion protocol the adenosine was started. Shortly after starting the adenosine the heart rate, which was initially 70 beats per minute, fell to less than 20 beats per minute. The patient was not symptomatic and I elected to continue the adenosine watching the heart rate. The lowest rate I observed was 17 beats per minute. The patient's blood pressure was adequate and she was alert and responsive. After 6 minutes the adenosine infusion was terminated and within 20–30 seconds the heart rate rebounded into the 60s. I do not recall ever doing another adenosine stress test in someone with atrial fibrillation but I recently saw a patient in the office who had a similar experience with another cardiologist.

Lesson Learned

In patients with atrial fibrillation and on rate control medicine (slowing atrio-ventricular (AV) node conduction) an additional rate controlling medicine working at the AV node, adenosine, may cause profound bradycardia. In most circumstances the stress examination can be continued with close observation.

H. Jack Pyhel

Case 10: When Not To Do an Exercise Test

Early in my career I was asked to do a physical on the 27-year-old brother of one of my residents. He had no insurance, but the physical was paid by a company that was sending him to work in Antarctica, to "winter over." I was to clear him medically and could do any tests I thought necessary. He was asymptomatic, without heart disease, but he requested an exercise test as he had an older uncle with coronary artery disease. His initial physical and electrocardiogram were normal. Unfortunately I consented to the exercise test without a good indication.

At 6:43 minutes into the test he started to develop inferior and mild lateral ST-segment depression (Fig. 20.6A). He was asymptomatic and the test was continued. At max exercise, at 8:57 minutes, he had about 2–2.5 mm of horizontal to upsloping inferior ST-segment depression and mild ST-segment depression in the lateral leads. See figure below (Fig. 20.6B). During recovery his ST-segment depression resolved quickly and was gone at 1:30 minutes in recovery. He remained asymptomatic. I felt his treadmill response was a false-positive test result, considering his age, asymptomatic status, and rapid resolution during recovery. I called the California company to say he was cleared medically to go, but he had a false-positive exercise test. They responded, he was not going. Next step, a Cardiolite. exercise test was ordered. The result was a reversible inferior perfusion defect suggesting ischemia. Next step, a cardiac catheterization showed normal coronary arteries. He went to work in Antarctica and did fine.

Lesson Learned

It is fine to do tests on healthy people as part of a demonstration, but do not test very low-risk patients when it involves work clearance or insurance. The chances are that a positive test will be a false positive. Unfortunately in this case, the nuclear scan was also a false positive. Nuclear scans have approximately half the false-positive rate of plain exercise tests but they definitely occur.

Corey H. Evans

Case 11: Diabetes Without Severe Heart Disease

WR was a 59-year-old Caucasian man with type 1 diabetes mellitus for 48 years. His diabetes was treated with continuous subcutaneous insulin infusion (insulin pump therapy) and he was under treatment for dyslipidemia. His basic metabolic index was 24.9 and he had no known diabetic complications. He maintained an active life style and cycled on a regular basis. An exercise stress test was recommended for evaluation. During his last exercise stress test (2 years previous) he completed Stage V of the Bruce protocol and the test was interpreted as normal. Most physicians would assume the presence of significant heart disease in such a patient.

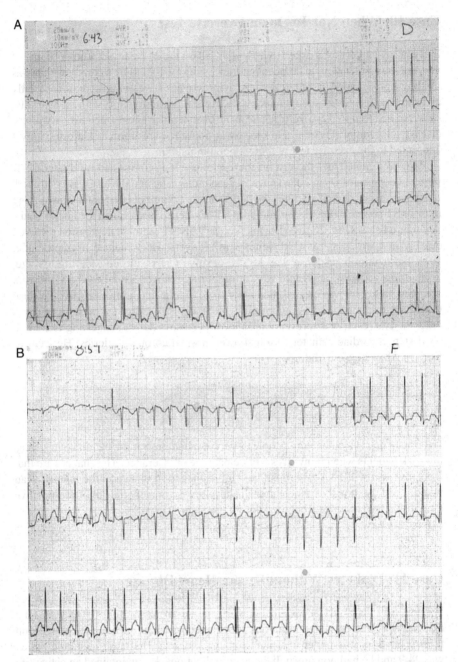

Fig. 20.6 (A) Despite baseline roll, there is inferior and lateral ST-segment depression. (B) At max exercise, electrocardiogram shows 2–2.5 mm of horizontal to upsloping inferior ST-segment depression and mild ST-segment depression in the lateral leads

His resting electrocardiogram revealed early repolarization and was within normal limits (Fig. 20.7A). He was begun on the Bruce protocol and reached Stage IV. His blood pressure was noted to be 240/80 (Fig. 20.7B). He continued the stress test until he reached maximum exercise in Stage V (13 minutes and 2 seconds) of the Bruce protocol (Fig. 20.7C). His maximum heart rate was 164 and his Borg scale was 10/10. Incidentally, the lead V_3 electrode lost connection at that point. He then entered recovery and at 1 minute into recovery his heart rate was 148 (Fig. 20.7D). At 5 minutes into recovery his BP was 230/50 and his heart rate was 112 (Fig. 20.7E).

Summary

1. This patient with long-standing diabetes performed well on the stress test and achieved 102% of his maximum predicted heart rate.
2. He did demonstrate an exaggerated blood pressure response and medication was prescribed.
3. He had no evidence of ischemic heart disease and he is in a low-risk group by achieving a heart rate of 160 or greater and completing Stage IV of the Bruce protocol. In addition, his Duke Treadmill Score is +13 which confirms a low-risk prognosis at 1 and 5 years.
4. Although no specific guidelines exist, most physicians would re-test this patient with diabetes again in 2 years unless new symptoms occur.

Lesson Learned

Not all patients with diabetes for nearly 50 years have severe heart disease.
Russell D. White

Case 12: A Patient with Atypical Chest Pain and Elevated Troponin

A 61-year-old man was evaluated by me, in the hospital, after presenting with somewhat atypical chest pain and a minimal elevation of his troponin, just slightly above the normal range. There was a history of hypertension but there were no electrocardiographic changes to suggest myocardial ischemia or left ventricular hypertrophy. His pain had been present a day before hospitalization and was short lived and not at all typical of myocardial ischemia. At the request of his physician I performed a treadmill stress examination.

Using the Bruce protocol he exercised for a total of 10 minutes. He achieved a heart rate just over 156 per minute and was noted to have some ST-segment depression in the absence of any chest pain (Fig. 20.8A). Three minutes into recovery the

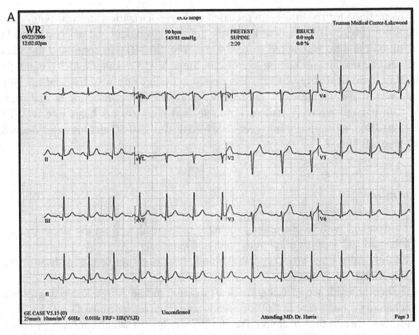

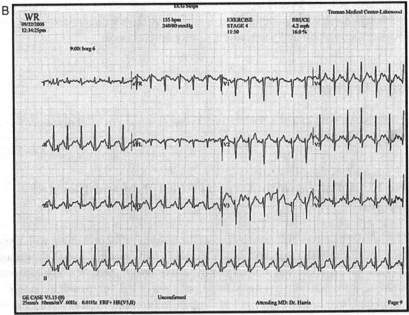

Fig. 20.7 (**A**) Resting electrocardiogram showing mild normal RT variant (early repolarization) and was within normal limits. (**B**) Normal exercise electrocardiogram at Stage IV. (**C**) Despite some baseline artifact and losing V₃ electrode, the tracing is normal. (**D**) Normal 1 minute recovery electrocardiogram. (**E**) Five minute recovery electrocardiogram is also normal

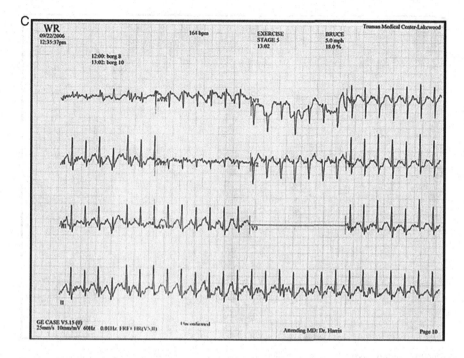

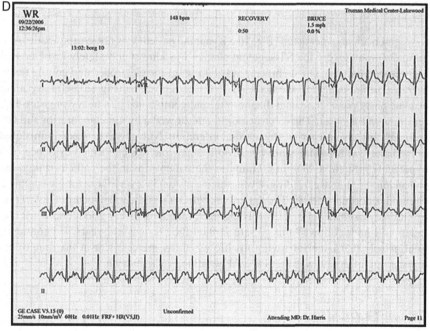

Fig. 20.7 (continued)

E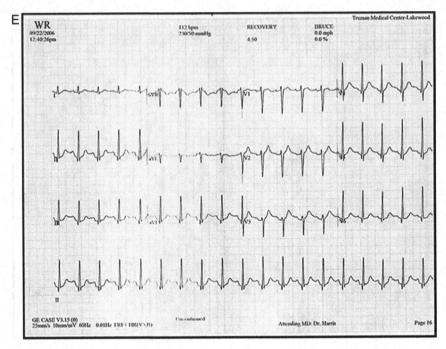

Fig. 20.7 (continued)

ST-segment change persisted (Fig. 20.8B) but the patient was not symptomatic. At 6 minutes into recovery the ST-segment change was almost completely resolved and I terminated the test. The technician was taking off the electrodes and getting ready to transport the patient to the floor. At 15 minutes post-test (Fig. 20.8C) the patient became pasty pale, somewhat diaphoretic, and complained of a heavy pressure-like sensation in the chest. The electrocardiogram showed a hyperacute inferior and lateral, possibly also posterior, myocardial infarction. Nitroglycerin was administered immediately with partial relief but several other tracings confirmed evidence of a hyperacute infarction. Within 60 minutes the patient was in the catheterization lab and an interventional cardiologist was placing a stent in a very large totally occluded circumflex coronary artery. The patient did suffer a significant myocardial infarction by cardiac enzymes but by echocardiography maintained very good left ventricular function. I have followed this patient in the office for several years. He continues to effusively thank me for saving his life when my greatest fear at the time of his myocardial infarction was that I would be talking to his lawyer.

Lesson Learned

Bad luck can happen to anyone, and I am not referring to the patient. Myocardial infarction and death on the treadmill are certainly infrequent and estimated at

A

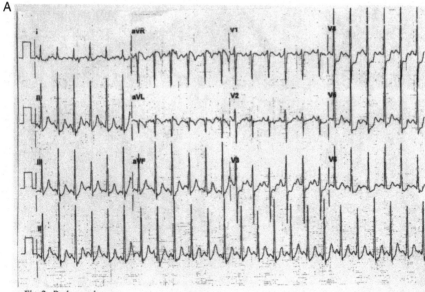

Fig. 2. Peak exercise.

B

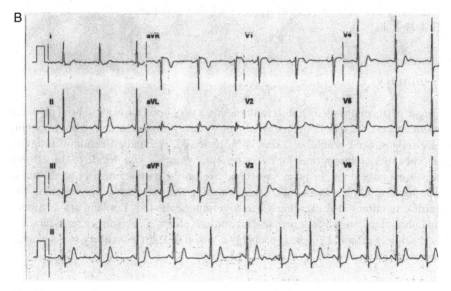

Fig. 20.8 (**A**) At peak exercise there is significant lateral upsloping to horizontal ST-segment depression (**B**) A 3 minute recovery electrocardiogram showing persistent lateral horizontal ST-segment depression. (**C**) Fifteen minute post-exercise electrocardiogram showing hyperacute inferior and lateral, possibly also posterior, ST elevation suggesting an acute myocardial infarction

C

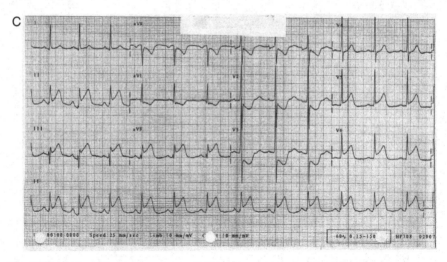

Fig. 20.8 (continued)

approximately 1 in 10,000 cases [5, 6]. I do not anticipate practicing long enough to do another 10,000 cases, and with any luck I should not experience another one.
H. Jack Pyhel

Summary

Before performing any treadmill examination a very good history and brief physical examination should be done. If any laboratory data is available, i.e., serum troponin, electrolytes, lipid profile, etc. should be reviewed. A standard treadmill protocol is probably not appropriate for every patient. Whatever you decide to do, always watch the patient carefully and keep one eye on the cardiac monitor at all times. The hardest part of a treadmill is not watching the patient walk or watching the cardiac monitor—it is deciding when to terminate the test. Looking at the patient and observing carefully the patient's breathing, color, gait, and any other symptoms is absolutely essential. There is probably a lesson to learn from every stress examination performed.

References

1. Come PC, Pitt B. Nitroglycerine-induced severe hypotension and bradycardia in patients with acute myocardial infarction. Circulation 1976; 54:624–28.
2. Lydakis C, Chaudary AY, Lip GY. The vasovagal effect of nitrates: an under-recognized complication of nitrate use. Int J Clin Pract 1998 Sep; 52(6):418–21.
3. Wuerz R, Swope G, Meador S, et al. Study of prehospital nitroglerine. Am Emerg Med 1994 Jan; 23(1):31–36.

4. Nemerovski M, Shah PK. Syndrome of severe bradycardia and hypotension following sublingual nitroglycerin administration. Cardiology 1981; 67(3):180–89.
5. Rochmis P, Blackburn H. Exercise tests: a survey of procedures, safety and litigation experience in approximately 170,000 tests. JAMA 1971; 217:1061.
6. Atterhog J, Jonsson B, et al. Exercise testing: a prospective study of complication rates. Am Heart J 1979; 98:572.

Index